Legal Aspects of Mental Capacity

To Austin

Legal Aspects of Mental Capacity

Bridgit Dimond

Emeritus Professor
University of Glamorgan
Wales
UK

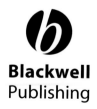

Blackwell
Publishing

Library of Congress Cataloging-in-Publication Data

Dimond, Bridgit.
The legal aspects of mental capacity / Bridgit Dimond.
p. ; cm.
Includes bibliographical references and index.
ISBN-13: 978-1-4051-3359-3 (pbk. : alk. paper)
1. Mental health laws—Great Britain.
2. Capacity and disability—Great Britain. I. Title.
[DNLM: 1. Great Britain. Mental Capacity Act 2005. 2. Mental Competency—legislation
& jurisprudence—Great Britain. 3. Informed Consent—legislation & jurisprudence—
Great Britain. W 32.5 FA1 D582L 2008]
KD737.D56 2008
344.4104′4—dc22
2007025761

A catalogue record for this book is available from the British Library.

Set in 10/12pt by Graphicraft Limited, Hong Kong
Printed in Great Britain by TJ International Ltd, Padstow, Cornwall

2 2008

Contents

Preface

The numbers of adults who are incapable of making their own decisions will never be known exactly but there are probably over 2 million. The number thought to be suffering from dementia is probably over 700 000, and this number is likely to rise as life expectancy increases. Mental incapacity covers a variety of conditions. Some may never have had capacity such as those with severe learning disabilities or who have been born with serious brain damage. Others may lose their capacity through deterioration and diseases such as Alzheimer's or through trauma such as road accidents. Some may suffer impairment temporarily, others lose mental capacity never to recover it. As a consequence significant decisions must be made on behalf of such diverse persons and for varying lengths of time. Such persons must be protected from exploitation and abuse. They are entitled to receive a good quality of life.

Legislation to provide a framework for the protection of mentally incapacitated and vulnerable adults and for decisions to be taken on their behalf has been in the pipeline for over 15 years. In the absence of statutory provision, the courts have had to fill the gaps and the common law (judge made law) has laid down the principles on when and how decisions are to be taken on behalf of such persons. The Mental Capacity Act 2005 has thus been long awaited and its effects will be felt across all fields of health and social care. Every health and social services professional will find that the Act and Regulations made under it will affect their work and the decisions they make. It is the intention of this book to assist practitioners in understanding the basic provisions of the Act and how it applies to their professional responsibilities. It is also intended to be of assistance to the many carers who are forced into or find themselves in the position of having to make decisions on behalf of mentally incapable relatives and friends. It has been decided not to include the full text of the Act as an appendix as originally planned, since all the legislation including the statutory instruments can be easily downloaded free of charge from the internet and references are given accordingly. Similarly the Code of Practice can be downloaded from the Department for Constitutional Affairs website.

A basic guide to the statutory provisions is set out in the first chapter. Each chapter setting out the basic provisions is followed by a series of Scenarios dealing with practical concerns, which are discussed in the light of the new legislation. The aim of these Scenarios is to show how the many facets of the Act and the regulations are likely to apply. Earlier cases are cited to illustrate how the new statutory provisions are likely to change or continue existing practice. In addition an extensive glossary and list of abbreviations are included to assist the reader who is not conversant with the law and its terminology. A list of useful websites is included for further information to be accessed. There is also a chapter dealing with some of the differences in Wales. Scotland passed its own Adults with Incapacity Act 2000, which came into force during the drafting of the provisions for the rest of the United Kingdom and undoubtedly had a strong influence on these. Unfortunately these provisions could not be included in this work, since they deserve a book in their own right.

The aim of the book is to make the law clearer and more understandable to the health and social services professional and to the informal carers. Inevitably as the Act is implemented, disputes over interpretation and application are likely to arise, which in turn will lead to a body of case law on its interpretation. It is hoped that future editions of this book can take on board the developing case law. This initial work is aimed at providing a useful foundation for an understanding of the law protecting those adults who lack mental capacity to make specific decisions and due to the speed of changes in this area, a website linked to the book is available at www.blackwellpublishing.com/dimond to highlight major developments.

In writing this book, I have had my nephew, a registered nurse for those with learning disabilities, very much in mind, and it is to him that this book is dedicated.

Acknowledgements

It is perhaps invidious to select a few names from the many who have assisted me in the preparation of this book, but I should like to recognise the assistance which I have received from Tessa Shellens and her colleagues, and from Penny Llewellyn, Gareth Barclay, Susan Elsmore, Peter Lawler, Dave Tomlin, Hugh Davies and Austin Dorrity. The copyright of The Stationery Office for Statutes and Statutory Instruments and of the various publishers for law reports is acknowledged. I should also like to express my appreciation of the conscientious work and assistance of my production editor Catriona Dixon and my proof reader Alison Morley.

I also wish to put on record my indebtedness to my family for their unceasing encouragement and in particular to Bette for her painstaking indexing of cases, statutes and contents, and her invaluable and constant support.

Table of Cases

Table of Statutes

Glossary

advance decision – when someone who has mental capacity (is able to make and understand a decision) decides that they do not want a particular type of treatment if they lack capacity in the future. A doctor must respect this decision if it is valid and applicable. An advance decision must be about treatment a person wants to refuse and when that person wants to refuse it.

appeal – when there is disagreement with a decision that has been made in court and an application is made for the case to be looked at again.

application to register – form that a *donor* or their *attorney* fill in to say that they want a *lasting power of attorney* to begin.

asset – something that a person owns.

attorney – (also know as *donee*) someone who has the *legal* right to make choices and decisions on behalf of someone else (the *donor*). The donor chooses who their attorney will be. Also known as donee or holder of the power of attorney.

attorney's authority – what a *donor* says in their *lasting power of attorney* that an *attorney* can do (including any restrictions or conditions provided on their authority).

best interests – anything done for people without *capacity* must be in their best interests (there is no legal definition of best interests but the criteria to be used are in Section 4 of the Mental Capacity Act 2005). Best interests means thinking about what is best for the person, not about what anyone else wants.

Bolam Test – the test laid down by McNair J in the case of *Bolam* v. *Friern HMC* on the standard of care expected of a professional in cases of alleged *negligence*.

Bournewood case – a case where the European Court of Human Rights held that w.k. law was in breach of Article 5.

Bournewood safeguards – legal provisions made to fill the gap revealed by the Bournewood case.

burden of proof – the duty of a party to litigation to establish the facts, or in criminal proceedings the duty of the prosecution to establish both the *actus reus* and the *mens rea* of the offence.

capacity – the ability to make decisions about a particular matter at a particular time (the legal definition of people who lack capacity is in Section 2 of the Mental Capacity Act 2005).

case citation – each case is reported in an official series of cases according to the following symbols: *Re F* (i.e. in the matter of F) or *F* v. *West Berkshire Health Authority* [1989] 2 All ER 545 which means the year 1989, volume 2 of the All England Law Reports, page 545. Each case can be cited by means of this reference system. In the case of *Whitehouse* v. *Jordan*, Whitehouse is the claimant, Jordan the defendant and 'v.' stands for versus, i.e. against. Other law reports include: AC Appeals Court; QB Queens Bench Division and WLR Weekly Law Reports.

case conference – a meeting to talk about a person's care or support.

certificate provider – an independent person who completes a Part C certificate to say that the *donor* understands the *lasting power of attorney* form and is not under pressure to make it.

Citizens Advice Bureau – provides free information and helps people sort out their legal or money problems (www.citizensadvice.org.uk)

civil action – proceedings brought in the civil courts.

civil partnership – a relationship between two people of the same sex which, when registered, gives certain *legal* rights and responsibilities (the legal definition of civil partnership is in Section 1 of the Civil Partnership Act 2004).

civil wrong – an act or omission which can be pursued in the civil courts by the person who has suffered the wrong (see *tort*).

claimant – the person bringing a civil action (originally *plaintiff*).

Code of Practice – separate, detailed statutory guidance on the Mental Capacity Act 2005.

common law – law derived from the decisions of judges, case law, judge made law.

condition to an LPA – tells an *attorney* to act in a particular way.

Court of Protection – specialist court for all issues relating to people who lack capacity (the Court of Protection is established under Section 45 of the *Mental Capacity Act 2005*).

Court of Protection visitor – someone who is appointed to report to the *Court of Protection* on a particular matter, for example, checking on *attorneys*. (Court of Protection visitors are established under Section 61 of the Mental Capacity Act 2005.)

criminal courts – courts such as magistrates and crown courts hearing criminal cases.

criminal wrong – an act or omission which constitutes an offence and can be pursued in the criminal courts by prosecution.

customary occasion – an occasion, for example, a birthday, on which presents are usually given.

declaration – a ruling by the court, setting out the legal situation.

deed of revocation – used to cancel *enduring powers of attorney* or *ordinary powers of attorney*.

Department for Constitutional Affairs – the Government department with responsibility for upholding justice, rights and democracy (www.dca.gov.uk). The department also has responsibility for policy on LPAs.

deputy – someone appointed by the *Court of Protection* to make decisions for a person who lacks capacity.

distinguished (of cases) – the rules of precedent require judges to follow decisions of judges in previous cases, where these are binding upon them. However in some circumstances it is possible to come to a different decision because the facts of the earlier case are not comparable to the case now being heard, and therefore the earlier decision can be 'distinguished'.

donor – person who makes a *lasting power of attorney*.

donee – a person appointed under a *lasting power of attorney*.

enduring power of attorney – is created under the Enduring Powers of Attorney Act 1985 and deals only with property and affairs.

F (Re) ruling – The House of Lords held that a professional who acts in the best interests of an incompetent person who is incapable of giving consent, does not act unlawfully if he follows the accepted standard of care according to the *Bolam Test*.

fee – money that a person has to pay for something.

good faith – when a person acts in good faith they act honestly, fairly and without any intention of taking unfair advantage.

independent advocate – a person who speaks up for someone else. The advocate will be independent of the person making a decision.

independent mental capacity advocate – an advocate appointed under the Mental Capacity Act 2005.

independent report – a report written by somebody who is not linked to the case.

informal – of a patient who has entered hospital without any statutory requirements.

joint attorneys – when a *donor* appoints more than one *attorney* and they are *joint attorneys*, they must always act together, for example all of them must sign every cheque made out.

joint and several attorneys – when a *donor* appoints more than one *attorney* and they are *joint and several attorneys* they can act together and they can act independently of each other.

judicial review – an application to the High Court for a judicial or administrative decision to be reviewed and an appropriate order made, e.g. declaration.

lack capacity – not being able to make or understand a particular decision or choice at a particular time.

lasting power of attorney (LPA) where a person (the donor) gives the other person (the attorney or donee) the right to make decisions about property, money or their well-being on their behalf in the future.

law of agency – law which applies when one person acts as an agent for another person, like an attorney does for a donor.

least restrictive intervention – anything done for people without *capacity* should be the least restrictive of their basic rights and freedoms.

legal – to do with the law.

legal aid and help – financial assistance and help with going to court.

legal profession – people who work with the law, such as solicitors and barristers.

legal representation – having someone who works with the law, like a solicitor, to tell a court your views.

life-sustaining treatment – treatment that is needed to keep a person alive.

litigation friend – needed when someone does not have capacity to tell a solicitor they want to go to court. It could be a relative or a friend or, when there is no one else appropriate, the Official Solicitor who then tells the solicitor what is wanted.

magistrate – a person (see *JP and stipendiary*) who hears summary (minor) offences or indictable offences which can be heard in the magistrates' court.

mediation – helping people come to an agreement.

mediator – a person who helps people come to an agreement.

mens rea – the mental element in a crime (contrasted with *actus reus*).

Mental Capacity Act 2005 / the Act – an Act of Parliament which makes the law about how to support and protect people who cannot make their own decisions. The Act makes it clear who can take decisions, in which situations, and how they should go about this. It lets people plan ahead for a time when they may lack capacity to make their own decisions about some things. It also creates new powers such as *lasting powers of attorney and deputies of the Court of Protection* and covers other issues to do with people who lack *capacity*.

named person / named people – people a *donor* chooses to be notified when the *application to register* is made.

negligence (1) – a breach by the defendant of a legal duty to take reasonable care not to injure the claimant or cause him loss.

negligence (2) – the attitude of mind of a person committing a civil wrong as opposed to intentionally.

Office of the Public Guardian / OPG – will help the Public Guardian carry out his duties. It will keep a register of *lasting powers of attorney* and check on what *attorneys* are doing amongst other things. (Section 57 of the Mental Capacity Act 2005 establishes the officer called the Public Guardian, and the functions of the Public Guardian are in Section 58.)

Official Solicitor – needed when someone does not have capacity to tell a solicitor they want to go to court and no one else can act for them. The Official Solicitor then acts for them or asks other solicitors to do it.

Ombudsman – a Commissioner (eg health, local government) appointed by the Government to hear complaints.

one-off decision by the court – a single decision by the *Court of Protection*.

ordinary power of attorney – a power of attorney under the Powers of Attorney Act 1971, which cannot be effective when the *donor* lacks capacity to make a decision.

out of pocket expenses – when an *attorney* spends their own money to pay for expenses incurred in doing the things that a *donor* has asked them to do in their *lasting power of attorney*.

personal welfare decisions – a person's day-to-day well-being and physical well-being, and includes decisions about where a person lives, what they wear and what they eat.

plaintiff – term formerly used to describe one who brings an action in the civil courts. Now the term *claimant* is used.

POVA – safeguard made to Protect Vulnerable Adults from abuse and exploitation.

Practice Direction – guidance issued by the head of the court to which they relate on the procedure to be followed.

pre-action protocol – Rules of the Supreme Court provide guidance on action to be taken before legal proceedings commence.

precedent – a decision which may have to be followed in a subsequent court hearing.

President – the head of the Court of Protection.

presumption of capacity – every adult has the right to make their own decisions and must be assumed to have *capacity* to do so unless it is proved otherwise.

prima facie – at first sight, or sufficient evidence brought by one party to require the other party to provide a defence.

professional attorney – someone who is paid for the services they provide as an *attorney*.

property and affairs – the things a person owns (like a house or flat) and the money they have.

prosecution – the pursuing of criminal offences in court.

Public Guardian – the head of the *Office of the Public Guardian*.

Public Guardian Board – a group of people who advise the Lord Chancellor on the work of the Public Guardian.

Public Guardianship Office – helps the Public Guardian carry out his duties, for example dealing with the registration of *lasting powers of attorney* and checking that *deputies* chosen by the Court of Protection are doing their job.

ratio – the reasoning behind the decision in a court case.

reasonable doubt – to secure a conviction in criminal proceedings the prosecution must establish 'beyond reasonable doubt' the guilt of the accused.

register of LPAs – a register of all *lasting powers of attorney* kept by the *Office of the Public Guardian*.

registration process – the *donor*, *attorney*(s) and *certificate provider* complete the *lasting power of attorney*, an *application to register* is filled in and sent to the *OPG* and the *OPG* checks the LPA and the *application to register*.

remit / remitting – remitting a fee means a person does not have to pay it.

replacement attorney – chosen by a *donor* to replace the original *attorney* if they are no longer able to act.

restriction to an LPA – tells an *attorney* they cannot do something.

revoke – cancel.

seal / sealing – once the *registration process* is complete, the *OPG* will seal each page of the *lasting power of attorney* to show it is valid.

solicitor – a lawyer who is qualified on the register held by the Law Society.

standard of proof – the level that the party who has the burden of proof must satisfy, e.g. on a balance of probabilities (civil courts); beyond all reasonable doubt (criminal courts).

statute law (statutory) – law made by Parliament, also known as Acts of Parliament.

Statutory Instrument – orders and regulations having binding force. They must usually be laid before Parliament and will usually become law if they are confirmed by a simple resolution of both Houses (affirmative resolution). Some become law after they have been laid for a prescribed period unless they are annulled by a resolution of either House (negative resolution).

stipendiary magistrate – a legally qualified magistrate who is paid (i.e. has a stipend).

Time out – a stage in the psychological treatment of a patient when he/she is temporarily excluded from social contact.

tort – a civil wrong excluding breach of contract. It includes: *negligence, trespass (to the person*, goods or land), nuisance, breach of statutory duty and defamation.

transition – a change in the law often preceded by interim temporary provisions.

trespass to the person – a wrongful direct interference with another person. Harm does not have to be proved.

trust corporation – a company which satisfies certain conditions, for example, the trustee department of a bank.

unreasonable – behaving in a difficult, unfair or awkward way.

vicarious liability – the liability of an employer for the wrongful acts of an employee committed whilst in the course of employment.

Abbreviations

A4A	Action for Advocacy
ACPC	Area Child Protection Committee
ACAS	Advisory, Conciliation and Arbitration Service
ACMD	Advisory Council on the Misuse of Drugs
Advice Now	Established by ASA to improve range and quality of information
AMHP	Approved Mental Health Professional
ANH	Artificial Nutrition and Hydration
ASA	Advice Services Alliance
ASW	Approved Social Worker
CEHR	Commission for Equality and Human Rights
CHAI	Commission for Healthcare Audit and Inspection (Formerly CHI)
CHC	Community Health Council
CHI	Commission for Health Improvement (Replaced by CHAI)
CHRE	Council for Healthcare Regulatory Excellence (Formerly CRHP)
COREC	Central Office for NHS Research Ethics Committees
CPS	Crown Prosecution Service
CRHP	Council for the Regulation of Healthcare Professionals (Now the CHRE)
CSCI	Commission for Social Care Inspection
CSIP	Care Services Improvement Partnership
CSIW	Care Standards Inspectorate for Wales
DCA	Department for Constitutional Affairs
DGH	District General Hospital
DH	Department of Health
DHA	District Health Authority
DHSS	Department of Health and Social Security (Divided in 1989 into DH and DSS)
DNA	Deoxyribonucleic Acid

DS	Director of Adult Services
DSS	Department of Social Security
DWP	Department for Work and Pensions
EC	European Community
ECHR	European Court of Human Rights
EEC	European Economic Community
EMI	Elderly Mentally Infirm
EPA	Enduring Power of Attorney
EWTD	European Working Time Directive
FHSA	Family Health Service Authority
GAfREC	Governance Arrangements for NHS Research Ethics Committees
GMC	General Medical Council
GP	General Practitioner
HFEA	Human Fertilisation and Embryology Authority
HIW	Healthcare Inspectorate Wales
ICAS	Independent Complaints Advocacy Service
IMCA	Independent Mental Capacity Advocate
ITP	Intention to Practise
IV	Intravenous(ly) or Intravenous infusion
IVF	In Vitro Fertilisation
JP	Justice of the Peace
LA	Local Authority
LHA	Local Health Authority
LHB	Local Health Board
LD	Learning Disabilities
LPA	Lasting Power of Attorney
LREC	Local Research Ethics Committee
LSA	Local Supervising Authority
LSAMO	Local Supervising Authority Midwifery Officer
LSSA	Local Social Services Authority
MCA	Mental Capacity Act 2005
MCIP	Mental Capacity Implementation Programme
MDA	Making Decisions Alliance
MHA	Mental Health Act 1983
MHAC	Mental Health Act Commission
MHRT	Mental Health Review Tribunal
MREC	Multi-Centre Research Ethics Committee
NAW	National Assembly for Wales
NCA	National Care Association
NHS	National Health Service
NHS SMS	NHS Security Management Service
NICE	National Institute for Clinical Excellence (up to 31 March 2005)
NICE	(from 1 April 2005) National Institute for Health and Clinical Excellence
NMC	Nursing and Midwifery Council
NPfIT	National Programme for Information Technology
NPSA	National Patient Safety Agency

NR	Nearest Relative
NSF	National Service Framework
OCN	Open College Network
OPG	Office of the Public Guardian
OS	Official Solicitor
PALS	Patient Advocacy and Liaison Services
PCC	Professional Conduct Committee
PCT	Primary Care Trust
PGO	Public Guardianship Office
PIAG	Patient Information Advisory Group
POVA	Protection of Vulnerable Adults
PPC	Preliminary Proceedings Committee
PPI	Patient and Public Involvement
PREP	Post-Registration Education and Practice
PVS	Permanent Vegetative State
QCA	Qualifications and Curriculum Authority
REC	Research Ethics Committee
RHA	Regional Health Authority
RMO	Responsible Medical Officer
RNLD	Registered Nurse for Learning Disabilities
RSCPHN	Registered Specialist Community Public Health Nurses
SCIE	Social Care Institute for Excellence
SCIG	Social Care Information Governance
SCT	Supervised Community Treatment
SHA	Strategic Health Authority
SI	Statutory Instrument
SOAD	Second Opinion Appointed Doctor
SSA	Site Specific Assessment
UKCC	United Kingdom Central Council for Nursing, Midwifery and Health Visiting
UKECA	United Kingdom Ethics Committee Authority
WAG	Welsh Assembly Government
WHO	World Health Organisation

1 Introduction: Anatomy of the Mental Capacity Act and its Terms

This introduction provides a simple guide to the legislation, the sources of further help, the terms used and the organisations involved.

The Mental Capacity Act 2005 has been awaited for over 15 years, and fills a huge gap in the statutory (i.e. by Act of Parliament) provisions for decision making on behalf of mentally incapacitated adults. This introduction sets out the main provisions of the Act in a nutshell and explains some of the terms used, the links with later Chapters and the Scenarios where these topics are considered in full.

Two basic concepts underpin the Act – the concept of capacity and the concept of best interests:

Mental capacity: only if an adult (i.e. a person over 18 years) lacks mental capacity can actions be taken or decisions made on his or her behalf. Capacity is defined in Sections 2 and 3 (see Chapter 4 and Scenario A). It is important to stress that the term 'mental capacity' is used in a specific functional way. A person may have the capacity to make one type of decision but not another. For this reason, the term 'requisite' mental capacity is used frequently throughout this book, to remind readers that it is the capacity in relation to a specific decision which is in question.

Best interests: if decisions are to be made or action taken on behalf of a mentally incapacitated adult, then they must be made or taken in the best interests of that person. The steps to be taken to determine 'best interests' are set out in Section 4. There is no statutory definition of 'best interests' (see Chapter 5 and Scenarios B).

Principles: Section 1 sets out five basic principles which apply to the determination of capacity and to acting in the best interests of a mentally incapacitated adult. These five principles are:

1. A person must be assumed to have capacity unless it is established that he or she lacks capacity.

2. A person is not to be treated as unable to make a decision unless all practicable steps to help him or her to do so have been taken without success.
3. A person is not to be treated as unable to make a decision merely because he or she makes an unwise decision.
4. An act done, or decision made, under this Act for or on behalf of a person who lacks capacity must be done, or made, in his or her best interests.
5. Before the act is done, or the decision is made, regard must be had to whether the purpose for which it is needed can be as effectively achieved in a way that is less restrictive of the person's rights and freedom of action.

These principles are considered in Chapter 3.

Human rights: in October 2000 the articles of the European Convention on Human Rights were incorporated into the laws of England, Wales and Northern Ireland (in Scotland they were incorporated on devolution) by the Human Rights Act 1998. As a consequence, any persons who claim that their human rights as set out in Schedule 1 to the Human Rights Act 1998 have been violated by a public authority can bring an action in the courts of the United Kingdom (UK) (Schedule 1 is discussed in Chapter 3).

The Convention on the International Protection of Adults is given statutory force by the Mental Capacity Act (MCA) and is set out in Schedule 3 to the MCA. Its provisions are considered in Chapter 3.

P is the person who lacks (or who is alleged to lack) capacity to make a decision(s) in relation to any matter.

Lasting power of attorney (LPA): the Act enables a person, known as P, when mentally capacitated to appoint a person known as the **donee** to make decisions about P's personal welfare, and property and affairs at a later time when P lacks mental capacity. The LPA may be general and not identify particular areas of decision making or it may specify the areas in which the donee can make decisions. It replaces the **enduring power of attorney** (EPA) which only covered decisions on property and finance. There are transitional provisions to cover the situation where a person has drawn up an EPA, and these are set out in Schedule 4 and discussed in Chapter 17. LPAs are considered in Chapter 6 and Scenarios C.

Court of Protection: a new Court of Protection replaces the existing Court of Protection, and has powers to make decisions on personal welfare in addition to property and affairs. (The previous Court could only consider matters relating to property and affairs.) Its powers, functions, constitution and appointment of **Court of Protection visitors** are discussed in Chapter 7 and Scenarios D.

Deputies: the Court of Protection has the power to appoint deputies to make decisions on the personal welfare, property and affairs of the mentally incapacitated adult. These powers and the restrictions upon them are considered in Chapter 7 and Scenarios D.

The Office of the Public Guardian is to be appointed by the Lord Chancellor to set up and maintain registers of LPAs, EPAs and deputies. It will supervise deputies and provide information to the Court of Protection. It will also arrange for visits by Court of Protection visitors. A **Public Guardian Board** scrutinises and reviews the way in which the Public Guardian discharges its functions. These offices are discussed in Chapter 7 and Scenarios D.

Independent mental capacity advocates: the Act makes provision for such persons to be appointed to represent and support mentally incapacitated adults in decisions about accommodation and serious medical treatment. These advocates are appointed under **Independent mental capacity advocate** services (IMCAs), which are established to provide independent advocates for mentally incapacitated adults in specified circumstances. They represent and support mentally incapacitated adults in decisions by NHS organisations on serious medical treatment, and in decisions by NHS organisations and local authorities on accommodation. The original remit of the IMCAs has been extended to cover care reviews and situations where adult protection measures are being taken. The arrangements for advocacy are considered in Chapter 8 and Scenarios E.

Advance decisions to refuse treatment (also known as living wills or advance refusals) are given statutory recognition, and special requirements are specified if these advance decisions are to cover the withdrawal or withholding of life-sustaining treatment. The definition of an advance decision and the statutory provisions are considered in Chapter 9 and Scenarios F.

Research on mentally incapacitated adults is subject to specific qualifications and unless these are complied with, the research cannot proceed. The provisions are discussed in Chapter 10 and Scenarios G.

Codes of Practice must be prepared by the Lord Chancellor, and their legal significance is considered in Chapter 17 and Scenarios M.

An offence of ill treatment or wilful neglect of a person who lacks capacity is created by the Act and this offence, together with other criminal offences in relation to a mentally incapacitated adult and the accountability of those who make decisions on their behalf, is discussed in Chapter 11 and Scenarios H.

Mental health and mental capacity

Treatments given to patients who are detained under the **Mental Health Act 1983** (as amended by the 2007 Act) are excluded from the provisions of the MCA. The distinction between the concepts of mental disorder and mental incapacity is considered in Chapter 13 and Scenarios J.

Coming into force of the MCA

The IMCA service came into force in England in April 2007 and will come into force in Wales in October 2007.

The criminal offence of ill-treatment or wilful neglect of a person lacking mental capacity came into force in April 2007.

Sections 1–4 covering the principles, definition of mental capacity and best interest and the guidance in the Code of Practice came into force in relation to IMCAs in April 2007.

All other provisions came into force in October 2007 (except for specific provisions relating to research – see Chapter 10).

Protection of mentally incapacitated adults provided in other statutory provisions is also included in this book to provide a comprehensive view, and is considered in Chapter 11 and Scenarios H.

Statutory law (made by Parliament) and **common law** (judge made or case law) are contrasted and explained in Chapter 2, which sets out the background to the passing of the Mental Capacity Act 2005.

Since devolution, Wales has enjoyed the ability to pass its own statutory instruments and issue its own guidance on health and social services law. Chapter 16 considers some of the differences in Wales. The Code of Practice drafted by the Department of Constitutional Affairs does however apply to Wales.

Scotland enacted an Adults with Incapacity (Scotland) Act in 2000, and the main differences between Scotland and England and Wales are not considered in this book.

The **Bournewood** case, sometimes referred to as the **Bournewood gap.** The European Court of Human Rights held that it was a breach of Article 5(1) for a person with learning disabilities to be kept in a psychiatric hospital under the common law doctrine of necessity (and therefore without being detained under the Mental Health Act 1983). As a consequence of this decision, it was apparent that the mental health law in England and Wales did not provide sufficient protection for those persons incapable of giving consent to admission to a psychiatric hospital, and who were being held outside the Mental Health Act 1983 in breach of Article 5(1). This gap in the law and the case itself, the Department of Health (DH) consultation paper on how the gap could be filled and the provisions made in the Mental Health Act to fill the gap, are considered in Chapters 3 and 13 and Scenarios J. The necessary changes to the MCA are known as the **Bournewood safeguards**.

Bolam Test: this is taken from a case heard in 1957[1] which was concerned with how negligence should be established. The judge held that the doctor must act in accordance with a responsible and competent body of relevant professional opinion. This is discussed in Chapter 11 on accountability and Scenarios H.

Protection of Vulnerable Adults (POVA): Government policy supported by several statutory provisions is designed to support vulnerable adults. See Chapter 11 and Scenarios H.

General authority: this was a concept used in earlier versions of the Mental Capacity Bill, to denote the power of a person to act out of necessity in the best interests of a mentally incapacitated adult. However it was considered to be misleading by the Joint Committee of the Houses of Parliament, and was not included in the MCA.

Children: the MCA applies to young persons over 16 years and adults. There are some provisions however which can apply to persons younger than that, and there are differences in law between the young person of 16 or 17 and an adult. These are considered in Chapter 12 and Scenarios I.

Human tissue and organ removal, storage and use: special protection is given to those lacking the requisite mental capacity to give consent to the removal, storage and use of human tissue and organs by the MCA and the Human Tissue Act, and regulations under both Acts. This topic is considered in Chapter 14 and Scenario K.

Sources of help

Any person trying to unravel the impact that the MCA has on their work or on the rights of the mentally incapacitated adult for whom they care will find extremely extensive resources for assistance. The main source of assistance is the website of the Department for Constitutional Affairs (DCA). The DCA has published many leaflets and booklets explaining the Act for a wide variety of readers, and these can be down loaded from its website.[2] These include: a users/clients or patients guide (*Making decisions about your health welfare or finance. Who decides when you can't?* (booklet 1)); a guide for family friends, and other unpaid carers (booklet 2); for people who work in health and social care (booklet 3); for advice workers (booklet 4), and an easy read guide (booklet 5).

The Mental Capacity Act 2005 itself can be downloaded from the DCA[3] and from the UK legislation site.[4] All the Statutory Instruments referred to can be downloaded from these sites. Hard copies of the legislation can be purchased from the Stationery Office.

The Code of Practice has been compiled by the Lord Chancellor across a significant number of areas (see Chapter 17). It can be accessed from the website of the DCA.[5] The Code of Practice should be followed by health and social services professionals and those listed in Section 42(4). However whilst it is not statutorily binding upon the informal or unpaid carer, there would be considerable benefit for such persons to follow the guidance in the code.

Explanatory Memorandum: accompanying the statute and available from the HMSO website is an Explanatory Memorandum which provides guidance in understanding some of the statutory provisions. It is not in itself the law, but could provide some help in comprehending some of the more difficult provisions.

Memorandum submitted to the Joint Committee on Human Rights in response to its letter of 18 November 2004: the Report of the Joint Committee of Parliament[6] provides further insight into the thinking behind the legislation, and is discussed throughout this book as appropriate. The report can be downloaded from the DCA website.

Professional guidance: many of the professional associations of those involved in the care of mentally incapacitated adults are drawing up detailed guidance for their members on the provisions of the Act and this is available from their websites (see websites list).

Protocols, procedures, guidance from the Healthcare Commission, Commission for Social Care and Inspection and other such institutions: during the next few years there is likely to be more guidance issued by some of the bodies involved in the inspection of health and social care institutions. Their recommendations following visits of inspection are not in themselves the law, but they could provide evidence of good practice. Similarly, conclusions and recommendations following inquiries carried out by the Health Service Commission or Ombudsman and the Ombudsman for Local Authorities may be extremely helpful to those involved in the care of those lacking mental capacity.

Protocols, procedures, guidance from employers: many National Health Service (NHS) trusts, primary care trusts and care trusts and social services departments are preparing protocols etc, to assist their staff in implementing the laws which apply to decision making on behalf of mentally incapacitated adults. These in general should be followed by staff, but registered practitioners also need to use their professional discretion and ensure that such guidance is in accordance with the basic principles of law and practice, as recommended in the codes of practice of their registered bodies.

Protocols, procedures, guidance and information from organisations involved in the care and protection of mentally incapacitated adults: many organisations which are involved in providing care and protection for mentally incapacitated adults gave advice and information to Parliament, and in particular to the Joint Committee during the progress of the Mental Incapacity and Mental Capacity Bills through Parliament. These organisations will continue to advise their members and other interested persons on the best practice in caring for and offering support and assistance to those lacking mental capacity. The websites of some of these organisations are set out in the list of websites at the end of the book.

Terms used

Many of the terms employed in the Act may alienate those who are seeking to obtain a greater understanding of the law. Many of the probably unfamiliar terms such as lasting power of attorney, donee, deputy and advance decision are considered in context, and are mentioned above with the chapters cited in which they are further discussed.

A **glossary** is also to be found on pages xvii–xxiv, which explains other legal terms with which the reader may not be familiar.

Organisations involved in the care and support of adults who lack mental capacity

The causes of mental incapacity are diverse. Some suffer from severe learning disabilities acquired as a result of brain damage or genetic causes, and would therefore never have enjoyed having capacity. Others may have lost their mental capacity as a result of deteriorating diseases such as Alzheimer's, or of a trauma such as a road accident. These persons once had capacity, and it is possible from discussions with family and friends to piece together a picture of that person's earlier beliefs, philosophy and likes and dislikes which can be used in determining 'best interests'.

The organisations providing support for such adults include the following:

Public authorities: NHS trusts, primary care trusts, care trusts, social services departments.

Charitable and voluntary organisations: these include many residential and care homes, community support homes, care agencies, and leisure organisations providing services for the disabled.

Profit making organisations: these provide many and varied services, often in contract with public authorities.

All such organisations may provide useful information on the care and support of those lacking mental capacity.

Scenarios are linked with each of the main chapters to illustrate some of the situations which may arise, and to assist in explaining how the new statutory provisions are likely to work.

Future changes: inevitably there will be disputes over the interpretation of some of the statutory provisions, and these disputes will result in court hearings and judgments which will set precedents on how the Act is to be interpreted, and thus become part of the common law (see Chapter 2).

References

1 *Bolam* v. *Friern Hospital Management Committee* [1957] 1 WLR 582.
2 www.dca.gov.uk
3 www.dca.gov.uk/legal-policy/mentalcapacity/index.htm
4 www.opsi.gov.uk
5 www.dh.gov.uk
6 House of Lords and House of Commons Joint Committee on the Draft Mental Incapacity Bill Session 2002–2003. H.L. paper 189–91; H.C. 1083–1.

2 Background to the Legal System and the Mental Capacity Act

Legislation relating to decision making on behalf of mentally incapacitated adults has been on the drawing board for over 15 years. This chapter explains the distinction between statutory and non-statutory law, discusses why statutory provision was considered necessary and looks briefly at the steps leading to the Mental Capacity Act 2005.

The legal system

The law derives from two main sources:

1. *Acts of Parliament and Statutory Instruments which are enacted under the powers given by the former*: these are known as statutory sources and include the legislation of the European Community. These take precedence over all other laws. Laws of the European Community automatically become part of the law of the United Kingdom. The Council and the Commission have law-making powers and this can be in the form of Regulations or Directives. The Human Rights Act 1998 is in a special position (see Chapter 3). Acts of Parliament and Statutory Instruments have Chapter numbers for each year, or a serial number. A website makes for easy access to Acts of Parliament and Statutory Instruments.[1]

2. *The common law (also known as case law or judge made law)*: this is made up of the decisions by judges in individual cases which are often, but not always, interpretations of statute law. The judge, in deciding a particular case, is bound by a previous decision on the law made by judges in an earlier case, if it is relevant to the facts before him and if that decision was made by a higher court than the one in which he is sitting. There is a recognised order of

precedence so that, for example, a decision by the House of Lords is binding on all other courts except itself, but would be subject to relevant precedents of the European Court of Justice. The decisions are recorded by officially recognised reporters, so that in a case similar to a previous one the earlier decision can be put before the court. If the facts and the situation are comparable and the decision was made by a court whose decisions are binding, then the earlier precedent will be followed. If there are grounds for distinguishing the earlier case (i.e. showing that there are significant differences from the earlier case) then the earlier case may not be followed.

Of vital importance to the system of precedence is a reliable procedure for recording the facts and decisions of any court case. Each court has a recognised system of reporting and the case is quoted by a reference which should enable the full report of the case to be found easily. An example is given in the glossary under *case citation*.

Changing the law

There are recognised rules for interpreting Acts of Parliament and in relation to the following of case precedents. Ultimately, however, if the law is unsatisfactory and fails to provide justice, the courts look to the Houses of Parliament to remedy the situation by new legislation. There is a right of appeal on matters of law to courts of higher jurisdiction. An appeal can be taken to the Court of Appeal and from there to the House of Lords, if permission is granted. Until the House of Lords has pronounced on a particular point of law, there may be considerable uncertainty as to what the law in a given situation is. A number of cases relating to mental capacity have been referred to the House of Lords in recent years.

Official guidance and advice

Department of Health (DH) circulars, Department of Social Security (DSS) circulars and Nursing and Midwifery Council (NMC) codes of practice are not legally binding, but they are recommended practice. Breach of these codes and guidance may be evidence of failure to follow the approved practice, but cannot in itself result in successful civil or criminal action.

Human rights

The rights recognised in the European Convention on Human Rights, which were brought into force in this country in October 2000, have also had a major impact on the rights and the protection of mentally incapacitated and vulnerable adults. This is considered in Chapter 3.

Judicial review

Administrative and other action can be challenged in the High Court by an application for judicial review. Public funding for legal costs in judicial review is available from legal professionals and advice agencies, which have contracts with the Legal Services Commission as part of the Community Legal Service.[2] Judicial review allows people with a sufficient interest in a decision or action by a public body to ask a judge to review the lawfulness of an enactment or a decision, action or failure to act in relation to the exercise of a public function. An example of a case where an application was made for judicial review of a decision by a local authority to reorganise its care homes with a private operator is shown in Box 2.1.

Box 2.1: an example of a judicial review.[3]

Care home residents applied for judicial review of a decision by the local authority to seek a private sector operator to accept a transfer of, operate and expand two care homes, and to close another two care homes once the residents had been transferred to suitable alternative accommodation. It was argued that the private operator was exercising functions of a public nature and that the residents' rights were protected under Article 8 of the European Convention on Human Rights (see Chapter 3). The application was refused on the grounds that the private operator was not exercising functions of a public nature. The transfer did not absolve the local authority of its duty to ensure that the residents' rights under Articles 3 and 8 were protected.

The law relating to trespass to the person and consent

It is a basic principle of the common law that a mentally competent adult is able to refuse even life saving treatment, for a good reason, a bad reason or no reason at all.[4] To act contrary to the wishes of a mentally competent person, in the absence of any legal justification such as the Mental Health Act 1983 or the Police and Criminal Evidence Act 1984, is known as a trespass to the person, i.e. a civil wrong. In certain circumstances it may also be a crime (see glossary under **trespass to the person**).

An action for trespass which belongs to a group of civil wrongs (known as 'torts') is one of the oldest remedies in law (known as a right of action in law); it includes an assault and a battery. An action for assault arises where the employee of the defendant (in this context normally the employer of the health professional, who would be sued because of its vicarious liability for the actions of the employee) causes a claimant reasonable apprehension of the infliction of a battery upon him/her; a battery arises where there is intentional and direct application of force to another person.

Assault and battery are also used to describe possible criminal actions, but when we are using the terms in relation to a trespass to the person, we are referring to a civil action brought in the civil courts (i.e. Small Claims Court, County Court, High Court) for compensation by a claimant. The fact that the defendant has acted out of good motives, e.g. the best interests of the claimant, is not a valid defence where the claimant is an adult, has the requisite mental capacity and has made it clear that he or she does not wish to have that intervention.

Unlike an action for negligence, harm does not have to be proved. The mere fact that a trespass has occurred is sufficient to bring an action. The legal action is known as actionable per se, i.e. actionable without proof of harm having been suffered.

An example of a case where a woman was able to refuse life saving treatment is shown in Box 2.2.

Box 2.2: *Re B* 2002.[5]

Miss B suffered a ruptured blood vessel in her neck which damaged her spinal cord. As a consequence she was paralysed from the neck down and was on a ventilator. She was of sound mind and knew that there was no cure for her condition. She asked for the ventilator to be switched off. Her doctors wished her to try out some special rehabilitation to improve the standard of her care and felt that an intensive care ward was not a suitable location for such a decision to be made. They were reluctant to perform such an action as switching off the ventilator without the court's approval. Miss B applied to court for a declaration to be made that the ventilator could be switched off.

The main issue in the case was the mental competence of Miss B. If she were held to be mentally competent, then she could refuse to have life saving treatment for a good reason, a bad reason or no reason at all. She was interviewed by two psychiatrists who gave evidence to the court that she was mentally competent. The judge therefore held that she was entitled to refuse to be ventilated. The judge Dame Elizabeth Butler-Sloss, President of the Family Division, held that Miss B possessed the requisite mental capacity to make decisions regarding her treatment, and thus the administration of artificial respiration by the trust against her wishes amounted to an unlawful trespass.

Dame Elizabeth Butler-Sloss restated the principles which had been laid down by the Court of Appeal in the case of St George's Healthcare Trust.[6]

- There was a presumption that a patient had the mental capacity to make decisions whether to consent to or refuse medical or surgical treatment offered.
- If mental capacity was not an issue and the patient, having been given the relevant information and offered the available option, chose to refuse that treatment, that decision had to be respected by the doctors. Considerations of what the best interests of the patient would involve were irrelevant.

- Concern or doubts about the patient's mental capacity should be resolved as soon as possible by the doctors within the hospital or other normal medical procedures.
- Meanwhile the patient must be cared for in accordance with the judgment of the doctors as to the patient's best interests.
- It was most important that those considering the issue should not confuse the question of mental capacity with the nature of the decision made by the patient, however grave the consequences. Since the view of the patient might reflect a difference in values rather than an absence of competence, the assessment of capacity should be approached with that in mind and doctors should not allow an emotional reaction to, or strong disagreement with, the patient's decision to cloud their judgment in answering the primary question of capacity.
- Where disagreement still existed about competence, it was of the utmost importance that the patient be fully informed, involved and engaged in the process, which could involve obtaining independent outside help, of resolving the disagreement since the patient's involvement could be crucial to a good outcome.
- If the hospital was faced with a dilemma which doctors did not know how to resolve, that must be recognised and further steps taken as a matter of priority. Those in charge must not allow a situation of deadlock or drift to occur.
- If there was no disagreement about competence, but the doctors were for any reason unable to carry out the patient's wishes, it was their duty to find other doctors who would do so.
- If all appropriate steps to seek independent assistance from medical experts outside the hospital had failed, the hospital should not hesitate to make an application to the High Court or seek the advice of the Official Solicitor.
- The treating clinicians and the hospital should always have in mind that a seriously physically disabled patient who was mentally competent had the same right to personal autonomy and to make decisions as any other person with mental capacity.

It was reported on 29 April 2002 that Miss B had died peacefully in her sleep after the ventilator had been switched off.

See Case Study H3 for discussion of the case in the context of the crimes of murder, manslaughter and assisted suicide.

Decisions relating to mental capacity

In the absence of statutory provision (i.e. prior to the bringing into force of the Mental Capacity Act 2005), disputes relating to the presence or absence of mental capacity and the decisions to be made in the event of capacity being seen to be lacking, have been made by the courts. In the leading case of Re F,[7] the House of Lords held that doctors could take action out of necessity, on behalf of a mentally incapacitated adult who was incapable of making her own decisions. The action had to be taken in her best interests and had to follow the reasonable standard of care. The facts of the case are shown in Box 2.3.

> **Box 2.3: Sterilisation of a mentally incapacitated adult (*Re F (Mental Patient: Sterilisation*) [1990]).**[7]
>
> F was 36 years old and had severe learning disabilities, with the mental age of a small child. She lived in a mental hospital and had formed a sexual relationship with a male patient. The hospital staff considered that she would be unable to cope with a pregnancy and recommended that she should be sterilised, considering that other forms of contraception were unsuitable. Her mother supported the idea of a sterilisation operation, but because F was over 18 years old did not have the right in law to give consent on her behalf. The mother therefore applied to court for a declaration that an operation for sterilisation was in her best interests and should be declared lawful.

The judge granted the declaration sought by F's mother. The Official Solicitor (who acts on behalf of the mentally incapacitated adult) appealed against the declaration to the Court of Appeal, which upheld the judge's order. The Official Solicitor then appealed to the House of Lords. The House of Lords held that there was at common law (i.e. judge made law or case law) the power for a person to act in the best interests of a mentally incapacitated adult. This power is derived from the principle of necessity.

The principle of necessity

Necessity may arise in an emergency situation, e.g. when an unconscious person comes into hospital, and the health professionals should do no more than is reasonably required in the best interests of the patient, before he/she recovers consciousness. Necessity may also arise in a situation where a person is permanently or semi-permanently lacking mental capacity. In such a situation, there is no point in waiting for the patient to give consent. According to Lord Goff:

> The need to care for him [the patient] is obvious; and the doctor must then act in the best interests of his patient just as if he had received his consent so to do. Were this not so, much useful treatment and care could, in theory at least, be denied to the unfortunate.

The doctor must act in accordance with a responsible and competent body of relevant professional opinion. This is known as the Bolam Test, taken from a case heard in 1957[8] (see Chapter 11 and Scenario H4).

In the case shown in Box 2.3, the House of Lords issued a declaration that sterilisation was in the best interests of F and could proceed. It did recommend that in future such cases of sterilisation for social reasons (as opposed, for example, to sterilisation which resulted from an operation to remove a cancerous growth) should be brought before the courts for a declaration to be made.

The courts have also had to decide on the appropriate treatment for sufferers from Creutzfeldt-Jakob disease (vCJD) which is shown in Box 2.4.

> **Box 2.4: Treatment for vCJD sufferers (*Simms* v. *an NHS Trust and the Secretary of State for Health*[9]).**
>
> JS a boy of 18 years and JA a girl of 16 years suffered from vCJD, and in each case the parents sought declaratory relief that each lacked capacity to make a decision about future treatment proposed for them, and that it was lawful in their best interests to receive it. The proposed treatment was new and so far untested on human beings. The judge concluded in the light of all the evidence and the circumstances that it was in the best interests of JS and JA to receive the treatment: JA as a 16-year-old came under the Children Act 1989 and the direct responsibility of the judge under Section 1 was to consider the child's welfare as the paramount consideration. (Subsequently the NHS Trust's two Committees, one on Clinical Governance and Quality and the other the Drugs and Therapeutic Panel, decided that the treatment could not be approved, and the DH was investigating other possible facilities for the provision of the treatment.)

Weaknesses of common law

The absence of statutory provisions has meant that the courts have had to make declarations on the absence of mental capacity, and to determine what actions appear to be in the interests of the mentally incapacitated person on the basis of existing case law or the common law. There was no statutory right for a person to make treatment or care decisions on behalf of a mentally incapacitated person over 18 years (apart from decisions on the treatment for mental disorder of patients detained under the Mental Health Act 1983). Parents or guardians have the right to make decisions on behalf of young persons and children up to the age of 18 years, but once the offspring are 18 years, parents no longer have the right at common law to make decisions on their behalf, even though the young person lacks the requisite mental capacity.

However the legal principles in the precedents set by the courts lack the clarity and detail that statutes and statutory regulations would provide, and there has been considerable pressure over many years for statutory provision for decision making on behalf of mentally incapacitated adults.

Law Commission

The ninth item of the Fourth Programme of Law Reform undertaken by the Law Commission in 1989[10] was the laws relating to decision making on behalf of mentally incapacitated adults. In the course of its work it published several consultation papers. The first was an overview of mentally incapacitated adults and decision making published in 1991.[11] This was followed by other papers[12] on specific topics such as medical treatment and research and the protection of vulnerable adults, and led ultimately to the Law Commission's Report on Mental Incapacity which included draft legislation, i.e. a Mental Incapacity Bill.[13]

Events since 1995

It would have been possible for the Law Commission's Mental Incapacity Bill printed at the end of its Final Report in 1995 to have been placed before Parliament for debate and enactment in 1995. However there was not the political will to progress at that time. The advent of the Labour Government in 1997 led to the publication of a new consultation paper, issued from the Lord Chancellor's Office, called *Who Decides?*.[14] It set out the issues which had been considered by the Law Commission between 1991 and 1995. *Who Decides?* was followed by a White Paper, *Making Decisions*,[15] in October 1999.

Subsequently draft legislation to bring the proposals set out in the White Paper into force was published in June 2003[16] and was the subject of scrutiny by a joint committee of the House of Commons and House of Lords. The Joint Committee published its report in November 2003 and made almost 100 recommendations on changes to the draft Bill, including the change of title to Mental Capacity Bill.[17] A revised Mental Capacity Bill was introduced into Parliament in 2004 and was the subject of considerable parliamentary debate, especially over the statutory provision for living wills or advance decisions (see Chapter 9). In Scotland the Adults with Incapacity (Scotland) Act 2000 has now been brought into force, and covers the situation of decision making on behalf of incapacitated adults.

Mental Capacity Act 2005

The Mental Capacity Bill received the royal assent in April 2005 but whilst some provisions came into force in April 2007, the rest was not due to be brought into force until October 2007 (see Chapter 17). Why the delay? Time was required for many consultation papers to be published including one on the draft Code of Practice and on the regulations to be drawn up under the Act. A new administrative organisation for the Court of Protection had to be established and the Office of Public Guardian set up. Regulations were required to be drafted under the powers set forth in the Act, to be consulted upon and approved by Parliament. In addition, of course, extensive training was required, not just of the health and social services professionals, but also of the judiciary and those allocated with the administration of the new provisions and charities and organisations concerned with the protection of vulnerable adults and the adults themselves.

Mental health legislation

There is a distinction between mental incapacity and mental disorder as defined in the Mental Health Act 1983. It is possible for a person to lack the mental capacity to make certain decisions but not to be suffering from mental disorder. Thus a person with learning disabilities may be incapable of making certain decisions, but would not necessarily come within the provisions of the Mental Health Act 1983. The definition of mental disorder under the 1983 Act as amended by the 2007 Act is considered in Chapter 13.

Mental health legislation must also be reviewed in the light of the Human Rights Act 1998. Article 5 of the European Convention on Human Rights recognises that:

> everyone has the right to liberty and security of person. No one shall be deprived of his liberty save in the following cases and in accordance with a procedure prescribed by law

This right is subject to specified exceptions including:

> the lawful detention . . . of persons of unsound mind

The Court of Appeal has held that where a patient refused to consent to treatment, the court would not give permission for the treatment to proceed unless medical necessity was convincingly shown.[18] The case is shown in Box 2.5.

Box 2.5: *R (N)* v. *Dr M and Others* (2002).

The responsible medical officer drew up for a detained patient (the claimant) a treatment plan, which included administering by injection anti-psychotic medicine for the prevention or alleviation of psychotic illness. The claimant did not consent to that treatment. A second doctor appointed under the provisions of the Mental Health Act 1983 to provide a second opinion issued a certificate that the patient was suffering from paranoid psychosis/severe personality disorder and required regular anti-psychotic treatment. The patient challenged those decisions. An independent psychiatrist advised that the claimant was very unlikely to be suffering from a psychotic illness and should not be given anti-psychotic medication. The Court of Appeal held that the judge had to be satisfied that the proposed treatment was both in the claimant's best interests and medically necessary for the purposes of Article 3 of the Human Rights Convention. The best interests test went wider than medical necessity: the standard of proof required was that the court should be satisfied that medical necessity had been convincingly shown. Provided the judge applied the correct approach to determining whether there had been a breach of a Convention right, the review of a decision which would otherwise violate a person's right under Article 6 would be sufficient for Convention purposes. The claimant lost her appeal.

In another case, the Court of Appeal held that the state had a duty to protect incompetent patients and that Section 2 of the Mental Health Act 1983 was incompatible with Article 5(4) of the European Convention on Human Rights.[19] The case is considered in Chapter 3.

Reform of the Mental Health Act 1983

Discussions on the reform of the Mental Health Act 1983 have been taking place for over eight years. An expert committee was set up by the Government in 1998 under the chairmanship of Professor Richardson to review the Mental Health Act 1983. Its terms of reference included the degree to which the current legislation needs updating, and to ensure that there is a proper balance between safety (both of individuals and the wider community) and the rights of individual patients. It was required to advise the government on how mental health legislation should be shaped to reflect contemporary patterns of care and treatment, and to support its policy as set out in *Modernising Health Services*.[20]

The Expert Committee presented its preliminary proposals, which set out the principles on which any future legislation should be based, in April 1999, and its full report was published in November 1999.[21] The Government presented its proposals for reform in 1999, with a final date for response by 31 March 2000.[22] The Consultation Paper was followed by a White Paper issued on 20 December 2000,[23] which proposed a new legal framework for the mentally disordered, and the second part made provision for high risk patients. The White Paper stated that new mental health legislation will provide a single framework for the application of compulsory powers for care and treatment, and that the new legislation will be compatible with the European Convention on Human Rights.

A draft Bill[24] was then published in 2002 for further consultation. This met with considerable criticism and provision for a new Mental Health Bill was not made in the Queen's speech in November 2003. However the Secretary of State for Health announced that a revised Mental Health Bill was to be brought forward for pre-legislative scrutiny. A further draft Mental Health Bill was published in November 2006 which, rather than introduce a new Mental Health Act (MHA), sought to amend the provisions of the Mental Health Act 1983.

The resultant Mental Health Act 2007 is very much a compromise on the radical proposals initially put forward in 1997. It amends the Mental Capacity Act 2005 to fill the gaps in the law revealed by the Bournewood case (see Chapters 3 and 13 and Scenario J10). It introduces a compulsory treatment order in the community and ensures that those with personality disorders can be compelled to be treated. It also provides rights to advocacy, safeguards on using electro-convulsive treatment and removes the right of a parent to overrule the refusal of a child of 16 and 17 years to be admitted to psychiatric hospital. The Act is considered in Chapter 13.

The future role of the common law

Inevitably disputes will arise over the interpretation of the Mental Capacity Act 2005 and the regulations enacted under it. It will be the task of the courts to lay down principles to be followed, possibly to fill gaps in the statutory provisions until such time as Parliament enacts amending legislation to fill those gaps. One significant gap which is being filled is known as the Bournewood gap. The Bournewood case and the problems which it has shown to exist in our present laws are discussed in the next chapter and in Chapter 13.

References

1   www. opsi.gov.uk/legislation
2   See Annex C to the *Pre-action Protocol for Judicial Review Civil Procedure Rules* available from the DCA website: www.dca.gov.uk/civil/procrules_fin/contents/protocols/prot_judicialreview

3   *R. (On the application of Johnson)* v. *Havering LBC* [2006] EWHC 1714; [2006] BLGR 631, QBD.
4   For more detailed discussion on the law relating to consent see Dimond, B. (2003) *The legal aspects of consent.* Quay Publishing, Dinton, Wiltshire.
5   *Re B (Consent to treatment: capacity),* Times Law Report, 26 March 2002; [2002] 2 All ER 449.
6   *St George's Healthcare NHS Trust* v. *S* [1998] 3 All ER 673.
7   *F* v. *West Berkshire Health Authority* [1989] 2 All ER 545; [1990] 2 AC 1.
8   *Bolam* v. *Friern Hospital Management Committee* [1957] 1 WLR 582.
9   *Simms* v. *an NHS Trust and the Secretary of State for Health* [2002] EWHC 2734.
10   Fourth Programme of Law Reform (1989) Law Com No 185 CM 800.
11   Law Commission (1991) *Mentally Incapacitated Adults and Decision-Making: An Overview.* Consultation Paper No 119. HMSO, London.
12   Law Commission (1993) *Mentally Incapacitated Adults and Decision-Making: A New Jurisdiction.* Consultation Paper No 128. HMSO, London; Law Commission (1993) *Mentally Incapacitated Adults and Decision-Making: Medical Treatment and Research.* Consultation Paper No 129. HMSO, London; Law Commission (1993) *Mentally Incapacitated and Other Vulnerable Adults: Public Law Protection.* Consultation Paper No 130. HMSO, London.
13   Law Commission (1995) *Mental Incapacity.* Report No. 231 TSO HMSO, London.
14   Lord Chancellor's Office (1997) *Who Decides?.* TSO.
15   Lord Chancellor's Office (1999) *Making Decisions: the Government's proposals for making decisions on behalf of mentally incapacitated adults.* TSO.
16   Department of Health (2003) Draft Mental Incapacity Bill, CM 5859; http://www.parliament.uk/parliamentary_committees/jcmib.cfmw
17   House of Lords and House of Commons Joint Committee on the Draft Mental Incapacity Bill Session 2002-3, HL paper 189-1; HC 1083-1.
18   *R (N)* v. *Dr M and Others,* Times Law Report, 12 December 2002; CA.
19   *R (MH)* v. *Secretary of State for Health,* Times Law Report, 8 December 2004, CA; [2004] EWCA Civ 1609.
20   Department of Health (1998) *Modernising Mental Health Services.* DH, London.
21   Department of Health (1999) *Review of Expert Committee Review of the Mental Health Act 1983.* DH, London.
22   Department of Health (1999) *Reform of the Mental Health Act 1983.* DH, London.
23   Department of Health (2000) *White Paper Reforming the Mental Health Act.* DH, London.
24   Draft Mental Health Bill 2002, CM 5538-1.

3 Human Rights and Statutory Principles for Governing Decision Making

Introduction

This chapter considers the underlying principles of law which apply to the making of decisions and acting on behalf of those who are incapable of making their own choices. Some of these principles are set out in the Mental Capacity Act 2005 itself; others are contained in the European Convention on Human Rights which has been incorporated into the laws of the United Kingdom (UK), and also in the Convention on the International Protection of Adults[1] which is given legal recognition by Section 63 of the Mental Capacity Act 2005. Chapter 2 of the Code of Practice gives guidance on the statutory principles and how they are applied.[2]

The Human Rights Act 1998

The UK was a signatory of the European Convention for the Protection of Human Rights and Fundamental Freedoms at the end of World War II. However, anyone who sought to bring an action for breach of their human rights, as set out in the Convention, was unable to take the case to the courts in this country but had to go to the European Court of Human Rights in Strasbourg. Please note that this is not the court of the European Community (i.e. the European Court of Justice), which meets in Luxembourg. It was estimated that to take a case to Strasbourg cost over £30 000 and took over five years. The Human Rights Act 1998 came into force on 2 October 2000 (it came into force in Scotland on devolution).

It has three main effects:

- First, it is unlawful for a public authority (or an organisation exercising functions of a public nature)[3] to breach the rights set out in the Convention.

- Secondly, from 2 October 2000 an allegation of a breach of the rights by a public authority can be brought in the courts of this country.
- Thirdly, judges can make a declaration that legislation which is raised in a case before them is incompatible with the articles of the Convention. The legislation will then usually be referred back to Parliament for reconsideration.[3]

The Act is not retrospective, but any person concerned about an infringement before 2 October 2000 could take a case to Strasbourg, depending upon time limits.

Action can be brought against a public authority or organisation exercising public functions for breach of the Convention articles in the courts of this country. An example of a declaration by a court that law is incompatible with the articles of the Convention on Human Rights is a declaration of the House of Lords,[4] which held that present marriage laws in the country which prevented a trans-sexual marrying following his gender change (because the law did not recognise the change of gender) were incompatible with the Convention on Human Rights. A Gender Recognition Act 2004 was then enacted which enables applicants who meet specified criteria to apply for a replacement birth certificate; they are then allowed to marry in their adopted sex.

European Convention on Human Rights[5]
Articles of the European Convention on Human Rights relevant to decision-making for persons lacking mental capacity

Article 2: Right to life

> Everyone's right to life shall be protected by law. No one shall be deprived of his life intentionally save in the execution of a sentence of a court following his conviction of a crime for which this penalty is provided by law. (See Protocols 6 and 13 which abolish the death penalty and were ratified by the UK.)

Diane Pretty failed in her attempt to secure an advance pardon for her husband, if he should assist her in securing a dignified pain-free death. Her argument that the Suicide Act 1961 was contrary to her human rights in making it illegal for anyone to aid, abet, counsel or procure the suicide of another or an attempt by another to commit suicide was not accepted by the English courts nor by the European Court of Human Rights in Strasbourg.[6] Article 2 does not include a right to end one's life.

In other cases it has been held that ending artificial feeding or ventilation of a patient in a persistent vegetative state was not contrary to Article 2 of the European Convention on Human Rights. For example, H a female patient had been in a permanent vegetative state for eight years, and a declaration was made that the health trust could withdraw hydration and nutrition from her and this was not contrary to Article 2 of the European Convention on Human Rights.[7] Article 2 imposed a positive obligation to give life sustaining treatment where that is in the best interests of the patient, but not where it would be futile.

Discontinuing treatment would not be an intentional deprivation of life under Article 2.

On Article 2 the House of Lords and House of Commons Joint Committee (hereafter 'the Joint Committee') stated that (Para 53):

> We are of the opinion that under the proper interpretation of Article 2, the State has a secondary obligation to protect life, but an individual can choose not to uphold that right. Accordingly the mechanisms under the draft Bill, which permit the refusal of consent to the carrying out or continuation of treatment, in accordance to the wishes of the patient, do not contravene Article 2 of the European Convention on Human Rights.

Article 3: Prohibition of torture

> No one shall be subjected to torture or to inhuman or degrading treatment or punishment.

The Mental Capacity Act 2005 includes principles to be followed in respecting the autonomy of a mentally competent adult (see below), and these go to the heart of the underlying concept behind Article 3. In the case cited above[8] the court held that the discontinuation of artificial hydration and nutrition to a person in a permanent vegetative state was not torture under Article 3, provided that withdrawing treatment was in line with a respected body of medical opinion and that the patient would be unaware of the treatment and not suffering.

The Joint Committee discussed whether the provisions on the use of restraint violated Article 3 and came to the conclusion, in agreement with the Joint Committee on Human Rights, that the draft Bill provided sufficient safeguards to ensure that the right to be free from degrading treatment was protected.

The amendments to the Mental Capacity Act resulting from filling the Bournewood gap (see below) have permitted a situation where loss of liberty may result from the provisions of the Act, but there are rigid conditions to be satisfied.

Article 4: Prohibition of slavery and forced labour

1. No one shall be held in slavery or servitude.
2. No one shall be required to perform forced or compulsory labour.
3. For the purpose of this Article the term 'forced or compulsory labour' shall not include:
    (a) any work required to be done in the ordinary course of detention imposed according to the provisions of Article 5 of this Convention or during conditional release from such detention;
    (b) any service of a military character or, in case of conscientious objectors in countries where they are recognised, service exacted instead of compulsory military service;
    (c) any service exacted in case of an emergency or calamity threatening the life or well-being of the community;
    (d) any work or service which forms part of normal civic obligations.

The courts have held that where trainee lawyers were required to undertake a certain amount of voluntary work as part of their training, that was not a violation of Article 4. However it is possible that where persons lacking mental capacity were compelled to work against their will, Article 4 rights could be seen as infringed, depending upon the circumstances.

Article 5: Right to liberty and security

1. Everyone has the right to liberty and security of person. No one shall be deprived of his liberty save in the following cases and in accordance with a procedure prescribed by law:
    (a) the lawful detention of a person after conviction by a competent court;
    (b) the lawful arrest or detention of a person for non-compliance with the lawful order of a court or in order to secure the fulfilment of any obligation prescribed by law;
    (c) the lawful arrest or detention of a person effected for the purpose of bringing him before the competent legal authority on reasonable suspicion of having committed an offence or when it is reasonably considered necessary to prevent his committing an offence or fleeing after having done so;
    (d) the detention of a minor by lawful order for the purpose of educational supervision or his lawful detention for the purpose of bringing him before the competent legal authority;
    (e) the lawful detention of persons for the prevention of the spreading of infectious diseases, of persons of unsound mind, alcoholics or drug addicts or vagrants;
    (f) the lawful arrest or detention of a person to prevent his effecting an unauthorised entry into the country or of a person against whom action is being taken with a view to deportation or extradition.
2. Everyone who is arrested shall be informed promptly, in a language which he understands, of the reasons for his arrest and of any charge against him.
3. Everyone arrested or detained in accordance with the provisions of Para 1(c) of this Article shall be brought promptly before a judge or other officer authorised by law to exercise judicial power and shall be entitled to trial within a reasonable time or to release pending trial. Release may be conditioned by guarantees to appear for trial.
4. Everyone who is deprived of his liberty by arrest or detention shall be entitled to take proceedings by which the lawfulness of his detention shall be decided speedily by a court and his release ordered if the detention is not lawful.
5. Everyone who has been the victim of arrest or detention in contravention of the provisions of this Article shall have an enforceable right to compensation.

The implications of Article 5 and the detention of a mentally disordered adult were considered in the Bournewood case (see below and Chapter 13). Its significance is far-reaching and applies to the many thousands of mentally incapacitated adults who are cared for in hospitals and residential and care homes, without being placed under the Mental Health Act 2007.

Restriction and loss of liberty

The distinction between a loss of liberty and a restriction on liberty were considered in a recent case, where the placement by a county council of a mentally incapable person in a care home was challenged as being a breach of Article 5 rights. The facts are shown in Box 3.1.

Box 3.1: Loss of liberty contrary to Article 5.[9]

Surrey County Council (SCC) placed DE in X residential care home in September 2005 and then transferred him to Y residential home two months later. JE, his wife, claimed that DE was being held against his wishes and that SCC was in breach of DE's rights under Article 5, and also DE's and her own rights under Article 8. The judge accepted earlier precedents from cases heard by the European Court of Human Rights that the difference between deprivation of and restriction upon liberty is merely one of degree or intensity, and not one of nature or substance.[10] The judge held that on the facts of the case the restrictions which SCC placed on DE (that he could not leave first X home and then Y home and return to live with JE) were in breach of his Article 5 rights.

It remains to be seen if the Bournewood safeguards (see below) introduced into the Mental Capacity Act 2005 by the Mental Health Act 2007 will enable a local authority to take appropriate action in such cases as the Surrey County Council without a breach of Article 5 rights.

Example of incompatibility between Ss2 and 29(4) of MHA and Article 5

In one case the Court of Appeal held that Sections 2 and 29(4) of the Mental Health Act 1983 were incompatible with Article 5(4) of the European Convention and the state had a duty to protect incompetent patients.[11] The case is shown in Box 3.2.

Box 3.2: *R (MH)* v. *Secretary of State for Health* (2004).

MH was 32 years old and suffered from Down's Syndrome. She was admitted to detention under Section 2 of the Mental Health Act 1983. Her mother applied for her discharge under Section 23, but this was barred by the responsible medical officer and an application was made under Section 29 to remove the mother as the nearest relative. This application had the effect of retaining the Section 2 detention beyond the 28 days until the application was heard by the court. MH maintained that her rights under Article 5.4 were violated since, because of her incapacity, she was unable to appeal to the Mental Health Review Tribunal under the statutory provisions. The Court of Appeal held that the state was obliged to make provision for referring to a court the case of a patient who was detained under the Mental Health Act 1983 who was incapable of exercising her right to apply to a mental health review tribunal on her own initiative. The Court of Appeal also held that Section 29(4) of the Mental Health Act 1983 was incompatible with Article 5(4) of the European Convention on Human Rights, since there was no provision for referral to court for a patient detained under Section 2 whose period of detention was extended under Section 29(4).

Restraint and loss of liberty

Several new clauses were added to the Mental Capacity Bill to ensure that where restraint was permitted subject to specified conditions this restraint could not amount to a loss of liberty under Article 5 (e.g. Section 6(5) of the Mental Capacity Act (MCA)):

> (5) But D does more than merely restrain P if he deprives P of his liberty within the meaning of Article 5(1) of the Human Rights Convention (whether or not D is a public authority).

However in order to make amendments to the MCA for the purposes of filling the Bournewood gap, the Mental Health Act 2007 Section 38(4)(a) has repealed Section 6(5) of the MCA and replaced it with new Sections 4A and 4B, which would justify the deprivation of liberty in specific circumstances (see Chapters 5 and 13). Sections 4A and 4B are set out in Boxes 3.3 and 3.4 respectively.

Box 3.3: Section 4A Restriction of deprivation of liberty.

Section 4A added under Section 45 of the Mental Health Act 2007:

(1)   The Act does not authorise any person (D) to deprive any other person (P) of his liberty.
(2)   But that is subject to:
    (a)   the following provisions of this Section, and
    (b)   Section 4B.
(3)   D may deprive P of his liberty if, by doing so, D is giving effect to a relevant decision of the court.
(4)   A relevant decision of the court is a decision made by an order under Section 16(2)(a) in relation to a matter concerning P's personal welfare (Power of Court of Protection to make decisions and appoint deputies on P's behalf – see Chapter 7).
(5)   D may deprive P of his liberty if the deprivation is authorised by Schedule A1 (hospital and care home residents: deprivation of liberty).

Box 3.4: Section 4B Deprivation of liberty necessary for life-sustaining treatment etc.

Section 4B added under Section 45 of the Mental Health Act 2007:

(1) If the following conditions are met, D is authorised to deprive P of his liberty while a decision as respects any relevant issue is sought from the court.
(2) The first condition is that there is a question about whether D is authorised to deprive P of his liberty under Section 4A.
(3) The second condition is that the deprivation of liberty:
   (a) is wholly or partly for the purpose of
      (i) giving P life-sustaining treatment, or
      (ii) doing any vital act, or
   (b) consists wholly or partly of
      (i) giving P life-sustaining treatment, or
      (ii) doing any vital act.
(4) The third condition is that the deprivation of liberty is necessary in order to:
   (a) give the life-sustaining treatment, or
   (b) do the vital act.
(5) A vital act is any act which the person doing it reasonably believes to be necessary to prevent a serious deterioration in P's condition.

A discussion of the human rights implications of the use of restraint can be found in Chapter 5.

As a consequence of the amendments to the Mental Capacity Act 2005 resulting from the need to fill the gap revealed by the Bournewood case, it would be possible for a person to lose their liberty under the MCA but only if the conditions laid down in the new proposed Sections 4A and 4B and the amending Schedules are satisfied (see Chapter 13).

Article 6: Right to a fair trial

1. In the determination of his civil rights and obligations or of any criminal charge against him, everyone is entitled to a fair and public hearing within a reasonable time by an independent and impartial tribunal established by law. Judgment shall be pronounced publicly but the press and public may be excluded from all or part of the trial in the interest of morals, public order or national security in a democratic society, where the interests of juveniles or the protection of the private life of the parties so require, or to the extent strictly necessary in the opinion of the court in special circumstances where publicity would prejudice the interests of justice.
2. Everyone charged with a criminal offence shall be presumed innocent until proved guilty according to law.

3. Everyone charged with a criminal offence has the following minimum rights:
    (a) to be informed promptly, in a language which he understands and in detail, of the nature and cause of the accusation against him;
    (b) to have adequate time and facilities for the preparation of his defence;
    (c) to defend himself in person or through legal assistance of his own choosing or, if he has not sufficient means to pay for legal assistance, to be given it free when the interests of justice so require;
    (d) to examine or have examined witnesses against him and to obtain the attendance and examination of witnesses on his behalf under the same conditions as witnesses against him;
    (e) to have the free assistance of an interpreter if he cannot understand or speak the language used in court.

The Joint Committee stated (Para 54) in its discussions on Article 6 that

> Although we have made recommendations that access to the Court of Protection should be further enhanced for persons lacking capacity we are of the opinion that there are sufficient mechanisms provided under the draft Bill to ensure that persons lacking capacity receive a prompt, fair and public hearing.

The role of the Court of Protection is discussed in Chapter 7 and Scenarios D.

Article 8: Right to respect for private and family life

1. Everyone has the right to respect for his private and family life, his home and his correspondence.
2. There shall be no interference by a public authority with the exercise of this right except such as is in accordance with the law and is necessary in a democratic society in the interests of national security, public safety or the economic wellbeing of the country, for the prevention of disorder or crime, for the protection of health or morals, or for the protection of the rights and freedoms of others.

The right to respect for private and family life is not an absolute right and there are several exceptions to it. There has to be a balancing act between the right itself and the interests of public safety, the protection of health or morals and the other circumstances set out in Para 2. For example it may be argued by a family where one member has severe learning disabilities, that the parents are entitled to take their own decisions about the care and treatment of that family member without any public interference. However, if it can be shown that the best interests of that family member are not being appropriately protected, then intervention in the decision making on behalf of that individual could be justified. Article 8 also covers the disclosure of information held about a person and their qualified right of access to it. In one case[12] the European Court of Human Rights (ECHR) held that the desire by a person born as a result of artificial insemination to know the details of their origin did engage Article 8 rights, and placed the state under a positive obligation.

Article 9: Freedom of thought, conscience and religion

1. Everyone has the right to freedom of thought, conscience and religion; this right includes freedom to change his religion or belief and freedom, either alone or in community with others and in public or private, to manifest his religion or belief, in worship, teaching, practice and observance.
2. Freedom to manifest one's religion or beliefs shall be subject only to such limitations as are prescribed by law and are necessary in a democratic society in the interests of public safety, for the protection of public order, health or morals, or for the protection of the rights and freedoms of others.

Article 9 protects rights in relation to a broad range of views, beliefs, thoughts and positions of conscience, as well as faith in a particular religion. It will be noted that in determining the best interests of a person who lacks the requisite mental capacity, the beliefs, views, values etc of that person must be taken into account in determining best interests, and relevant people must be consulted over what these values etc might be.

Article 10: Freedom of expression

1. Everyone has the right to freedom of expression. This right shall include freedom to hold opinions and to receive and impart information and ideas without interference by public authority and regardless of frontiers. This Article shall not prevent States from requiring the licensing of broadcasting, television or cinema enterprises.
2. The exercise of these freedoms, since it carries with it duties and responsibilities, may be subject to such formalities, conditions, restrictions or penalties as are prescribed by law and are necessary in a democratic society, in the interests of national security, territorial integrity or public safety, for the prevention of disorder or crime, for the protection of health or morals, for the protection of the reputation or rights of others, for preventing the disclosure of information received in confidence, or for maintaining the authority and impartiality of the judiciary.

This Article has to be balanced against the qualified privacy rights recognised by Article 8. The Court of Protection has the power to determine whether a hearing involving a person lacking mental capacity should be heard in private and to make an order prohibiting any disclosure of the names (see Chapter 7).

Article 14: Prohibition of discrimination

The enjoyment of the rights and freedoms set forth in this Convention shall be secured without discrimination on any ground such as sex, race, colour, language, religion, political or other opinion, national or social origin, association with a national minority, property, birth or other status.

Even though Article 14 does not explicitly mention mental capacity or age, both could be the subject of unlawful discrimination since the list of forms of discrimination is preceded by the words 'such as' and ends with 'or other status'. The list is not meant to be exhaustive. At present Article 14 does not stand in its own right: it has to be used in conjunction with the alleged violation of another article. There are however suggestions that it should be amended to this effect.

The Department for Constitutional Affairs (DCA) has provided a guide to the Human Rights Act which can be downloaded from its website. The third edition was published in October 2006.[13]

Statutory principles governing decision making

The earlier draft of the Mental Capacity Bill did not specify basic principles which should apply to decision making on behalf of others. The Joint Committee pointed out that unlike its Scottish counterpart (Adults with Incapacity (Scotland) Act 2000) the draft Bill did not have a specific statement of the fundamental principles on which it is based. Para 37 quoted the five general principles in the Scottish Act. The Joint Committee noted the principles set out in Section 1 of the Children Act 1989 and the specific considerations applying to the exercise of powers in Section 1 of the Adoption and Children Act 2002. The Joint Committee (Para 43) welcomed

> the Department's commitment to give further consideration to the possibility of incorporating a statement of principles on the face of the Bill. We believe that such a statement inserted as an initial point of reference could give valuable guidance to the courts, as well as helping non-lawyers to weigh up difficult decisions. Evidence given to us indicates that this would be welcome to a wide range of those who have to deal with the problems of substitute decision-making in practice. We also believe that such a statement would be valuable in helping to frame the Codes of Practice based on the Bill.

The Joint Committee suggested five principles which could be included in the Bill and with some minor modifications these were incorporated into the Bill.

The principles were for the most part already contained in common law rulings, but they are now given statutory effect. The five principles are set out in Section 1 and are discussed below.

Principle one: presumption of capacity

> A person must be assumed to have capacity unless it is established that he lacks capacity.

A person is one over 16 years (see Section 2(2)). The presumption of capacity could be rebutted on a balance of probabilities. The burden of establishing lack of capacity would be upon a person alleging it. The presumption and determination of capacity are considered in Chapter 4 and Scenarios A. The presumption of capacity has been a basic provision at common law[14] and Section 1(2) now puts this in statutory form.

Principle two: practical steps to assist capacity

> A person is not to be treated as unable to make a decision unless all practicable steps to help him to do so have been taken without success.

Interestingly, the Act uses the term 'all practicable steps'. The absence of the word 'reasonably' places a much higher duty on health professionals and carers to promote the capacity of the individual to make decisions. This is further discussed in Chapter 4 and Scenarios A.

Principle three: unwise decisions

> A person is not to be treated as unable to make a decision merely because he makes an unwise decision.

The impact of this principle, clearly established at common law, can be seen in the case of *Re B*,[15] which is discussed in Chapter 2 (see Box 2.1). Miss B's refusal to accept ventilation for her paralysed condition clearly troubled the President of the Family Division, but she accepted that since Miss B's competence had been established, then it was her right to make a decision that would eventually lead to her death. It is thus a principle of law that a mentally competent person can make a decision which is contrary to his or her best interests. It follows therefore that where an individual has signed an advance decision refusing life saving treatment, a person nominated by him to carry out his wishes does not have to act in the best interests of that individual, but in accordance with the advance decision (see Chapter 9 and Scenarios F on advance decisions).

Principle four: best interests

> An act done, or decision made, under this Act for or on behalf of a person who lacks capacity must be done, or made, in his best interests.

Once lack of capacity has been established, then any decisions must be made in the best interests of the person lacking the requisite mental capacity. This is further discussed in Chapter 5 and Scenarios B.

Principle five: least restrictive options

> Before the act is done, or the decision is made, regard must be had to whether the purpose for which it is needed can be as effectively achieved in a way that is less restrictive of the person's rights and freedom of action.

Examples were given in the parliamentary debates on the implications of choosing the least restrictive option, and these are discussed in Chapter 5 and Scenarios B.

Convention on the International Protection of Adults

Section 63 provides that Schedule 3 gives effect in the private international law of England and Wales to the Convention on the International Protection of Adults, signed at The Hague on 13 January 2000 (Cm 5881) (in so far as this Act does not otherwise do so). (Scotland implemented the Convention in Schedule 3 of the Adults with Incapacity (Scotland) Act 2000.) The Convention provides international protection for adults who cannot protect their interests. For example it determines which jurisdiction should apply when a national of one country is in another country. The Convention on the International Protection of Adults defines an adult with incapacity as being a person who is over 16 years, and as a result of an impairment or insufficiency of his personal faculties cannot protect his interests. Protective measures for such adults can include the determination of incapacity and the institution of a protective regime, placing the person under the protection of an appropriate authority, guardianship, curatorship or any corresponding system, designation and functions of a person having charge of the adult's person or property or representing or otherwise helping him, placing the adult in a place where protection can be provided, administering conserving or disposing of the person's property and authorising a specific intervention for the protection of the person or his or her property.

The central authority in relation to the protection of mentally incapacitated adults in England and Wales is the Lord Chancellor. Part 2 of Schedule 3 sets out the scope of the jurisdiction of the competent authority, and Part 3 considers the appropriate jurisdiction when a mentally incapacitated adult becomes habitually resident in another country. Part 4 covers the recognition and enforcement of protective measures of other Convention countries in appropriate circumstances. Part 5 covers cross-border placement of adults lacking mental capacity, and requires co-operation between Convention member countries. Part 6 makes provision for a certificate given by a Convention country under Article 38 of the Convention to be regarded as proof of the matters contained in it, and enables regulations to be made by the Lord Chancellor and for the commencement of the different paragraphs of the Schedule. The Convention can be accessed through the internet.[16]

Disability discrimination

The House of Commons Select Committee[17] considered the relationship between the Mental Capacity Bill and disability discrimination legislation. The point was noted in the parliamentary discussions on the Bill that there is no specific reference to the Disability Discrimination Act (DDA) in the Mental Capacity Bill, and the DDA does not specifically cover discrimination on grounds of age. However any person over 16 years who was discriminated against in relation to mental capacity would be protected by the Mental Capacity Act 2005, the Disability Discrimination Act 1995 and also the Human Rights Act 1998 Schedule 1 Article 14 linked with Article 3 or any other relevant article.

The Equality Act 2006 provides for the Commission for Equality and Human Rights (CEHR) to be established in October 2007, when it will take over the work of the existing three Commissions: Disability Rights Commission, Commission for Race Equality and the Equal Opportunities Commission.[18] Trevor Philips has been appointed as the CEHR chair.

In December 2006 public bodies were placed under a new disability equality duty to ensure that their organisations had a policy to identify and eradicate discrimination against disabled people. Public authorities are required to carry out six duties:

- to promote equality of opportunity between disabled and other persons
- to eliminate discrimination that is unlawful under the DDA 1995
- to eliminate harassment related to their disabilities
- to promote positive attitudes
- to encourage participation in public life, and
- to take account of their disabilities, even where that involves them more favourably than other persons.

The Bournewood case

An example of the impact of the European Convention on Human Rights can be seen in the Bournewood case.[19] In this case the House of Lords considered the question of whether a mentally incapacitated person, incapable of giving consent to admission, could be held at common law in a psychiatric hospital rather than being placed under the Mental Health Act 1983. It decided that Section 131 of the Mental Health Act 1983 did not require a mentally disordered person to have the capacity to consent to admission as an informal patient, and there was no breach of Article 5 of the European Convention on Human Rights when a person with severe learning disabilities was detained by common law powers and not placed under the Mental Health Act 1983.

The claimants subsequently took the case to the European Court of Human Rights[20] where they succeeded, the court holding that there was a breach of Article 5 and the right to liberty. As a consequence of this decision the UK Government was compelled to draft legislation to fill the gap revealed by the Bournewood case. The case itself, the results of this consultation and the consequential amendments are further considered in Chapter 13.

Conclusions

The inclusion of statutory principles in the primary legislation rather than just in the Code of Practice is crucial to the protection of the interests of those who lack the requisite mental capacity. Even though many of the statutory principles were already accepted at common law (judge made or case law), setting them at the heart of the MCA with an enforceable obligation has created a new situation. The duty to obey the statutory principles which is placed on all those making decisions or acting on behalf of others should clarify the rights of and the duties to those who require protection. This clarity should be reinforced by the Code of Practice.

References

1   Convention on the International Protection of Adults signed at The Hague on 13 January 2000. CM 5881.
2   Code of Practice for the Mental Capacity Act 2005. Department of Constitutional Affairs February 2007. TSO, London.
3   The House of Lords decided, in a majority decision, in June 2007 that private care homes under contract with local authorities for the provision of places were not exercising functions of a public nature for the purposes of the Human Rights Act. This has led to an understandable reaction from many charities concerned with the care of vulnerable adults that overriding legislation be passed. See: *YL* v. *Birmingham City Council* Times Law Report, 21 June 2007, HL.
4   *Bellinger* v. *Bellinger* [2003] UKHL 21; [2003] 2 WLR 1174.
5   Schedule 1 to the Human Rights Act 1998 sets out those articles of the European Convention on Human Rights which were incorporated into the laws of the UK. The Human Rights Act can be accessed via www.opsi.gov.uk/legislation
6   *R. (Pretty)* v. *Director of Public Prosecutions and another, Medical Ethics Alliance and others, interveners*, Times Law Report, 23 October 2001; *R. (on the application of Pretty)* v. *DPP Secretary of State for the Home Department intervening*, Times Law Report, 5 December 2001; [2001] UKHL 61; [2001] 3 WLR 1598; *Pretty* v. *UK ECHR*, Current Law 380 June 2002 2346/02; [2002] 35 EHRR 1; [2002] 2 FLR 45.
7   *NHS Trust A* v. *H* [2001] 2 FLR 501.
8   *NHS Trust A* v. *H* [2001] 2 FLR 501.
9   *Re DE (an adult patient), JE and Surrey County Council* [2006] EWHC 3459.
10 *Guzzardi* v. *Italy* (1980) 3 EHRR 333; *Ashingdane* v. *United Kingdom* (1985) 7 EHRR 528.
11 *R. (MH)* v. *Secretary of State for Health*, Times Law Report, 8 December 2004, CA; [2004] EWCA Civ 1609.
12 *Rose and another* v. *Secretary of State for Health and the Human Fertilisation Authority* [2003] EWHC 1593.
13 Department for Constitutional Affairs (2006) *A Guide to the Human Rights Act 1998* 3rd edn. DCA, London.
14 *MB(re) (Adult Medical Treatment)* [1997] 2 FLR 426.
15 *Re B (Consent to treatment: capacity)*, Times Law Report, 26 March 2002; [2002] 2 All ER 449.
16 www.hcch.net/index_en.php?
17 HoC Select Cttee, 21 Oct 2004.
18 www.cehr.org.uk
19 *R.* v. *Bournewood Community and Mental Health NHS Trust ex p L* [1998] 3 All ER 289; [1999] AC 458.
20 *HL* v. *United Kingdom (Application No 45508/99)*, Times Law Report, 19 October 2004.

4 Definition of Mental Capacity

Why is capacity important?

If a person over 18 years has the necessary mental capacity, then his or her right to make his or her own decisions is protected. If however he or she lacks the requisite mental capacity then action has to be taken on his or her behalf. The existence or non-existence of the requisite mental capacity is central therefore to the law on decision making. The adult person who has the requisite capacity can make any decisions no matter how unwise; the adult person who lacks the requisite capacity cannot make those decisions, but someone will act in his or her best interests.

Presumption that capacity exists

It was a basic presumption of law that every adult is presumed to have mental capacity, and this presumption has now been given statutory effect in the Mental Capacity Act 2005. Section 1(2) recognises as a basic principle that:

> A person must be assumed to have capacity unless it is established that he lacks capacity.

This presumption can however be rebutted (i.e. replaced) by evidence to the contrary, as Scenario A1 illustrates. The standard of proof for the rebuttal is on a balance of probabilities (S.2(4)). This is known as the civil standard of proof, and contrasts with the criminal standard of proof which requires the judge or jury to be satisfied beyond reasonable doubt that the accused is guilty of a crime. The civil standard is therefore a lower standard of proof and can be more easily satisfied than the criminal standard.

How is mental capacity defined?

There is a two-stage process for determining whether a person lacks the requisite mental capacity to make a specific decision. The first stage is to determine whether there exists an impairment or disturbance in the functioning of the mind or brain. The second stage is to determine if this impairment or disturbance results in an inability to make or communicate decisions.

Stage 1 Existence of an impairment, or a disturbance in the functioning of, the mind or brain

Mental capacity is defined in Section 2 of the Act as:
   For the purposes of this Act

   (1)   a person lacks capacity in relation to a matter if at the material time he is unable to make a decision for himself in relation to the matter because of an impairment of, or a disturbance in the functioning of, the mind or brain.
   (2)   It does not matter whether the impairment or disturbance is permanent or temporary.
   (3)   A lack of capacity cannot be established merely by reference to:
       a.   a person's age or appearance, or
       b.   a condition of his, or an aspect of his behaviour, which might lead others to make unjustified assumptions about his capacity.
   (4)   In proceedings under this Act or any other enactment, any question whether a person lacks capacity within the meaning of this Act must be decided on the balance of probabilities.

These factors are illustrated in Scenario A2.

   The assessment has to be made 'at the material time'. This would mean that where a person is suffering from intermittent capacity which can sometimes occur with Alzheimer's disease, if there are interludes of capacity and during that time the person is able to understand the information and can make and communicate the relevant decision, then for the purposes of the MCA that person does not lack the requisite capacity. The Act specifically provides that the fact that a person is able to retain the information relevant to a decision for a short period only does not prevent him from being regarded as able to make the decision (see below – S.3(3)).

Superficial judgments

The factors set out in Section 2 for determining capacity are significant considerations in the determination of mental capacity, since it is easy to make superficial judgments based on irrelevant criteria such as 'The man looks like a tramp: he must lack mental capacity'.

   The Joint Committee was concerned that there may be too easy an assumption of incapacity and failure to make the time and support available to enable people with learning disabilities to contribute to the decision making process. The Joint Committee therefore recommended that:

> Codes of Practice should set out clearly the need for evidence on both 'impairment of or disturbance in mental functioning' and of lack of capacity, as defined in the draft Bill, and the appropriate means of determining that evidence in the best interests of the person concerned so that the criteria against which an appeal might be judged are transparent. [Para 76] . . . and
> we recommend that the Codes of Practice should make clear that those acting under the General Authority [a concept now set aside – see Chapter 5] or an LPA [Lasting Power of Attorney] must appreciate the concept of capacity/incapacity and be fully aware of the responsibilities thus placed on them when carrying out or assisting decision-making on behalf of any person who is considered incapacitated. . . . The Codes of Practice must set out a framework on these matters which is readily understandable to lay persons. [Para 77]

The Code of Practice Chapter 4 gives guidance on the definition and application of the concept of mental capacity.

Children and young persons. Why only adults of at least 18 years?

Persons under 16 years are excluded from the provisions of the Act (Section 2(5)), apart from the provisions of Section 18(3), which enables the exercise of powers under Section 16 in relation to property and affairs, even though P has not reached 16 but the court considers it is likely that P will still lack capacity to make decision in respect of the matter when he is 18 years (see Chapter 12 and Scenarios I).

Young persons of 16 and 17 have a statutory right to give consent to treatment.[1] However judges have ruled that at common law it is possible to overrule the refusal of a person of 16 or 17 who is refusing life saving treatment, if that treatment is in his or her best interests.[2] In contrast, the refusal of a person over 18 years to receive even life saving treatment cannot be overruled, provided that they have the requisite mental capacity. This difference explains why an advance decision or living will can only be drawn up by an adult over 18 years: as the law stands at present a young person of 16 and 17 cannot refuse life sustaining treatment if that is in his or her best interests.

However Section 40 of the Mental Health Act 2007 amends the Mental Health Act 1983 so that a parent cannot give consent to the admission of his child of 16 or 17 to psychiatric hospital if that child has the requisite capacity and does not consent to the making of the arrangements for admission. This may lead to a change in the law relating to overruling the refusal of a 16- or 17-year-old in other specialities apart from psychiatry.

Stage 2 Ability to make decisions

Once it has been established that there exists an impairment of, or a disturbance in the functioning of, the mind or brain, then the next stage is to determine whether this prevents P from making a specific decision.

What is meant by inability to make decisions?

The phrase 'unable to make decisions for himself' used in Section 2 is subsequently defined in Section 3:

A person is unable to make a decision for himself if he is unable:

a. to understand the information relevant to the decision
b. to retain that information
c. to use or weigh that information as part of the process of making the decision, or
d. to communicate his decision (whether by talking, using sign language or any other means).

This follows very closely the common law decision set in the Broadmoor case by Thorpe J[3] and subsequently expanded by the Court of Appeal in the case of *Re MB*.[4] The case of MB was followed in a case involving a detained patient at Broadmoor Special Hospital who was refusing treatment for his bipolar affective disorder. He denied that he was mentally ill. The judge held that he lacked the mental capacity because he was not able to appreciate the likely effects of having or not having the treatment, and his decision was upheld by the Court of Appeal.[5]

The statutory definition covers both the actual mental inability to make decisions, and also the situation where the individual may have the requisite mental competence, but be unable to communicate his or her views. However every effort must be made to facilitate communication.

Facilitating communication. What steps must be taken to assist P in having the requisite capacity, e.g. in being able to communicate?

The Act requires information to be communicated in an appropriate way.
    Subsection 3(2) provides that:

A person is not to be regarded as unable to understand the information relevant to the decision if he is able to understand a general explanation of it given to him in a way that is appropriate to his circumstances (using simple language, visual aids or any other means).

This would require ensuring that any appropriate technical equipment or speech therapy aids were utilised in order to facilitate communication with the patient. In addition it must be remembered that one of the basic principles of the Act (see Chapter 2 and Section 1(3)) is that:

A person is not to be treated as unable to make a decision unless all practicable steps to help him to do so have been taken without success.

This is of particular significance in situations such as those where a patient has brain damage which results in their only being able to communicate through technological means. There is no qualification in the section such as that only **reasonably practicable** means need be used. The consequence is, that if through technology and equipment it is possible to communicate with a brain damaged/ speech impaired person, then those facilities must be made available. 'Appropriate to his circumstances' could therefore have significant resource implications as Scenario A3 illustrates.

Temporary retention of information

Mental capacity can exist even if the relevant information is retained for only a short period. Subsection 3(3) provides that:

> The fact that a person is able to retain the information relevant to a decision for a short period only does not prevent him from being regarded as able to make the decision.

Clearly however the decision must be made at the time the information is still retained in the person's mind. Intermittent competence provides real problems for those assessing mental competence. This is discussed in Scenario A5.

What kind of information is relevant?

The Act further specifies that the information relevant to the decision includes:

> Information about the reasonably foreseeable consequences of deciding one way or another or failing to make the decision (S.3(4)).

The Code of Practice[6] gives the following guidance on giving relevant information to a mentally incapacitated adult to assist him or her in making a decision:

- Take time to explain anything you think might help the person make the decision. It is important that they have access to all the information they need to make an informed decision.
- Try not to give more detail than the person needs – this might confuse them. In some cases, a simple, broad explanation will be enough. But it must not miss out important information.
- What are the risks and benefits? Describe any foreseeable consequences of making the decision, and of not making any decision at all.
- Explain the effects the decision might have on the person and those close to them – including the people involved in their care.
- If they have a choice, give them the same information in a balanced way for all the options.
- For some types of decisions, it may be important to give access to advice from elsewhere. This may be independent or specialist advice (for example from a medical practitioner or a financial or legal adviser). But it might simply be advice from trusted friends or relatives.

Functional approach to mental capacity

Central to the definition of mental capacity is that a person's mental capacity is defined in terms of the decision which has to be made. Thus a person with severe learning disabilities may be able to make decisions about the food to eat, the clothes he or she wishes to wear and social outings to be made. However that same person may be unable to make a decision about the extraction of a tooth or similar treatment. This is known as the functional approach to defining mental capacity or the specific issue approach, and is considered further in Scenario A3.

Issues arising in defining if a person has mental capacity

Who carries out the assessment of capacity?

On a day-to-day basis for routine decisions it would be the health professional or carer who is deciding whether a patient/client has the requisite mental capacity to make decisions. The existence of the mental capacity to make routine decisions such as choice of food, clothing and activities will be determined by the carer. Clearly their training should include how such judgments are to be made. In practice the person making the assessment would be the person who is requiring the decision to be made: for example if a care assistant in a residential home for the older person was handing out medication, then it would be the care assistant who would decide if that resident had the capacity to understand what was being offered and decide whether or not he or she should take it. For everyday situations the immediate carer would automatically be deciding on whether or not a person had the capacity to make their own decisions.

When is help brought in for the assessment?

However it is important that where significant decisions are to be made, where there could be disputes and where there may be formal hearings over the decisions to be made, then independent professional assistance should be brought in to determine whether a patient/client has the requisite mental capacity. Psychiatrists and clinical psychologists are the professions most frequently used to provide an expert opinion on whether the patient/client has mental capacity, but other health professions with the necessary training could also undertake this activity. Records should be kept of any assessment relating to mental capacity. Bringing in an expert to determine capacity is considered in Scenario A6.

How often must the assessment be carried out?

The assessment is a functional assessment (see **Functional approach to mental capacity**) and therefore any assessment of capacity must be linked with the specific decision which is to be made. It follows that any new decision requiring a different level of capacity should lead to a fresh assessment. In addition any change in the patient's/client's mental condition would require another assessment to determine his or her level of capacity for decision making. This poses considerable problems where a patient has fluctuating capacity. To carry out the full assessment of the requisite mental capacity for each and every decision would appear to involve considerable time and could result in a bureaucratic nightmare.

Procedures and policy would have to emphasise when the full assessment was required. It would appear impracticable for a full assessment to be carried out each and every time there is a decision or action which in theory could be construed as a trespass to the person, if the patient/client/resident fails to give consent.

For example a person with Alzheimer's disease may in the early stages ebb in and out of an understanding of their environment. At one moment they may resist having their clothes put on or their face washed and yet, at another, appear to consent to taking medication. The care plan should set out specifically how the care assistant should determine whether that person is capable of giving consent to the care and/or treatment which is being offered, and the action to be taken if the patient appears to lack the capacity to give consent to the proposed activity.

Assessment when P has fluctuating capacity is made more difficult when there is a high turnover of care staff and considerable pressure on staff because of understaffing. Unjustified assumptions might be made too easily. Strong and constant supervision and clear care planning is essential to ensure that the MCA is correctly implemented and the principles followed.

What if there is a dispute over the assessment?

Normally carers would make the assessment as specific decisions arose to be made or specific action required to be taken. If there is a dispute as to whether or not the resident/patient had the requisite capacity, then an independent expert able to make an assessment may have to be brought in to determine if capacity exists.

What role do relatives play in the assessment?

Often relatives are the main carers of the adult whose capacity is in question, and they would therefore be determining capacity on a day-to-day basis. However for critical decisions such as serious medical treatment, accommodation decisions and other significant decisions, they may be encouraged to bring in experts to carry out the assessment. This would depend upon the mental condition of the person, since in some situations there may be no doubt as to the presence or absence of capacity. The implications of needing to determine capacity in everyday situations is illustrated in Scenario A8, where there is an argument for ensuring that care assistants or health care support workers receive a basic understanding of the legislation.

Has guidance been provided on the assessment?

The Joint Committee emphasised the importance of the Code of Practice in advising on the assessment of capacity:

> Given the diverse range of situations which will be covered by the statutory framework for decision-making imposed by the Bill, we consider that the processes and requirements relating to the assessment of capacity would be most appropriately dealt with in a Code of Practice, as required under Clause 30(1)(a).[7]

The Code of Practice has thus provided general guidance on the assessment of capacity and suggested several methods of supporting a person in making his or her own decisions. These include: reducing the stress level of P; if it is a situation of temporary loss of capacity, then waiting for capacity to be recovered; using specialist persons such as a speech therapist or family members to assist in communication with P, and being aware of any cultural, ethnic or religious factors which may have a bearing on the person's way of thinking, behaviour or communication.[8]

The British Medical Association and the Law Society have published a guide to the assessment of mental capacity for health and legal professionals, carers and all those involved in looking after people with suspected mental impairment.[9]

Is the assessment a medical one or does it involve social, and other types of assessment?

Since capacity is determined on a specific issue basis, it is important to ensure that the correct experts are brought in to determine P's capacity in the light of the type of decision to be made.

The more serious the decision, the more formal the assessment of capacity may need to be. The assessor must be prepared to justify findings and clearly records must be kept.

What happens if P does not accept the assessment of a lack of capacity?

It may be that P challenges a decision that he or she is lacking the requisite capacity. In such circumstances, P should be assisted in refuting that assessment and if necessary taking a case to the Court of Protection. Scenario A7 considers a situation where there is a dispute over the assessment of capacity.

Unwise decisions

The fact that making unwise decisions is not conclusive of a lack of mental capacity has now been given statutory effect in Section 1 of the Mental Capacity Act 2005, where the basic principles are set out. Principle No. 3 is:

> A person is not to be treated as unable to make a decision merely because he makes an unwise decision.

Self-determination is the opposite of paternalism. Health professionals may find it difficult to accept when a mentally competent patient refuses life-saving treatment, but that is the competent adult's right in law. It follows therefore that provided the patient is defined as having the mental capacity to make a specific decision, according to the approved tests, the fact that the decision is irrational or unwise or contrary to the best interests of the patient, is not relevant.

This principle was brought out clearly by the President of the Family Division, Dame Elizabeth Butler Sloss, in the case of *Re B:*[10]

It was most important that those considering the issue should not confuse the question of mental capacity with the nature of the decision made by the patient however grave the consequences. Since the view of the patient might reflect a difference in values rather than an absence of competence the assessment of capacity should be approached with that in mind and doctors should not allow an emotional reaction to, or strong disagreement with, the patient's decision to cloud their judgment in answering the primary question of capacity.

The Law Commission in its report in 1995[11] recommended (Para 3.19):

A person should not be regarded as unable to make a decision by reason of mental disability merely because he or she makes a decision which would not be made by a person of ordinary prudence.

On the issue of making unwise decisions the Joint Committee stated that:

We considered carefully the dilemma created when a person with apparent capacity was making repeatedly unwise decisions that put him/her at risk or resulted in preventable suffering or disadvantage. We recognise that the possibility of over-riding such decisions would be seen as unacceptable to many user groups. Nevertheless, we suggest that such a situation might trigger the need for a formal assessment of capacity and recommend that the Codes of Practice should include guidance on:

- whether reasonable doubt about capacity and the potentially serious consequences of not intervening indicated the need for an appropriate second opinion
- circumstances in which the statutory authorities should be responsible for providing a level of support as a safeguard against abuse and
- where there was genuine uncertainty as to capacity and an urgent decision was required to prevent suffering or to save life, the benefit of doubt would be exercised to act in that person's best interests in relation to any assessment of capacity (Para 78).

The Code of Practice points out that a person who was hitherto extremely rational but who is repeatedly making unwise decisions may be demonstrating a lack of capacity, and this should be explored. This is considered in Scenario A4, which is taken from the Code of Practice.

The fact that unwise decisions should not be regarded as evidence of mental incapacity is an extremely important provision, and it determines the order in which the assessment must be made:

First there must be a definition following reasonable criteria on whether a person satisfies the statutory definition of mental competence.

Second the requisite mental capacity is established according to that definition, then the person can make their own decision, no matter how foolish they would appear to the majority of persons.

The dangers of making an assessment of incapacity on the basis of the wisdom of the decision making is obvious. To those who see blood transfusions as a basic natural part of life saving medicine, the refusal by Jehovah Witnesses to accept blood transfusions may seem very unwise, but to say such lack of wisdom is therefore evidence of mental incapacity would be contrary to the human rights of those who held that belief.

Dangers in making assumptions

In psychiatric care there has been a tendency in day-to-day care and treatment to assume that if the patient agrees with what is proposed, then the patient has the necessary mental capacity, but if the patient disagrees with what is proposed then that disagreement brings the issue of capacity into question, and at that point an assessment is made. There should be an awareness of a person's mental capacity at all times. However the presumption that mental capacity exists can be rebutted if there is evidence to the contrary. That evidence must be more than the mere fact that the patient has refused to co-operate with treatment schemes.

Conclusions

The determination of capacity is at the heart of the Mental Capacity Act 2005. Once it is concluded that an individual has the requisite mental capacity to make a specific decision, then at that point carers, relatives, health and social services professionals must be prepared to leave that specific decision to the individual. There is no room in the law for paternalism where a person can exercise his or her own autonomy. However if the conclusion of the assessment is that the person lacks the requisite mental capacity, then actions and decisions must be taken in the best interests of that individual, and it is to this that we turn in the next chapter.

References

1   Family Law Reform Act 1969 Section 8.
2   *Re W (a minor) (medical treatment)* [1992] 4 All ER 627.
3   *Re C (adult: refusal of medical treatment)* Family Division [1994] 1 All ER 819.
4   *Re MB (an adult: medical treatment)* [1997] 2 FLR 426.
5   *R (on the Application of B)* v. *S (Responsible Medical Officer, Broadmoor Hospital; sub nom R. (on the Application of B)* v. *SS* [2006] EWCA Civ 28, Times Law Report, 2 February 2006, CA.
6   Code of Practice for the Mental Capacity Act 2005. Department of Constitutional Affairs February 2007 para 3.9. TSO, London.
7   House of Lords and House of Commons Joint Committee on the Draft Mental Incapacity Bill Session 2002–2003. HL Paper 189–1; HC 1083–1 para 245.
8   Code of Practice for the Mental Capacity Act 2005. Department of Constitutional Affairs February 2007 para 3.10. TSO, London.
9   British Medical Association and Law Society (2004) *Assessment of Mental Capacity* 2nd edn. BMA, London.
10   *Re B (Consent to treatment: capacity)*, Times Law Report, 26 March 2002; [2002] 2 All ER 449.
11   Law Commission (1995) *Mental Incapacity*. Report No. 231. TSO, London.

Scenarios A
Capacity

Presumption of capacity

Scenario A1: The presumption of capacity is rebutted.

Bob, 21 years, has learning difficulties and has lived in residential accommodation for the past six years. He has been suffering very badly from toothache, but hates anyone looking into his mouth. His paid carers decide that he should see a dentist and possibly have an extraction. Bob is not prepared to go to the dentist. Can he be forced to attend?

As a 21-year-old there would be a presumption that Bob had the mental capacity to make his own decisions, but a test may well establish that he lacks the capacity to understand the implications of not attending the dentist and the possibility that if he had an infection it could spread to the rest of his body and that, if treatment were not to be given, his situation could become extremely serious if not life threatening. If following an assessment it was concluded that Bob was incapable of realising the seriousness of his situation and lacked mental capacity to make a decision, the presumption that he had mental capacity would be rebutted. Actions would then have to be taken in his best interests (see Chapter 5).

Stage 1 An impairment or disturbance?

> **Scenario A2: Situation: a tramp.**
>
> Denis is found wandering the streets on a cold, rainy windy winter night. He is invited to take refuge in accommodation for the homeless. He accepts the offer and is given food and a bed and offered a shower. An assistant helps him prepare for the shower and notices that he has an extremely serious abscess on his ankle which looks as though it could be gangrenous. Denis agrees to see the doctor who visits the home each week and is advised that he may have to have an amputation of his leg, since the gangrene could be fatal, and that he should be examined by a specialist. Denis refuses any such examination, consultation or treatment. Could he be compelled to undergo treatment?

Working through the statutory definition of capacity the following steps could be used:

- What is the decision to be made?
- The answer to this is: has Denis the capacity to make a decision on whether he should consent to or refuse possibly life saving treatment?
- There is a presumption that Denis has the capacity to make this decision: is there evidence that this presumption should be challenged?
- Does Denis have an impairment of, or a disturbance in the functioning of, the mind or brain?
- If so, does this impairment or disturbance mean that he is unable to make a decision for himself in relation to whether or not he should have treatment?
- Denis's state of clothing and appearance and tramp condition should be ignored for the purpose of determining whether or not he has capacity to make that specific decision.

If the conclusion is that Denis does not have an impairment or disturbance in the functioning of his mind or brain, or alternatively, he does have such an impairment or disturbance, but it does not affect his ability to make that particular decision, then the conclusion will be that Denis does not lack mental capacity and can decide himself whether to have that treatment. That conclusion means that his refusal to have the amputation could not be overruled in his best interests. As an adult with the requisite mental capacity to make that particular decision, he is entitled to make that decision and he therefore can make an unwise decision, i.e. a decision which would appear to be contrary to his best interests (see page 48).

Explanation of 'appropriate to his circumstances'

> **Scenario A3: Situation: capacity and communication.**
>
> Anna, aged 34 years, has cerebral palsy and has spent most of her life in residential accommodation with residents who have similar conditions. She is asked if she

would like to move into a new care home that is just being opened. The decision is critical since she has several friends in the present home and there is a dispute amongst the carers over the move, since some feel that it would not be in her best interests. She has considerable difficulty in communicating and has in the past had regular speech therapy to assist her in using sign language. Unfortunately there is a shortage of speech therapists in the area and one is not available to assist Anna in communicating her wishes about the proposed move. The manager is proposing that the move should take place on the grounds that Anna is incapable of communicating her wishes, that it is not practical to do any more and that it is in her best interests to go into the new accommodation. Some of the carers dispute these proposals. What action can be taken and what is the law?

The following steps must be taken in determining whether Anna has the mental capacity to make a specific decision.

1. Does she have an impairment or a disturbance in the functioning of her mind or brain?

    This question would be decided on a balance of probabilities. (This is the lighter test – used in civil proceedings – to determine liability and contrasts with the tougher test – beyond reasonable doubt – which is used in criminal proceedings.)

    From the facts given it is clear that Anna has cerebral palsy and this would constitute an impairment or disturbance in the functioning of her mind or brain. For Anna this is a permanent impairment or disturbance, but this does not affect the definition of mental capacity (though, if she was deemed to lack the requisite mental capacity, it could have affected how her best interests were decided – see Scenarios B).

    In addition, in determining whether Anna had the requisite mental capacity, her age, appearance, or a specific condition or aspect of her behaviour should not be used as the basis for superficial judgments about her capacity. For example if Anna had constant uncontrollable limb movements and was continually dribbling, this should not be seen as implying that she was incapable of having the requisite mental capacity to make a decision on her accommodation.

2. Is Anna over 16 years? The answer to this is that she is 34 and so the powers under the Act can apply to her.

3. Does the impairment or disturbance in the functioning of the brain or mind result in Anna being unable to make a decision for herself?

    The statutory test to be applied to answer this question is:

    a. Does Anna understand the information relevant to the decision?
    b. Does she retain that information?
    c. Can she use or weigh the information as part of the process of making the decision?
    d. Can she communicate her decision (whether by talking, using sign language or any other means)?

a. Does Anna understand the information relevant to the decision?

Before this question can be answered, it must be clear what information has been given to Anna. The Mental Capacity Act 2005 requires her to be told information about the reasonable foreseeable consequences of deciding whether to stay in the present home, or of deciding to move to the new accommodation, or the consequences if she fails to make the decision. She should, if possible, be shown the new accommodation, where she would sleep, who would be her fellow residents, what different facilities would be available to her, how the location would be different from the existing home, and be given a good idea of her new life were she to move – i.e. all the relevant information which is likely to affect her decision making, so that she would be in a position to make a realistic decision.

Her capacity to understand this information should be checked out by the person or persons who have taken on the duty of ascertaining her ability to make this decision. There are considerable advantages in using a person for this task, whether informal or paid carer, who knows Anna well and can discern Anna's ability to understand the information given to her. The fact that the information has to be put to her in very basic terms, perhaps using simple language, visual aids, or any other means does not count against her having the necessary mental capacity. The Act makes it clear in S.3(2) that:

> A person is not to be regarded as unable to understand the information relevant to a decision if he is able to understand an explanation of it given to him in a way that is appropriate to his circumstances (using simple language, visual aids or any other means).

If the answer to this first question is that Anna does seem to be able to understand the information given to her, the next question is:

b. Does she retain that information?

She needs to retain the information about the implications of moving home for as long as it takes her to make the decision. If, for example, she were to visit the new home one week and a fortnight were to elapse before she was asked by the carer or social worker or health professional whether she wanted to move, she would need to remember the information and understand the significance of her decision. The Act states in S.3(3) that:

> The fact that a person is able to retain the information relevant to a decision for a short period only does not prevent him from being regarded as able to make the decision.

The information needs to be retained as long as is necessary to the making of the decision. It may be that the information would need to be repeated if any significant length of time were to elapse before Anna made the decision.

c. Can she use or weigh the information as part of the process of making the decision?

This third question requires an analysis of her cognitive skills. It might be thought that only a clinical psychologist or psychiatrist could determine this, and certainly in the event of a Court of Protection hearing such expert evidence may be necessary for the court purposes (see Scenario A6). However for day-to-day matters, where there is not a dispute, the carers, whether paid or informal, would have the responsibility of deciding if Anna had the ability to weigh all the information she had received and come to a decision. It might for example be that Anna, having seen the wonderful facilities available in the new accommodation, decided that she would prefer to stay in the present house because she had grown fond of her fellow residents and the staff, and would not want to leave them. However if she learnt that some of the existing residents and a few of the staff would be moving to the new accommodation, she might change her mind. Once again, in deciding if Anna had the cognitive skills to make this decision the appropriate means of communication should be used.

d. Can she communicate her decision (whether by talking, using sign language or any other means)?

This is the final question to be asked in determining whether Anna's brain or mind impairment or disturbance results in her being unable to make a decision for herself in relation to a particular matter.

On the facts given in Scenario A3 it would appear that Anna does have the ability to understand the information, retain and make a decision using it, but there are problems associated with her communicating her answer. She needs a speech therapist to assist her in the communication and one is not available. Can those responsible define her as lacking the requisite mental capacity and therefore make the decision in her best interests?

The answer would appear to be 'No.' The second principle to govern the implementation of the Mental Capacity Act is that:

A person is not to be treated as unable to make a decision unless all practicable steps to help him to do so have been taken without success. (S.1(3))

If Anna can only express her decision if she is given the assistance of a speech therapist then the decision making may have to wait until a speech therapist can attend. This is preferable to a decision being made on the assumption that Anna lacked the capacity. Of particular significance is the wording of Section 1(3). All **practicable steps** must be taken to help her to make the decision. There is no use of the word '**reasonable**'. Had only reasonable steps been required, then the cost, the practicality, the delays and other factors could have been taking into consideration in determining what was reasonably practicable. However by requiring all practicable steps to be taken, the Act is ignoring the cost, time and other considerations. If it can be done, then it should be done, i.e. if Anna can understand and communicate with the assistance of a speech therapist, then a speech therapist's help should be secured and Anna's decision should wait until that time.

An unwise decision

Once it has been decided that Anna does have the capacity to make a decision on her future accommodation and to communicate it, then it is irrelevant if she makes a decision which to her carers would appear to be an unwise decision. This is because the third principle is:

> A person is not to be treated as unable to make a decision merely because he makes an unwise decision.

It is however important that the analysis of mental capacity follows the correct order. Mental capacity to make a specific decision must be determined first. Mental capacity must not be inferred because a person makes unwise decisions.

The Code of Practice considers the problem of a person constantly making unwise decisions and the possibility that this might become evidence of a lack of capacity.[1]

There may be cause for concern if somebody:

- repeatedly makes unwise decisions that put them at significant risk of harm or exploitation or
- makes a particular unwise decision that is obviously irrational or out of character.

These things do not necessarily mean that somebody lacks capacity. But there might be need for further investigation, taking into account the person's past decisions and choices. For example, have they developed a medical condition or disorder that is affecting their capacity to make particular decisions? Are they easily influenced by undue pressure? Or do they need more information to help them understand the consequences of the decision they are making?[1]

Scenario A4: Too many unwise decisions?[2]

Cyril, an elderly man with early signs of dementia, spends nearly £300 on fresh fish from a door-to-door salesman. He is very fond of fish but there is far too much to fit into his freezer. Before the onset of dementia, he was always very thrifty and careful with his money and would never have dreamt of buying such a quantity of expensive fish or spending this amount in one go.

This decision alone may not automatically mean he now lacks capacity to manage all aspects of his property and affairs, but his daughter makes further enquiries and discovers Cyril has overpaid his cleaner on several occasions (something he has never done in the past). He has also made payments from his savings that he cannot account for.

His daughter decides it is time to use the registered Lasting Power of Attorney her father made in the past. This gives her the authority to manage Cyril's property and affairs whenever he lacks the capacity to manage them himself. She takes control of Cyril's chequebook to protect him from possible exploitation, but she can still ensure he has enough money to spend on his everyday needs.

Functional approach to capacity

It will be noted that in discussing Scenario A3 and Anna's capacity to make a decision, the phrase 'requisite mental capacity' has been used. This is because the Mental Capacity Act (MCA) defines capacity in terms of a specific matter to be decided.

As Section 2(1) of the MCA states:

> a person lacks **capacity in relation to a matter** if at the material time he is unable to make **a decision for himself in relation to the matter** because of an impairment of, or a disturbance in the functioning of, the mind or brain.

As can be seen from the words which the author has put in bold, capacity is decision-specific. In Scenario A3 for example, it might be found that Anna is able to make her own decisions on what to wear or what to eat, but is unable to understand the decision about moving accommodation, and therefore lacks the capacity required for that decision.

The fact that the MCA uses a functional definition of capacity has been seen as an important protection of the rights of vulnerable adults. Criticisms were made in the consultation on the draft Code of Practice that the language suggested that a person lacked mental capacity, and needed to be revised to emphasise the functional and decision-specific principles that are central to the Act. The Department for Constitutional Affairs (DCA) undertook to rewrite the draft with this consideration in mind and to seek for an appropriate phrase. It could be suggested that the phrase 'X has or lacks the requisite mental capacity' should cover the situation, and this is the phrase used in this book.

The Joint Committee in its discussion of the definition of capacity[3] made the following point:

> This functional approach to capacity implies that a person may be capable of making one decision but not another (perhaps more complex) one, or may be capable of making a particular decision at one point in time but not at another. [Para 65]
>
> We note the functional approach adopted by the draft Bill when allied to Best Interests is intended to provide protection to those lacking capacity. In this context, we believe that every effort should be made in both the Bill and in the Codes of Practice to ensure that this Bill is seen as enabling rather than restricting. [Para 66]

The House of Lords also saw the need to recognise the issue of general incapacity in a way that would not undermine the primacy of the functional approach.

The issue of a functional test of capacity was also considered in the House of Commons[4] where Mr. Burstow stated:

> Capacity is the underlying basis on which the Bill is intended to operate and is both specific to the decision that is being made and specific to the time at which a decision is taken. A person's capacity may vary; it may well vary as a result of the way in which capacity was lost – due to a head injury, for example. It may vary due to the nature of the medical condition. So it is important that we state specifically in the Bill that that is how the principles should be read and

understood. That will guard against the people who take decisions assuming that a person is incapacitated because he cannot make decisions about a specific matter. In other words, the person may be unable to make a decision about complex medical treatment, but can certainly make decisions about the clothes and shoes he wants to wear, the type of recreation that he wants to take and the type of food that he wants to eat, which goes very much to the argument advanced by the I Decide coalition.

Intermittent capacity

It would appear that Anna's condition in Scenario A3 is stable, but there are many situations where the person has fluctuating capacity. This is considered in Scenario A5.

Scenario A5: Intermittent incapacity.

Amy is in the early stages of Alzheimer's and is becoming increasingly forgetful and confused. However she does enjoy lucid moments. Her daughter, Joan, is advised that Amy should have an operation for her hiatus hernia which has ulcerated. During an apparently clear thinking moment, Amy tells Joan that she would not want to have any operation. She felt that at 86 she had enjoyed her life, and did not now want to undergo such treatment. Joan felt that Amy was mentally capable and meant what she said. She told the nurses, but the surgeon was not prepared to accept such a refusal and considered that an operation was in Amy's best interests. What is the legal position?

It is unfortunate that Joan did not ensure that an advance decision was drawn up to reflect Amy's wishes (see Chapter 9 and Scenarios F for further discussion of this). It may be possible during a future bout of mental competence for Amy to be asked to repeat her wishes and these should be binding upon all the multi-disciplinary team. Only when incapacity is clearly established is there room to apply the best interests test to the decision to be made on behalf of Amy (see Chapter 4 and Scenarios B).

Use of experts in determining if the requisite capacity exists

As noted above, for most day-to-day decisions the determination of capacity will be carried out by the paid or informal carer. However in certain circumstances expert opinion will be required, as illustrated in the following Scenario A6.

Scenario A6: Expert assessment of capacity.

Florie was pregnant and being treated for a panic attacks. She also suffered from needle phobia, which meant that she was terrified of having an injection. Her midwifery team were concerned that she might need to have a Caesarean and therefore wondered whether she would be considered to have the necessary mental capacity to make a decision. The team members were divided upon whether or not she would be able to make a decision. A clinical psychologist was asked to assess Florie's mental capacity to make a decision about a Caesarean and she decided that Florie's needle phobia rendered her mentally incapable of making such a decision. Subsequently it became apparent that a Caesarean section would be needed to save Florie's and the baby's lives. An application was then made by the National Health Service (NHS) Trust to the Court of Protection for a declaration that a Caesarean could be carried out in Florie's best interests since she lacked the mental capacity to make her own decision. The psychologist gave evidence to the court of her assessment and the basis for her conclusion that Florie lacked the capacity to make that decision.

There are considerable advantages in bringing in a person who is independent of the multi-disciplinary team caring for the patient but has the expertise to make a determination on whether or not capacity exists. In Scenario A6 a situation is considered where it would appear essential to seek the views of an expert on whether the requisite capacity exists. It would be open to the person representing Florie to ask for another expert opinion on Florie's competence to make the decision and, if that expert agreed with the psychologist, then the court could make a declaration that Florie lacked the requisite capacity and then go on to determine what action should be taken in her best interests (see Chapter 5).

Dispute over the assessment

If it were decided that Anna in Scenario A3 did not have the requisite capacity to make the decision over accommodation, Anna might be encouraged to appeal against that decision. (The use of the Independent Mental Capacity Advocacy Service is considered in Chapter 8 and Scenarios E.) Scenario A7 illustrates a situation where the absence of capacity is disputed.

Scenario A7: Dispute over assessment of capacity.

Beryl is eight months pregnant and has made it clear that she would not want to have any surgical intervention. She believes on religious grounds that such intervention is immoral and contrary to God's will. The midwives have reasons to believe that she lacks the mental capacity to make such a decision and consider that, in the event of her lack of capacity being confirmed, she should, if necessary, have a Caesarean section. The obstetrician supports the midwives. Beryl claims that she does have the capacity to refuse such intervention.

In such a situation as Scenario A7 an application should be made to the Court of Protection, where the issue of the presence or absence of mental capacity can be heard. Clearly both Beryl and the NHS Trust will require to have expert witnesses who can give evidence on the issue of her capacity. Beryl's relatives may also wish to be represented at the hearing. (See Scenarios D for discussion over a Court of Protection application and hearing, and see Scenarios E for discussion of the role of the Independent Mental Capacity Advocate.)

Assessment of capacity in an everyday situation

As discussed above there will be situations where experts are brought in to assess whether an individual is capable of making a specific decision, but often in a day-to-day context it will be those persons who are in regular attendance on the patient/client who have to make decisions over a person's capacity. This is illustrated in Scenario A8.

Scenario A8: Who determines capacity?

Angela, 75 years, was admitted to hospital following a fall at home. She had recovered, but it was considered inadvisable for her to return to live on her own and a place was being sought in a care home. There were times on the ward when she appeared to be lucid and able to make her own decisions. At other times she appeared to be confused and disorientated. The health care support worker bringing the tea trolley to the ward shouted at the door asking if anyone wanted a drink. One person responded. Angela had a friend Dawn with her. Dawn asked her if she would like a drink. Angela seemed confused, but was persuaded that it seemed a good idea and Dawn chased after the trolley and obtained a cup of tea for Angela. Angela drank it in one go and was clearly very thirsty. It was apparent to Dawn that Angela was unable to identify when she was thirsty or hungry and, had Dawn not been present, Angela would have been incapable of obtaining a drink for herself. Whose responsibility should it have been to ensure that Angela had food and drink?

The simple answer to the question posed in Scenario A8 is that the nursing staff should on Angela's admission and on a regular basis thereafter have decided on Angela's ability to take reasonable care of herself, and ensure that she received appropriate drinks. The care assistant should have been briefed as to which patients should be helped to have drinks. Where a patient was assessed as lacking the capacity to determine her own thirst, the support worker should have been told not to rely upon the patient responding. There would be considerable justification in ensuring that all staff who had contact with patients were aware of the basic provisions of the Mental Capacity Act 2005. Unfortunately Scenario A8 is all too common in the NHS. A survey by Age Concern reported in August 2006 that nurses were often too busy to assist patients who need help with eating. It surveyed 500 nurses and found that 90% said that they did not always have the time to help, despite evidence that malnutrition is common among older patients.[5] In March 2007, it was reported that Age Concern was seeking an army of volunteers to feed elderly patients who might otherwise go hungry because nurses are too busy to sit with them at mealtimes.[6]

Conclusions

In these Scenarios we have considered how the mental capacity of a person to make a requisite decision has been determined. The same principles would apply to other causes of mental capacity besides cerebral palsy. In taking Anna's situation in Scenario A3 we came to the conclusion that she did have the requisite mental capacity to make her own decision about accommodation. What would happen however if it was decided that she lacked the requisite capacity? We turn to Chapter 5 and Scenarios B, which consider how best interests are determined.

References

1   Code of Practice for the Mental Capacity Act 2005. Department of Constitutional Affairs February 2007 para 2.11. TSO, London.
2   Code of Practice for the Mental Capacity Act 2005. Department of Constitutional Affairs February 2007 para 2.11. TSO, London.
3   The Joint Cttee. Chapter 6 paras 62–78.
4   HoC Select Cttee. 19 Oct 2005.
5   News item: 'Old left hungry'. *The Times*, 29 August 2006.
6   Womack, S. 'Volunteers needed to feed elderly'. *The Daily Telegraph*, 14 March 2007.

5 Making Decisions in the Best Interests of Others

Best interests

Where decisions have to be made on behalf of a person who lacks the requisite mental capacity, then they must be made in the best interests of that person (unless there have been instructions by the person before he or she lost capacity, e.g. in an advance decision or in appointing a donee under a lasting power of attorney).

It is the fourth principle of the Mental Capacity Act 2005 (S.1(5)) that:

> An act done, or decision made, under this Act for or on behalf of a person who lacks capacity must be done, or made, in his best interests.

An exception to acting in the best interests is the situation where P has drawn up an advance decision which applies to the situation which has arisen. In this case the advance decision will prevail, even though this may be contrary to P's best interests (see Chapter 9). Similarly, if in a lasting power of attorney P has given the donee specific instructions about personal welfare or property or financial decisions these must be followed, even if they are contrary to P's best interests.

What is meant by best interests?

Best interests is not defined in Section 4, but this section provides a checklist of the considerations which must be taken into account in determining what are P's best interests. An example of how the courts have determined 'best interests' in the case of a boy of 18 years with severe learning disabilities and renal failure who may need a kidney transplant, is shown in Case B1[1] on page 69.

Section 4 sets out the steps to be taken in deciding best interests. These include briefly:

- do not make unjustified assumptions (4(1))
- consider all the relevant circumstances (4(2))
- consider whether capacity is likely to be recovered (4(3))
- support P's ability to participate (4(4))
- in life saving treatment, a desire to bring about death should not be the motivation (4(5))
- consider P's wishes and feelings, beliefs and values and other factors P would consider (4(6))
- consult views of specified others about what is in P's best interests and P's wishes, feelings etc. (4(7))

These specified steps also apply to others taking decisions on behalf of P, such as those exercising a lasting power of attorney (see Chapter 6) and deputies of the Court of Protection (see Chapter 7).

The criteria used to determine best interests

1 Unjustified assumptions (4(1))

The person who is making the decision must not make it merely on the basis of the person's age or appearance, or a condition of his or an aspect of his behaviour which might lead others to make unjustified assumptions about what might be in his best interests. In other words, just as in the determination as to whether or not someone lacks mental capacity, so in the determination of what is in that person's best interests a superficial judgment cannot be made (see Scenarios B1 and B2). There is evidence from recent research that has been carried out by the Disability Rights Commission[2] that those with learning disabilities are likely to have higher rates of unmet health needs, higher rates of respiratory disease, likely to be more obese than the rest of the population, and that generally their access to health provision is poorer than those without disabilities. Often the recording in primary care of those with learning disabilities is inadequate, and the proportion of people with learning disabilities who are known to the service is estimated at around one-quarter of actual prevalence. People with learning disabilities are less likely to receive health interventions, for example, in the treatment of diabetes. This research would suggest that too often those making decisions on behalf of those who lack the requisite capacity are making unjustified assumptions about their best interests, and not taking the necessary action to ensure that they are not disadvantaged in the receipt of healthcare.

Advocacy clearly has a very important role to play in such situations (see Chapter 8). Unfortunately however the advocate is only likely to be involved when serious medical treatment is already being considered. There may be no advocate when a hip replacement is a possibility but is not raised by the surgeon, because of the perceived lack of capacity of the patient. The new disability equality duty, placed on public bodies in December 2006 to eradicate institutional discrimination against disabled people, should lead to clearer identification and meeting of the health needs of disabled people (see Chapter 3).

2 Consider all the relevant circumstances (4(2))

It is a statutory requirement that all the relevant circumstances must be taken into account. Relevant circumstances are defined as:

> those of which the person making the decision is aware and which it would be reasonable to regard as relevant.

What is relevant will vary from person to person and the kind of decision which has to be made: financial decisions will require different kinds of information than medical or social ones. Clearly health and social services professionals must ensure that full documentation is completed on the relevant circumstances that they have taken into account in making a decision on behalf of P. There would also be advantages if the informal carer also kept records as to the basis of some of the significant decisions they might have to make on a person's behalf (see Chapter 15 and Scenarios L).

3 Consider whether capacity is likely to be recovered (4(3))

Temporary or permanent

There is a statutory requirement (S.4(3)) that the decision maker must consider whether it is likely that the person will at some time have capacity in relation to the matter in question and, if it appears likely that he will, when that is likely to be. (See Scenario B3 and contrast this with Scenario B4.)

4 Support P's ability to participate (4(4))

Participation

It is a statutory requirement that the decision maker should, so far as is reasonably practicable, permit and encourage the person to participate, or to improve his ability to participate, as fully as possible in any act done for him and any decision affecting him.

Participation may require mechanical aids. There may be considerable resource implications in facilitating participation of the client in decision making.

Reasonably practicable however enables cost, value, time and other considerations to be taken into account in achieving that participation. Had the word 'reasonable' not been included, then if participation was scientifically or practically possible, it would have to take place. (This contrasts with the second principle contained in Section 1(3) that:

> A person is not to be treated as unable to make a decision unless **all practicable steps** to help him to do so have been taken without success.

where there is no 'reasonable': see Scenario B5.)

5 In life saving treatment, a desire to bring about death should not be the motivation (4(5))

Continuation of life

It was of concern to those debating the Bill that the decision maker could make life and death decisions and decide that the mentally incapacitated adult could be allowed to die, whilst notionally acting in the best interests of the patient/client. If life-sustaining treatment is being considered, then the decision maker must begin by assuming that it will be in the person's best interests for his life to continue. Life-sustaining treatment is defined in Section 4(10) as:

> Treatment which in the view of a person providing health care for the person concerned is necessary to sustain life.

If the mentally incapacitated person had drawn up, when mentally capacitated, an advance decision which applied to the particular circumstances, then this would take precedence in the decision making (see Chapter 9). There may be circumstances where letting die is in the best interests of the patient. For example where the patient is in the terminal stages of cancer and suffers a cardiac arrest, doctors treating the patient may consider that resuscitation is not in the best interests of the patient. The statute does not require health professionals to carry out treatment which in their professional judgment is not in the best interests of the patient, and this is in accordance with the common law, the decision by the United Kingdom (UK) courts and the European Court of Human Rights in the Burke case.[3] This case is considered in Chapter 9.

Nor does the statute permit voluntary euthanasia to take place. A doctor would be permitted in law to provide pain relieving treatment for the patient, even though this may, incidentally, shorten the patient's life, but the doctor cannot give an overdose of pain relieving medication to bring about the patient's death. This is in keeping with existing statute (Suicide Act 1961) and common law (the law of murder) and, since the failure of the Assisted Suicide Bill in the House of Lords, will continue to be the law for the foreseeable future (see Chapter 11).

6 Consider P's wishes and feelings, beliefs and values and other factors P would consider (4(6))

Modified best interests

The effect of the statutory provisions of determining best interests is a modified best interests test, close to what has been described as a substituted judgment test. Scenario B6 illustrates the difference between a simple best interest test and a modified one.

This modified best interest test is possible when a person once had the mental capacity and evidence of their earlier wishes and feelings can be provided. However if a person has never had the requisite mental capacity, such as those with severe learning disabilities or serious brain damage from birth, then it is difficult to apply any test other than the simple best interests test.

Circumstances to be taken into account

There could have been a requirement that best interests were determined on an objective basis: what would any reasonable person wish to be decided for them or what action would any reasonable person want? However the statutory provisions allow for a subjective test, so that the particular characteristics of the client/patient can be taken into account in determining what is in their best interests.

Past and present wishes and feelings

The decision maker must consider, so far as is reasonably ascertainable, the person's past and present wishes and feelings. This is more realistic where a person once had mental capacity, such as a person who now has Alzheimer's and is at the present time incapable of making any decisions. A profile can be built up of that person's personality and character. Scenarios B6 and B7 provide examples of how this statutory provision would work.

Beliefs and values

The decision maker must also take into account any beliefs and values that P once had. This is discussed in Scenario B7. The fact that these beliefs and values are contrary to those held by the decision maker is irrelevant, as Scenario B13 shows.

Any other factors

Any other factors that the client/patient would be likely to consider if he were able to do so may include a wide variety of topics. For example it may be that the client was a very altruistic person, generous with charities. The fact that he always contributed to a particular charity could be taken into account in decisions relating to the use of his income or capital. It may be that the person once had particular hobbies and interests, and this fact may be taken into account in determining his accommodation or his expenditure.

Scenario B8 illustrates a situation where risks to P are an important factor in determining best interests.

7 Consult views of specified others (4(7))

Consultation with others

The decision maker is obliged to take into account the views of others who are specified in the Act. This requirement is qualified by the words,

'if it is practicable and appropriate to consult them'.

Interestingly there is no 'reasonably' qualifying practicable. This means that every effort must be made to contact the specified persons. However the use of the word 'appropriate' signifies that the decision maker could decide that certain persons need not be consulted. This may for example include a person with whom the client/patient had fallen out, or with whom they have not had contact over a long period. Those the Act requires to be consulted include:

A nominated person

It may be that the client/patient has named a person as someone to be consulted on the matter in question or on matters of that kind. The decision maker would need to clarify the fact of the nomination, as well as the area over which they could be consulted. Thus a relative may have been nominated to be consulted over the client's care and treatment, but not over any financial matters.

Carer

Anyone engaged in caring for the person or interested in his welfare must be consulted by the person making the decision (S.4(7)(b)).

The Act does not specify whether or not the carer is paid, and therefore the views of both informal and paid carers could be obtained over what is considered to be in the best interests of the mentally incapacitated person.

Donee of a lasting power of attorney and deputy appointed for the person by the court

If either of these appointments have been made, then the decision maker has a duty to consult them if he or she considers it practical and appropriate. The donee of a lasting power of attorney (LPA) may for example have had a long acquaintance with P prior to P's loss of mental capacity, and can provide the decision maker with information about P's wishes and feelings, beliefs and values.

Content of consultation

The decision maker would discuss with those persons to be consulted what would be in the person's best interests and, in particular, would ascertain the client/patient's wishes, feelings, beliefs and values and other factors that he would be likely to consider if he had the capacity. Those consulted could provide the decision maker with the personal history of the client/patient, together with information on their personality, character, individual wishes, feelings, beliefs and values, so that a picture can be drawn up of what that person would have wanted for himself or herself.

Scenarios B9 and B10 illustrate situations dealing with consultation in the determination of best interests.

Application of the best interests criteria

These statutory requirements on how best interests is to be decided must be followed by anyone exercising powers under a lasting power of attorney, or any other powers exercised on behalf of a person who is reasonably believed to lack capacity (S.4(8)). (An exception to this would be where an LPA specifies action which must be taken by the donee of the power, which could be contrary to P's best interests.)

Thus, whenever decisions are to be made on behalf of a person who lacks capacity the principles set out in Section 4 must be applied. However where an advance decision (see Chapter 9) has been drawn up, is relevant and applies to the decision, then the best interests criteria would not be relevant. Those acting under the advance decision must carry out the refusal of P (if it is valid and relevant to the circumstances), since those wishes were recorded at a time when P had the requisite mental capacity.

It must be emphasised that the use of the best interest criteria only comes into play when the decision has been made that P lacks the requisite mental capacity to make a specific decision. As long as P has the mental capacity, P can make his or her own decisions, whether or not they are in his or her best interests.

Who decides? What role does the family play?

For day-to-day decisions the immediate carer would be deciding whether a person lacks the requisite capacity and if so, what is in the person's best interests. However for more serious decisions, such as medical treatment or accommodation, the health professionals and social services personnel would be making the decision, but would involve informal and paid carers and family members in the decision making process.

Disputes over what is in a person's best interests

Where there are disputes over the decision and there is no local resolution of the dispute, then an application could be made to the Court of Protection which might appoint a deputy to assist in the resolution of the problem (see Chapter 7).

Standard of compliance

Where an act is done or decision made by a person other than the court, then there is sufficient compliance with Section 4 (best interests) if the person complies with steps to be taken in determining best interests and in taking into account all the specified considerations (S.4(1) to (7)), and he reasonably believes that what he does or decides is in the best interests of the person concerned (S.4(9)).

This means that any civil or criminal proceedings brought against the decision maker can be defended on the grounds that there was compliance with the statutory provisions. However in the event of a dispute the decision maker would have to produce evidence that the statutory provisions were followed, and therefore documentation on the persons who have been consulted, the information which has been taken into account, and what has been decided as relevant would be essential evidence. Records of such information are essential for health and social services professionals, but they would also be of great value to the unpaid carer.

Thus even informal carers and decision makers would be well advised to keep records of some of the significant decisions made on behalf of the mentally incapacitated person (see Chapter 15).

Decisions in relation to care and treatment (S.5)

Further provisions are made by Section 5 in relation to acts carried out in connection with the care and treatment in the best interests of the adult who lacks the requisite mental capacity.

The following stages must take place:

1. A person (D) has taken reasonable steps to determine if P lacks capacity in relation to the matter in question, and
2. he reasonably believes that P does lack capacity, and
3. he reasonably believes that it will be in P's best interests for the act to be done

Then D (the person carrying out the activity) does not incur any liability in relation to the act that he would not have incurred if P had had the capacity to consent in relation to the matter and had consented to D's doing the act.

In other words, if the statutory provisions are followed, the absence of consent by P does not create a trespass to the person in relation to D's actions. This section puts in statutory form the protection recognised at common law and set out in the case of *Re F*.[4] It provides legitimacy for all those activities by lay persons, health and social services professionals taken out of necessity in the best interests of a mentally incapacitated adult. Only two conditions are required: that there should have been reasonable steps taken to ascertain that P lacks capacity and that these steps led to the conclusion that P was mentally incapable in relation to that matter, and secondly that the acts should be in the best interests of P. The principles set out in Section 1 apply to this situation, as does the definition of capacity in Sections 2 and 3 and the definition of best interests in Section 4.

However this protection is limited, since Section 5(3) explains that nothing in Section 5 excludes a person's civil liability for loss or damage, or his criminal liability, resulting from his negligence in doing the act (see Chapter 11). The provisions are illustrated by the example in Scenario B13.

Exclusions from Section 5

The power recognised in Section 5 to take action in relation to the care and treatment of a mentally incapacitated adult does not authorise a person to act contrary to a donee of a lasting power of attorney granted by P, or a deputy appointed for P by the court (S.6(6)). However this would not prevent a person providing life-sustaining treatment or doing an act which he reasonably believes to be necessary to prevent a serious deterioration in P's condition whilst awaiting a decision from the courts (S.6(7)).

Restraint

Where the decision maker acts with the intention of restraining the client/patient, it does not come under the protection of Section 5 unless two further conditions are satisfied. These are:

- that the decision maker must reasonably believe that it is necessary to do the act in order to prevent harm to the client/patient and
- that the action is a proportionate response.

Proportionate means that the act of restraint is proportionate to both the likelihood of harm to the client/patient and the seriousness of the harm.

The use of restraint is defined as including both the decision maker using or threatening to use force to secure the doing of an act which the client/patient resists, or resisting P's liberty of movement, whether or not P resists. This is illustrated in Scenario B11. Scenario B13 considers a situation where an intimate procedure was carried out under anaesthetic at the same time as surgery for a fractured ankle.

Restraint and loss of liberty

Concern was expressed by both the Joint Committee of Parliament and the Joint Committee on Human Rights that, as originally drafted, the clause covering restraint did not make sufficiently clear that the restraint provisions could not justify a deprivation of liberty contrary to Article 5 of the European Convention on Human Rights.

Lord Goodhart[5] drew the Committee's attention to the report of the Joint Committee on Human Rights published the day before.[6] In discussing this issue, Para 4.8 states:

> The Government states that the Bill's provisions about restraint 'do not permit deprivations of liberty within the meaning of Article 5 ECHR. Restraint is defined as including restriction of liberty. The Government has never intended this to include actions which would amount to a deprivation of liberty for Article 5 purposes'. This makes clear that the power to restrain is not intended to be interpreted as authorising deprivation of liberty and therefore engaging Article 5.

In its response to the comments by the Joint Committee on Human Rights on the Mental Capacity Bill that the Government had not expressly confined the use or threat of force to strictly emergency situations, the Government agreed that any restriction of liberty should be the shortest and least restrictive possible. Definition of restraint would include pulling someone away from a busy road, putting a seatbelt on someone in a car, or administering sedatives in order to undertake treatment. Sometimes it is not always in a person's best interests for matters to be left until it is an urgent situation. For example restraint may be necessary in order to undertake a diagnostic procedure. The example was also given of a bad tooth where restraint was needed before it became an emergency situation.

There are strict safeguards surrounding the use of restraint:

- the minimum level of restraint must be used
- the principle of the least restrictive option applies to the use of restraint.

The matter can always be referred to the Court of Protection.

A new subsection was added to the Bill to make it absolutely clear that the Mental Capacity Act 2005 would not authorise a loss of liberty:

> But D does more than merely restrain P if he deprives P of his liberty within the meaning of Article 5(1) of the Human Rights Convention (whether or not D is a public authority) (S.6(5)).

However this subsection was repealed by the Mental Health Act 2007 as a result of the amendments to the Mental Capacity Act (MCA) to fill the Bournewood gap. Under these amendments, if the specified strict conditions are followed, it would be lawful to detain a person in his or her best interests and deprive him or her of liberty (see Chapter 13).

The Mental Health Act 2007 repealed Section 6(5) of the MCA and replaced it with new Sections 4A and 4B, which would justify the deprivation of liberty in specific circumstances (see Chapters 3 and 13). Sections 4A and 4B are set out in Boxes 3.3 and 3.4 respectively on pages 24 and 25.

Restraint and lasting power of attorney

The donee of a lasting power of attorney giving powers in relation to personal welfare is only authorised to restrain P if the three conditions laid down under Section 11 are satisfied. See Chapter 6 for further discussion of this.

Payment for necessary goods and services

Under Section 7 if necessary goods and services are supplied to a person who lacks capacity to contract for the supply, he must pay a reasonable price for them. 'Necessary' is defined as meaning suitable to a person's condition in life, and to his actual requirements at the time when the goods or services are supplied. See Scenario H2.

Expenditure

Under Section 8 if an action relating to care and treatment (covered by Section 5) involves expenditure, then it is lawful for D to pledge P's credit for the purpose of the expenditure, and to apply money in P's possession for meeting the expenditure. If D bears the expenditure on P's behalf, then it is lawful for D to reimburse himself out of money in P's possession, or to be otherwise indemnified by P. These subsections do not affect any power under which a person has lawful control of P's money or other property, and has power to spend money for P's benefit.

Whether D is a paid or informal carer, it would be wise for records to be kept of any moneys taken from P by D to reimburse himself, so that if challenged D can provide evidence of the justification for the reimbursement. See Scenario B12 on reimbursement.

Decisions relating to organ and tissue removal and retention are considered in Chapter 14.

Decisions about sexual activity

If the principles of *Valuing People*[7] (Rights, Independence, Choice and Inclusion (see Chapter 11)) are followed, the care plan for a person with learning disabilities may include the achievement of a sexual relationship. This may present difficulties for those paid carers who have strong beliefs in sexual relations only taking place within marriage. Scenario B14 illustrates some of the potential problems.

Intimate care

Problems can arise in the care of those who lack the capacity to give consent over their intimate care. Screening breasts for lumps, cervical screening, washing of the genitalia and similar procedures can all pose problems when the patient/client is unable to understand the justification for what is proposed, is unable to give consent, and furthermore may resist any intimate touching of his or her person. A typical situation is discussed in Scenario B15.

Decisions excluded from the Act

The MCA excludes some decisions being made under the Act on the basis that these are so personal to the person making them that they cannot be delegated to another person and that specific mental capacity is required for these kinds of decisions to be made. The excluded decisions are specified in Section 27.

Excluded decisions (S.27(1))

> Nothing in this Act permits a decision on any of the following matters to be made on behalf of a person:
> a.   consenting to marriage or a civil partnership
> b.   consenting to have sexual relations
> c.   consenting to a decree of divorce being granted on the basis of two years' separation
> d.   consenting to a dissolution order being made in relation to a civil partnership on the basis of two years' separation

e. consenting to a child's being placed for adoption by an adoption agency
f. consenting to the making of an adoption order (as defined in the Adoption and Children Act 2002)
g. discharging parental responsibilities in matters not relating to a child's property
h. giving a consent under the Human Fertilisation and Embryology Act 1990.

In certain of these specified situations there will be lawful alternatives to the giving of consent. For example under Section 27(1)(e) and the consenting to a child being placed for adoption, if the birth mother lacked the capacity to give consent to that adoption taking place, the rules on dispensing with consent in the adoption legislation would apply. The possibility of the Court of Protection giving consent or giving a deputy powers to consent on behalf of the mentally incapacitated person is precluded by Section 27(1)(e).

A marriage is void if one or other parties to the marriage lacks the capacity to give consent, and thus Section 27(1)(a) prevents consent being given on behalf of a mentally incapacitated person.

Exclusion of Mental Health Act matters (S28(1))

Nothing in this Act authorises anyone to give a patient medical treatment for mental disorder, or to consent to a patient's being given medical treatment for mental disorder, if, at the time when it is proposed to treat the patient, his treatment is regulated under the Mental Health Act 2007. (Medical treatment and mental disorder and patient have the same meaning as in that Act.)

This exclusion is considered further in Chapter 13 on mental health and mental capacity and is discussed in Case B2.

Exclusion of voting rights (S29(1))

Nothing in this Act permits a decision on voting at an election for any public office, or at a referendum, to be made on behalf a person.

The definition of referendum is as set out in Section 101 of the Political Parties, Elections and Referendums Act 2000, and means a referendum or other poll held in pursuance of any provision made under an Act of Parliament on one or more questions specified in or in accordance with any such provision. The decision on how to exercise the right to vote is intensely personal and is non-delegable. It is a right which is effectively lost in the event of a person losing mental capacity and could not be covered by an advance decision.

Advance decisions

Where P had created a valid advance decision, then Section 5 would not apply to any care and treatment specified in the advance decision. The best interests test does not apply where a person has the mental capacity to make their own decisions or where they have by means of an advance decision made clear, at a time when they had the requisite mental capacity, what care and treatment they would not want if they were in the future to lack that capacity (see Chapter 9). The Code of Practice suggests that under Section 5 an advance directive cannot exclude basic care for the patient: it can only cover treatment. However there is no statutory definition of care, and the definition of treatment states that 'treatment' includes a diagnostic or other procedure. Case law will ultimately be required to determine what comes within the definition of care (and therefore cannot be refused by an advance decision) and what comes within the definition of treatment (and therefore can be refused by an advance decision). (See Chapter 9 and Scenario F8.)

Accountability is considered in Chapter 11.

Conclusions

The concept of best interests is at the heart of decision making under the MCA, and the Act provides no simple test for defining best interests. It sets out the steps to be taken and the considerations to be used in determining it. It is highly subjective and, as case law develops over the outcome of the test in individual cases, we may discern a move away from the medical model which has dominated decision making in care and treatment disputes since the case of *Re F*.

References

1   *An Hospital NHS Trust and S (by his litigation friend the Official Solicitor) and DG (S's father) and SG (S's mother)* [2003] EWHC Fam 365.
2   Disability Rights Commission (2006) *Equal Treatment: Closing the Gap*. DRC.
3   *R. (on the application of Burke)* v. *General Medical Council and Disability Rights Commission and the Official Solicitor to the Supreme Court* [2004] EWHC 1879; [2004] Lloyd's Rep Med 451.
4   *F* v. *West Berkshire Health Authority* [1989] 2 All ER 545.
5   House of Lords 25 January 2005. Hansord column 1247.
6   Joint Committee on Human Rights. W.K. Pasl. 24 January 2005.
7   Department of Health (2001) *Valuing People: A New Strategy for Learning Disability for the 21st Century*. White Paper CM 5086. DH, London.

Scenarios B
Making Decisions in the
Best Interests of Others

Introduction

Once it has been decided that P lacks the requisite mental capacity to make a specific decision, then decisions must be made for him in his best interests. The following Scenarios consider some of the issues which can arise in making this determination.

Unjustified assumptions

> **Scenario B1: Unjustified assumptions.**
>
> Ralph had been sleeping on the streets for several months and was dishevelled and dirty. He was brought to a Salvation Army hostel and seen by a doctor, who considered that he was suffering from severe kidney failure and would require immediate dialysis and possibly ultimately a kidney transplant. Ralph made it clear that he was refusing any such treatment.

The first question which arises here is, does Ralph have the mental capacity to make the decision for himself, after being given all the relevant information? If the answer to that is yes, then he is entitled to refuse any treatment. If however it is determined according to the principles set out in Section 1 and in relation to the definition of mental capacity set out in Sections 2 and 3 that he lacks the requisite mental capacity, then the decision must be made in his best interests. In deciding what is in his best interests, the fact that he has been a tramp for some time and does not appear to enjoy a very high quality of life is irrelevant. However his ability to keep to the strict post-transplant regime of anti-rejection medication would be relevant to the priority assigned to him for a transplant operation.

Scenario B2: Too old for treatment.

Angela is 84 years old and has been in a care home for five years. One winter, following her 'flu injection, she appeared to be suffering from a severe chest infection. Her relatives, who seldom visited her, advised the home manager that at her age they did not consider that there was any point in a doctor being called or in antibiotics being prescribed. The manager was uncertain what action to take.

The first issue to arise in Scenario B2 is the question of Angela's mental capacity. Is she able to understand the information given to her, retain it and make a decision in the light of it? If Angela is reasonably believed to have the requisite mental capacity, then she can decide for herself what treatment to have. On the other hand if the manager and the relatives decide that Angela does not have the requisite mental capacity, then action has to be taken in her best interests.

Section 4(1) makes it clear that the determination of her best interests must not be made merely on the basis of her age, appearance or any condition or behaviour of hers. The fact that Angela is 84 years old, lacks mental capacity and is in a care home is irrelevant for the purposes of determining her best interests. (It could be, of course, that the relatives are thinking of their best interests were Angela to die in the near future and they would benefit financially from her death.) In addition, where the decision relates to life-sustaining treatment the decision maker must not, in considering whether the treatment is in Angela's best interests, be motivated by a desire to bring about her death. Life-sustaining is defined as:

> Treatment which in the view of a person providing health care for the person concerned is necessary to sustain life. (S.4(10))

It is highly probable that the doctor called in to examine Angela would consider that in her situation antibiotics are a life-sustaining treatment. Such treatment could therefore not be withheld on the grounds that it was in Angela's best interests to die, and therefore it was concluded that the antibiotics should not be prescribed and administered.

Example of a case which decided what were 'best interests'

The Mental Capacity Act (MCA) sets out the factors to be taken into account in determining what are the best interests, but it does not actually give a definition of the term. Guidance on how the courts have determined best interests will be used in the implementation of the MCA. One such example is shown in Case B1, where in a potentially life saving situation the court had to decide whether it was in the best interests of a boy of 18 years to be given a kidney transplant.

> **Case B1: Is a transplant in the best interests?** *A Hospital National Health Service (NHS) Trust and S* 2003.[1]
>
> S was born with a genetic condition, velo-cardiac facial syndrome and had a number of major problems including severe learning disabilities and bilateral renal dysplasia. He was 18 at the time of the court hearing in 2003. He had been admitted to hospital in 2000 with acute renal failure and had been on haemodialysis ever since. There was a dispute between some of the health professions and the parents over his continuing treatment, including whether a kidney transplant should eventually be carried out.

Dame Elizabeth Butler-Sloss, President of the Family Division, had to decide how S's best interests were to be determined. She quoted her statement in *Re A (Male Sterilisation):*[2] 'best interests encompasses medical, emotional and all other welfare issues'. She also quoted Thorpe LJ in the same case, where he suggested that the judge with the responsibility to make an evaluation of the best interests of a claimant lacking capacity should draw up a balance sheet.

> The first entry should be of any factor or factors of actual benefit. . . . Then on the other sheet the judge should write any counterbalancing dis-benefits to the applicant . . . then the judge should enter on each sheet the potential gains and losses in each instance making some estimate of the extent of the possibility that the gain or loss might accrue. At the end of that exercise the judge should be better placed to strike a balance between the sum of the certain and possible gains against the sum of the certain and possible losses. Obviously only if the account is in relatively significant credit will the judge conclude that the application is likely to advance the best interests of the claimant.[3]

In deciding what was in S's best interests, the judge accepted the principle that just because a person cannot understand treatment it is wrong to say that he cannot have it. If there is a quality of life then, even if it is necessary to go through a traumatic period, it would be worthwhile in the long term. She noted that all parties agreed that haemodialysis should continue and if necessary be followed by peritoneal dialysis. In addition she concluded that AV fistula should be attempted if medically indicated, even though he disliked needles, since it was not at all clear that he was seriously afraid of needles and there was no evidence that S had a needle phobia. In relation to the kidney transplant, which at the present time was hypothetical, the mother was prepared to offer her kidney. The judge ruled that whilst there were significant medical difficulties, that his severe learning disability militated against explanations about the transplant, and that the hospital were concerned about the consequences of emergency surgery on an autistic boy, she considered that it should be possible to manage him post-operatively. She stated that:

> On balance, if the medical reasons for a kidney transplantation are in his favour, and alternative methods of dialysis are no longer viable, in my judgement,

a kidney transplantation ought not to be rejected on the grounds of his inability to understand the purpose and consequences of the operation or concerns about his management.[4]

Temporary or permanent incapacity

Whilst the temporary or permanent nature of the person's condition is irrelevant to the definition of mental capacity for making a specific decision, it is relevant in determining the best interests of the patient. In determining what are in the best interests of the person lacking the required mental capacity, the decision maker must decide if the person is likely to recover mental capacity in relation to the matter in question and if so, when that recovery is likely to be. It follows that if the making of a serious decision can be delayed without harm to the person until such a time as that individual can decide for himself or herself, then the delay would be in the best interests of the individual. The two situations are illustrated by Scenarios B3 and B4.

Scenario B3: Road accident 1.

Following a road traffic accident, Mike, aged 33 years, is brought unconscious into Accident and Emergency (A&E). His right arm is badly injured and surgeons believe that although they could save it, in the long term Mike might be better served with a prosthesis. It is likely that Mike will recover consciousness in a few hours and the surgeons consider that they could wait to discuss all the options with him then before any decision to amputate is made.

The situation in Scenario B.3 contrasts with that in Scenario B.4.

Scenario B4: Road accident 2.

Mavis, aged 33 years, comes into A&E following a road accident. She is unconscious. She has severe learning difficulties and would be unable to understand that her right arm is so badly injured that it might have to be amputated. The surgeons discuss all the options with her parents and the manager of the care home in which she lives and decide that it is in her best interests that the amputation should take place immediately and there would be little justification in waiting until she regained consciousness.

The length of the delay until the requisite mental capacity is restored is of course relevant, and if in Scenario B3 the doctors decided that an operation on the arm could not wait till the recovery of Mike's mental capacity, then action would have to be taken in his best interests whilst he was still unconscious.

Encouraging participation in decision making

Scenario B5: Reasonable practicable support.

Glen received severe injuries at birth, as a consequence of which he is unable to communicate effectively. He has been cared for at home by his elderly parents but there is now a possibility that he could be transferred to a home for young people with physical disabilities. It is possible that he could participate in the decision making but only with extremely expensive high tech equipment which neither health nor social services consider they have the resources to provide. What is the law?

In determining Glen's mental capacity to make a decision about his transfer to another home, all practicable steps must be taken to help him achieve the necessary capacity and the ability to communicate (see Scenario A3). Once it is concluded that Glen does not have the requisite capacity, then reasonable steps must be taken to assist him in having the requisite mental capacity to participate in the decision making process.

> He must, so far as reasonably practicable, permit and encourage the person to participate, or to improve his ability to participate, as fully as possible in any act done for him and any decision affecting him. (S.4(4))

What should health and social services do for Glen which would be seen as 'so far as reasonably practicable'? In answering this question, the cost, the time, the value to Glen and other priorities could be taken into account. Each organisation may come up with a different answer depending upon their resources and the demands upon those resources. They must act reasonably, which would mean it would be unjustified to treat two clients with identical needs in different ways. Documentation would be required of how a particular decision was reached, and all the considerations which were taken into account in deciding what facilities and services Glen would be able to have and what facilities and services were refused.

The basic questions to be answered by health and social services are:

1. Does Glen have the requisite mental capacity?
2. If not, could any practicable steps be taken to assist in his having the requisite mental capacity?
3. If the answer to 2 is 'Yes', then those steps must be taken.
4. If the answer to 2 is 'No', then the decision must be taken by others.
5. How could Glen be assisted so that he could participate in the decision making process?

6. Is this assistance available?
7. If so, what is the cost of this assistance, and is the expenditure justified in terms of the benefit that it would bring to Glen's active participation and in comparison with other priorities? It could be for example that there were available a highly expensive computer activated by touch, but it would take considerable time for Glen to be taught how to use this equipment and the decision over accommodation would have to be made in the near future.

Modified best interests

If an objective test were used to determine the best interests of a person lacking the required mental capacity, then their past and present wishes and feelings, what they once believed in, and their earlier values before they lost mental capacity could be ignored for the purposes of determining their best interests. However the Mental Capacity Act 2005 requires a subjective assessment of what is in P's best interests.

How would P decide if he or she now had the capacity to make the specific decision?

Where P once had the requisite mental capacity, there would be evidence of how they once acted, their values, beliefs, feelings and wishes. Where P has never had mental capacity for this kind of decision, it is more difficult to ascertain what he or she would want if they now had the capacity to decide.

Scenario B6: Modified best interests test.

Mavis was by family background a strong member of the Jehovah's Witness faith and had always made it clear that in the event of her requiring a blood transfusion and her lacking the capacity or ability to make a decision, she would not want to be given blood. She had not however completed the Jehovah's Witness card to that effect. In her late 60s she suffered dementia and was moved to a residential home. Her physical health weakened and she was diagnosed as suffering from chronic leukaemia and required a blood transfusion. She lacked the mental capacity to make any decision about having a blood transfusion.

If a simple best interests test is used in the case of Mavis in Scenario B6, then it could be argued that Mavis would die without a blood transfusion, and therefore it is in her best interests to have a transfusion. However if a modified best interests test is used, then account can be taken of what she would have said had she still retained the mental capacity to make a decision. On this basis, assuming that she still kept her beliefs, and had not changed her mind about having a transfusion, then the blood transfusion could be withheld on the grounds that looking at her previous wishes and feelings, she would have refused it when she had the mental capacity, and therefore would continue to have refused it at a time when she lacked the capacity. Scenarios B6 and B7 illustrate the issues.

> **Scenario B7: Previous wishes and feelings.**
>
> Audrey has severe Alzheimer's and has been in a residential home for several years. The home is due to be demolished and residents are being moved to other homes. There are two principal choices for Audrey: an inner city home with close access to shops, restaurants and cinemas, and a rural home surrounded by gardens and fields. Audrey's daughter explains to the home manager that Audrey had always lived in the city, and would prefer to be close to public activities and city life than to be banished to the countryside.

Clearly Audrey's life and preferences made at an earlier time when she had capacity should be taken into account in making the decision over which home would be in her best interests.

Closely linked with past and present wishes and feelings are the beliefs and values which she once had, and would be likely to influence her decision if she now had capacity. In the situation in Scenario B6 account has been taken of the previous beliefs and values of Mavis. The Code of Practice uses the example of a young girl, brain injured in a road accident, who had previously been politically active and whose father, when making investment decisions on her behalf, was able to take into account to what investment choices her beliefs and values would have led her.[5]

Risk taking

Scenario B8 illustrates a situation where risks to P are an important factor in determining best interests.

> **Scenario B8: Risk taking.**
>
> Harry has severe learning disabilities and also suffers from epilepsy, which is not entirely under control with medication. He loves swimming but has been told that because of the risk of his suffering an epileptic fit whilst in the water, it is too dangerous.

Scenario B8 first raises the question: can Harry make his own decision about going swimming? If the answer to that is 'no', then the decision must be made in his best interests. The decision maker must follow the steps outlined in Chapter 5, and also carry out a risk/benefit analysis taking into account Harry's own wishes and feelings. Harry's quality of life would obviously be improved if he were able to undertake those activities he enjoys, and the decision maker would have a duty to see if the risks could be managed to reduce the possibility of harm arising in the water: more staff in attendance, the use of harnesses (see Scenario B11) and other methods of ensuring Harry's safety whilst he is the water should be considered. The assumption that it would be safer for him to stay at home should not be made without rigorous examination.

Consultation with others

Whoever is making the decision, and this would apply to an informal carer as well as a health or social services professional, there must be consultation with others so that their views can be taken into account. The Act requires taking into consideration:

> if it is practicable and appropriate to consult them, the views of –
>
> (a)   anyone named by the person as someone to be consulted on the matter in question or on matters of that kind,
> (b)   anyone engaged in caring for the person or interested in his welfare,
> (c)   any donee of a lasting power of attorney granted by the person, and
> (d)   any deputy appointed for the person by the court,
>
> as to what would be in the person's best interests and, in particular, as to the matters mentioned in subsection (6).

The following Scenarios illustrate the effect of this consultation.

Scenario B9: The views of others on P's best interests.

Ruth has been in a care home for two years and seems unsettled and unhappy. She appears to lack short term memory and is diagnosed as being in the early stages of dementia. However she is able to work the key pad for the door locks and frequently walks out of the front door onto a busy road. She has four children. Three of them visit her when they can. The fourth lives abroad and only sees Ruth once a year. Her younger daughter, Jane, is proposing to move to a larger house and turn the garage into a downstairs self contained flat for Ruth. The other siblings who are not on good terms with Jane are opposed to this move. They consider that it is in Ruth's best interests to remain in the care home, where they feel that she is well cared for. They do not consider that she is capable of living in self contained accommodation, and do not believe that the younger sister would be able or would be prepared to give Ruth the time and support that she needs. They also suspect that Jane is more interested in Ruth's personal assets and would exploit her financially. There is no evidence that Jane visits Ruth more frequently than the other two siblings who live in this country.

It is probable that social services would take the lead in determining how this decision was to be made and what was in Ruth's best interests. Let us assume the following.

Brenda Thomas is the social worker appointed to carry out an assessment of Ruth.

- She has evidence from the home manager and from the general practitioner (GP) who attends Ruth at the home that Ruth lacks the mental capacity to decide for herself where she should live.
- She therefore obtains all the relevant information necessary to determine Ruth's best interests.
- This would include finding out whether it was possible to assist Ruth in participating in the decision. For example could a speech therapist or a specialist in the care of the elderly be of any assistance?
- She would take medical advice in deciding if Ruth was likely to recover capacity so that she could make her own decisions. If there was no such likelihood, she would have to make the decision in Ruth's best interests.
- She would ascertain if it were appropriate to arrange for the appointment of an independent mental capacity advocate (see Chapter 8 and Scenario E1).
- She would consult with the three members of the family who visited Ruth, and ascertain when the fourth child was likely to be in the country, so he or she could also be consulted on their views on what is in Ruth's best interests.
- She would also ascertain if there were other relatives who would have relevant views as to what was in Ruth's best interests.
- She would also consult with the carers in the home, the GP and others involved in her present care and treatment.
- All these people would be asked what they knew of Ruth's past and present wishes and feelings, and if Ruth has any written statements (made when she had the requisite mental capacity) which are relevant to her future accommodation.
- They would also be asked about any beliefs and values that would have influenced Ruth had she had the requisite mental capacity, and any other factors which Ruth would have considered had she been able to do so.
- In the light of these views as to what was in Ruth's best interests, and the views of the independent mental capacity advocate (if appointed), Brenda would make her decision over what was in Ruth's best interests.

Let us assume that Brenda decided in the light of the information that she had obtained that it was in Ruth's best interests to remain in the care home. She may have discovered, for example, that Ruth had never been very close to her younger daughter Jane, but that Ruth had always been meticulous in treating each of her children equally. Brenda also found out that Jane was in serious financial difficulties, and that Ruth paid the full home fees from the considerable capital that was left to her from the death of her husband and the sale of her house. Brenda also found out that Ruth appeared to be friendly with several fellow residents in the care home and would sit with them for meals and when watching television. Ruth also appeared to enjoy the outings from the home.

Brenda's decision that Ruth should remain in the care home was challenged by Jane, who was prepared to apply to the Court of Protection for an order enabling Ruth to be transferred to her house. It is possible that a deputy would be appointed by the Court of Protection to make the decision (see Chapter 6 and Scenario D1).

Brenda should have the records which show the views that she had received and all the data which informed her decision. It is important that those she has consulted give their views on what would appear to be in Ruth's best interests, and their views as to Ruth's wishes and feelings, beliefs and values rather than their own views as to what they would want. Even in this apparently simple decision there is a lot to be taken into consideration, and there are considerable resource issues for social services in this decision making process, particularly where there are disputes within a family or between clinicians and informal carers.

Independence

Scenario B10 presents another situation comparable to Scenario B9, when the views of others may prevent the best interests of P taking priority.

Scenario B10: A sexual relationship.

Geoffrey suffered brain damage at birth and has always been cared for by his parents. They gave up work at his birth and spent their lives devoted to him. A speech therapist has worked with Geoffrey in developing his communication and encouraged him to participate in activities outside the home. He enjoys going to the pub and has met up with a girl in similar circumstances with whom he would like to have a sexual relationship. His parents are horrified at this development and do not consider it is in Geoffrey's interests to have these outside interests, since false expectations may be set up and he may eventually want to move into other accommodation, where he would be unable to cope.

The starting point in this Scenario is Geoffrey's mental capacity to decide if he wishes to take part in these activities and, ultimately, if he wishes to leave home. Only if an assessment is made which confirms that Geoffrey lacks the requisite mental capacity, is it necessary to determine what is in his best interests. There is a danger here that his parents, who have seen the dependent, disabled side of Geoffrey, have not taken on board the potential he has for developing his independence and for enjoying activities outside the home. Geoffrey may well find it difficult to represent himself against the wishes of his parents to whom he owes so much. He may need support from an advocate in such a situation (see Chapter 8).

Use of restraint

Additional factors have to be taken into account when the decisions and action taken on behalf of a person who lacks the required mental capacity involve restraint. The person must believe that restraint is necessary to prevent harm to P, and the restraint must be proportionate to the likelihood of P suffering harm and the seriousness of that harm.

Section 6(4) defines a person as using restraint if he:

(a)   uses, or threatens to use, force to secure the doing of an act which P resists, or
(b)   restricts P's liberty of movement, whether or not P resists.

The MCA originally provided that if D goes beyond this mere restraint and deprives P of his liberty, then this would be unlawful and contrary to Article 5(1) of the European Convention on Human Rights (S.6(5)). However this subsection was repealed by the Mental Health Act 2007 as a consequence of the amendments made to the MCA to make provisions to fill the Bournewood gap (see Chapter 3).
Scenario B11 illustrates the use of proportionate restraint.

Scenario B11: Restraint or loss of liberty?

Bob had received a serious head injury in a road traffic accident and had little thought for his own safety. He enjoyed shopping, but would dart across roads in front of traffic. His carers decided that they could only take him shopping safely if he were to wear a harness. He disliked this restraint, and fought to have it taken off, but the carers insisted he wore it when he went out. Could he argue that it was unlawful?

Taking Bob shopping is an act in connection with the care and treatment of Bob, and therefore comes within Section 5 provisions. If reasonable steps have been taken to assess Bob's mental capacity to go shopping and it is concluded that he lacks the ability to make a decision, but it would be in his best interests to go, then the use of the reins would come within the provisions of Section 6 and the use of restraint.
The carers must answer the questions:

1.   Does Bob lack the requisite mental capacity to make his own decisions?
2.   If the answer to Q. 1 is 'yes', do they reasonably believe that it is necessary to restrain Bob in order to prevent harm to him?
3.   Is the use of the reins a proportionate response to the likelihood of Bob suffering harm and the seriousness of that harm?

In addition they must ensure that the principles set out in Section 1 are followed, that it is in the best interests of P to go shopping, and that the least restrictive option is being taken.
On the assumption that Bob lacks the requisite mental capacity, the next two questions must be answered. Since the use of the reins is to prevent Bob running into the road and possibly being killed, it would seem that questions 2 and 3 could be answered in the affirmative. Other alternatives could be not going at all, and thus reducing the quality of life of Bob, or of taking more than one carer, with resource implications which may lead to no further or much fewer shopping trips.

Loss of liberty

The amendments made to the Mental Capacity Act to enable persons to be deprived of their liberty if certain specified conditions exist are considered in

Chapter 13. Where such authorisation exists for a deprivation of liberty the principles set down in Section 1 would still apply.

Expenditure

If the act of care and treatment involves the expenditure of money, then Section 8 permits P's credit to be used for such expenditure and any money spent by D in connection with P's care and treatment to be reimbursed. These sections apply even though D does not have a lasting power of attorney.

Scenario B12 illustrates the principle of reimbursement.

Scenario B12: Reimbursement.

Max was subject to extreme bouts of mood, from severe depression to hyper mania. In the latter mood he became very extravagant and spent wildly. Subsequently he regretted his generosity and wild spending and refused to pay the bills. His carer Sally bought, out of her own money, food and household goods for Max. He then refused to reimburse her.

Sally is entitled to have her expenditure reimbursed. She would have to produce receipts and also be able to show that the expenditure was on Max's behalf. It is hoped that local discussion, negotiation or mediation would resolve the dispute, but if not she could apply to the Court of Protection for a declaration that Max owed moneys to her, which she was entitled to receive.

Standard of compliance

If the decision maker has followed the requirements of the MCA in determining whether or not the requisite mental capacity existed, and if it did not, in determining the best interests of the person according to the criteria set out in Section 4(1)–(7), then the MCA says that there has been sufficient compliance with the Act. Clearly documentation would be necessary if a person's compliance with the Act was disputed. However there could be compliance with the MCA but still evidence of criminal behaviour or negligence, which could be followed by civil proceedings for compensation, as Scenario B13 illustrates.

Scenario B13: Consent but negligence.

Ruth had severe learning disabilities and was cared for in a community home. She was incapable of giving consent to even the basic forms of care. Every Thursday afternoon she was bathed by a care assistant. Unfortunately, at one bathing session, the care assistant failed to test the water before putting Ruth in the bath, and Ruth screamed out in pain and was scalded.

Under Section 5 the bathing of Ruth would be considered to be an act in connection with the care and treatment of P. The care assistant, manager or supervisor would have assessed Ruth's inability to give consent to having a bath and determined that it was in Ruth's best interests to have a bath. These activities would have been protected by Section 5. However the failure to ensure that the water was of the correct temperature and the harm that it caused to Ruth would be both an act of negligence in civil law (a breach of the duty of care which caused harm to the person – see Chapter 11 and Scenarios H3 and H4) and also a criminal offence. Were Ruth to die as a result of the scalding, the care assistant or her managers could be prosecuted for manslaughter.

Decision making and persons detained under the Mental Health Act

It is a principle of the Mental Capacity Act that where the provisions of the Mental Health Act apply in relation to a detained person's treatment, then the MCA does not authorise treatment (Section 28 of the MCA – see Chapter 13). However treatment under the Mental Health Act only covers treatment for mental disorder, and a case heard in 2006 and shown in Case B2 illustrates what happens when a detained patient who lacks capacity requires treatment for a physical disorder.

Case B2: Detained patient requiring treatment for a physical disorder.[6]

A Primary Care trust and NHS trust applied to court for a declaration that H, a detained patient under Section 3 of the Mental Health Act 1983, could be treated for her ovarian cyst (which appeared to be cancerous) with a hysterectomy. H refused the operation because she wished to have children. She also refused more limited surgery for the removal of the cyst. Medical experts were of the view that it was in her best interests to undergo the proposed surgery. Declarations were sought that she lacked the capacity to make decisions, that it was in her best interests to undergo a total hysterectomy and it was lawful to provide sedation and reasonable physical restraint in order to administer treatment.

The President of the Family Division of the High Court granted the application. He reiterated the principle that no medical treatment could be given without the consent of a mentally competent adult. A person lacked capacity if some impairment of mental function rendered that person unable to make a decision whether to consent to treatment. He decided that H had delusional beliefs about her circumstances. It was clear that she did not appreciate the seriousness of her condition and the sense of threat to life that it presented if unalleviated. She therefore lacked the capacity to decide. The court was not tied to the clinical assessment of what was in a patient's best interests. It was obliged to take into account a broad spectrum of medical, social, emotional and welfare issues before reaching its own conclusion. In balancing the benefits and disadvantages of the proposed treatment, the judge decided that the hysterectomy was in her best interests.

The judge made the declarations sought but also declared that forcible administration of post operative chemotherapy was not covered by these declarations.

Following the implementation of the MCA, if a similar situation to Case B2 were to arise after October 2007, the application would go to the new Court of Protection. The definition of mental capacity in Sections 2 and 3 of the Act (see Chapter 4) would be applied, and the criteria for best interests as set down in Sections 4 of the Act would also be applied (see Chapter 5).

Serious medical treatment

Where the decision relates to whether serious medical treatment should be undertaken, the possibility of appointing an independent mental capacity advocate should be considered (see Chapter 8). This only arises where there is no appropriate person who could be consulted on behalf of the patient/client to determine what was in his or her best interests. The question however arises as to whether other treatments, not normally seen as serious, could be carried out at the same time. Scenario B14 provides an example.

Scenario B14: What treatments?

Barbara had mild learning disabilities and lived in a community home. She was a very keen walker and on one trip stumbled and fractured her ankle badly. She needed to have surgery with a general anaesthetic. It was not clear that she understood what was required, and an expert was brought in to determine her ability to give a valid consent to the operation. The expert was of the view that whilst she wanted her ankle to heal, she did not understand the nature and effects of the anaesthetic and could not give a valid consent. It was therefore decided that she should be seen as a person lacking the specific capacity to give consent to the treatment, and the MCA would therefore apply. Her mother was consulted about Barbara's views, beliefs and values, and she said that she considered that it was in Barbara's best interests to have the surgery. An independent mental capacity advocate was not required, since the mother could be consulted. The mother also asked if Barbara could have a cervical smear at the same time, as she had been unable to get her to agree to a smear in the clinic and the doctor was not prepared to use force.

There would appear to be no problem in ensuring that the operation to repair the ankle took place in the best interests of Barbara. What however of the cervical smear? Could it be done whilst Barbara was under the anaesthetic? The first question to be asked is: did Barbara have the requisite mental capacity to give or refuse consent to the cervical smear? If the answer to that question is 'yes', then it could not be done without her consent. If on the other hand the answer was 'no', she did not have the requisite capacity to make a decision about a cervical smear, then taking the smear whilst she was under the anaesthetic would appear to be in her best interests. The alternative would be to carry it out whilst she was conscious and therefore possibly resisting, which would be more traumatic for her. Unfortunately the easy way out is to fail to take the cervical smear, which probably accounts in part for the low health screening undertaken on those with learning disabilities (see Chapter 5).

Decisions about sexual activity

Scenario B15: Sexual activity.

Ken had been in a care home for over ten years. He had mild learning disabilities. Staff discussed with him a care plan following the principles of *Valuing People*.[7] Ken made it clear that he wanted to experience a sexual relationship. Brenda his key worker stated that she was not prepared to assist him in this. In particular, she believed such an intimate relationship should not be encouraged with any of the women who lived in the care home. John, a care assistant, suggested that they should arrange to take Ken to Amsterdam to visit a prostitute. It was agreed by the care team that Ken would be able to give consent to having sex, but would be incapable of organising the trip. By a majority decision, with Brenda dissenting, it was agreed that Ken would be taken to Holland by a single care worker, and the costs would come out of Ken's personal moneys.

The circumstances in Scenario B15 are perhaps a little extreme, but it is a well recognised fact that a care plan for a person with learning disabilities should include sexual health and activity where that is appropriate. Whilst Ken may have had the capacity to consent to having sex with a prostitute, he may not have been able to appreciate some of the risks which went with that such as venereal disease, and the care workers would have a duty to ensure that all reasonable care was taken to prevent that. Brenda's personal beliefs and values are irrelevant in determining what is in Ken's best interests. Only if what is proposed is contrary to the law or an affront to public decency would she be justified in protesting against the planned trip. Following the implementation of the MCA she could of course seek a declaration from the Court of Protection that what is being proposed for Ken was contrary to his best interests. The chances of her succeeding are by no means certain.

Intimate care

Scenario B16: A necessary protocol.

Karl had Down's syndrome and was cared for by his elderly parents. When they were in their 70s they agreed that Karl should move to a care home, where he could get to know people of his own age. He visited the care home several times for short stays for respite and then moved in. The care staff were concerned that he resisted any attempt to have intimate areas washed, and he was not prepared to wash himself. They were particularly concerned at the possibility of infections developing under his foreskin. His key worker Fred discussed the problems with his mother, who said that she alone bathed him and made sure that all areas were properly cleaned, but she could understand that Karl would not want any one else to interfere with him. The care team discussed the problem with Karl's GP, who said that it was not his concern and he could not help. The care team considered the possibility of inviting his mother to come once a month to wash Karl, but this was considered inappropriate and a lapse of their own professional duties. They then devised a protocol which stated that once a month, Karl should have a full cleaning session: two members of staff were required to be present and all efforts would be made to persuade Karl to wash himself and to assist him. If necessary minimal restraint would be used. The care would be documented and reviewed as appropriate.

Scenario B16 presents an example of the everyday activities necessary for the care and treatment of those incapable of giving consent to what could be seen (in the absence of the statutory provisions) as a trespass to their person. Nail cutting, hair washing and such hygienic procedures can all present difficulties, especially when the client resists any such care. Individually their lack is not a life and death question, but over time a lack of hygiene or nail cutting can become a life saving necessity. Where the client is incapable of giving consent and physically resisting any intervention, the restraint provisions of the MCA must be complied with and all reasonable care taken. Documentation is essential to show the circumstances and the fact that what was done was in the best interests of the client.

Check list for determining best interests on behalf of P

- Is there a reasonable belief that P lacks the requisite mental capacity for the decision in question?
- If the answer is 'yes', have superficial factors – such as age, appearance, condition or aspects of behaviour – been discounted as the sole basis for making the decision?
- Is the mental incapacity temporary or permanent, and if temporary, how long before capacity is likely to be recovered and if so, could the decision making

await, without harmful effects for P, that recovery, so that P could make his or her own decisions?

- Have all relevant circumstances, of which the decision maker is aware and which it would be reasonable to regard as relevant, been taken into account?
- What reasonably practicable steps to encourage P to take part in the decision making exist?
- Have these reasonably practicable steps been taken?
- Is life-saving treatment under consideration?
- If so, is it clearly understood that the decision maker must not be motivated by the desire of bringing about P's death?
- Have the following been taken into account:
  a. P's past and present wishes and feelings and any written statements of P?
  b. P's beliefs and values that would have influenced his decision had he had the capacity?
  c. Other factors that P would have taken into account had P been able to do so?
- Have the following (if relevant) been consulted:
  a. Anyone named by P as someone to be consulted on the matter in question or matters of this kind?
  b. Anyone engaged in caring for P or interested in his welfare?
  c. Any donee of a lasting power of attorney granted by P?
  d. Any deputy appointed for P by the court?
- Have records been kept of the answers to the above questions and the action and discussions which have taken place?
- What is the balance of the risks and benefits of the proposed action?

In addition to the above, if restraint has been used, the following questions should also be asked:

- Does D reasonably believe that it is necessary to do the act in order to prevent harm to P?
- Is the proposed act a proportionate response to the likelihood of P's suffering harm and the seriousness of that harm?

References

1   *An Hospital NHS Trust and S (by his litigation friend the Official Solicitor) and DG (S's father) and SG (S's mother)* [2003] EWHC Fam 365.
2   *Re A (Male Sterilisation)* [2000] 1 FLR 549 at 555.
3   *Re A (Male Sterilisation)* [2000] 1 FLR 549 at 560.
4   *An Hospital NHS Trust and S (by his litigation friend the Official Solicitor) and DG (S's father) and SG (S's mother)* [2003] EWHC Fam 365.
5   Code of Practice for the Mental Capacity Act 2005. Department of Constitutional Affairs February 2007 para 5.46. TSO, London.
6   *Trust A & Trust B v. H (An adult patient)* [2006] EWHC 1230.
7   Department of Health (2001) *Valuing People: A New Strategy for Learning Disability for the 21st Century.* White Paper CM 5086. DH, London.

6 Lasting Powers of Attorney

Introduction

The original power of attorney, whereby a person appointed an attorney or donee to act on his behalf in a matter of property or finance, was of limited value since it ended whenever the person appointing the attorney became mentally incapable of handling his or her affairs. For many this would be the very point at which an attorney would be required. The Enduring Power of Attorney Act 1985 was therefore enacted to cover this gap. The person had to have the requisite mental capacity to draw up the enduring power, which would continue in spite of the fact that the donor had lost his or her mental capacity, at which point the attorney could exercise the powers granted on behalf of the donor. There was one major limitation however about the Enduring Power of Attorney (EPA) as provided for under the 1985 Act: it only covered property and financial decisions. It did not cover matters of personal welfare. As a consequence one of the significant creations of the Mental Capacity Act 2005 was provision for a lasting power of attorney, under which the donor, when mentally capable, could grant powers of attorney covering care and treatment decisions, as well as, or instead of, property and finance decisions.

What about existing EPAs?

The Enduring Power of Attorney Act 1985 is repealed by Section 66(1)(b) of the Mental Capacity Act (MCA) and no enduring power of attorney within the meaning of the 1985 Act is to be created after the commencement of the MCA on 1 October 2007 (S.66(1)(b) and S.66(2)). However Schedules 4 and 5 to the Act apply to any enduring power of attorney that was created before then. In addition Regulation 23 and Schedule 7 to the Regulations[1] set out the form of notice to be given to the donor and to his relatives, when an attorney under an enduring power intends to apply for registration. Regulations 24–28 and Schedule 8 to the Regulations specify other requirements applying to the registration process for EPAs.

Thus existing enduring powers of attorney created before the repeal of the 1985 Act are still valid and integrated into the new scheme as a result of Section 66(3) and Schedule 4. Schedule 4 applies to any enduring power of attorney created under the 1985 Act and before the commencement of the Mental Capacity Act 2005 (S.66(3)).

Schedule 5 also contains transitional provisions in relation to the 1985 Act (see Chapter 17 on implementation of the MCA).

It would always be open to a person who has set up an enduring power of attorney to end it and create instead a lasting power of attorney, provided he still has the requisite mental capacity. However this is not necessary if he only wishes to delegate property and financial matters and, under the transitional provisions, the EPA will continue to be effective. Of course if the donor of the EPA no longer has the requisite mental capacity, it is not possible for him to replace it with a lasting power of attorney (LPA).

Section 44 creates a criminal offence if a donee of an enduring power of attorney (and also a donee of a lasting power of attorney) ill-treats or wilfully neglects P (see Chapter 11).

The Office of the Public Guardian (OPG) (see Chapter 7) has provided guidance on the transitional provisions relating to enduring powers of attorney.[2] A leaflet on the differences between an EPA and an LPA is available from the Public Guardianship web site. It emphasises that an EPA must be made before 1 October 2007, and notes: the differences in the decisions which can be made by an attorney under an EPA in contrast to an LPA; the duties of the attorney under an EPA compared with an LPA, and registering the powers and revoking the powers of each.

What is a lasting power of attorney?

An LPA is a new statutory form of power of attorney recognised in Section 9 of the MCA. By means of this power of attorney the donor (P) confers on the donee (or donees) or the attorney(s) authority to make decisions about all or any of the following:

a.   P's personal welfare or specified matters concerning P's personal welfare, and
b.   P's property and affairs or specified matters concerning P's property and affairs.

This includes authority to make such decisions in circumstances where P no longer has capacity.

Different forms are available for the two kinds of LPA, i.e.:

a.   a property and affairs LPA and
b.   a personal welfare LPA

The 'donor' is the person granting the power, (known in the legislation as 'P'); and the 'donee' or the 'attorney' is the person who is given the power. The 'instrument' is the document granting the power and the conditions on which it is given.

The power only comes into force, for care and welfare decisions, when the donor no longer has the mental capacity to make his or her own decisions. This contrasts with the donation of powers in relation to finance and property, where the actual delegation can take place when the donor still has the requisite mental capacity.

To create a valid LPA, the conditions laid down in Section 10 must be complied with.

Firstly, it must be registered in accordance with the provisions of Schedule 1.

Secondly, it must be registered at the time when P:

- executes the instrument
- has reached 18, and
- has capacity to execute it.

These conditions are considered in more detail below.

Any instrument which purports to convey authority but does not comply with Section 9 or 10 or Schedule 1 confers no authority. The authority conferred by the LPA is subject to the provisions of the MCA and in particular the principles laid down in Section 1 (see Chapter 3), Section 4 and the definition of best interests (see Chapter 5). In addition any conditions or restrictions specified in the instrument must be complied with.

Consultation on LPAs

In January 2006 a consultation paper was published which invited views and comments on:

- the draft LPA forms for property and affairs and for personal welfare and the prescribed information
- the draft guidance to accompany the forms
- the certificate process and who should be able to provide certificates, and
- the registration process.

The consultation ended on 14 April 2006, and a response to the consultation on the forms and guidance for making a Lasting Power of Attorney was issued on 17 July 2006.

The January 2006 consultation paper did not cover the fees payable when registering an LPA. The Department of Health (DH) noted that work was under-way to cost the new processes and procedures fully that would govern LPAs, and it was its intention to consult formally on the fees and fees policy later in 2006. It would also have the LPA forms fully designed at a later stage, to include the prescribed information in the body of the form, and would discuss the design of the forms with user groups in due course.

Forms to be used

The consultation proposed the creation of two prescribed forms – one for making an LPA in relation to property and affairs and one for making an LPA in relation to personal welfare. It accepted that there would be people who wished the same person to act in relation to both their personal welfare and their property and affairs. Under these proposals two separate forms (and two separate certificates) would be required, one for each area of delegation. The consultation considered that a single form would be too cumbersome in practice, and confusing for those simply wishing to make an LPA in relation to one area or the other. In addition a single form for both types of LPA could be misleading, as an LPA for property and affairs can be used both when the donor has capacity and also when the donor lacks capacity, whereas an LPA for personal welfare can only be used when the donor lacks capacity.

The consultation stated that creating a third form had been considered for use when someone wished to appoint the same person as an LPA with powers in respect of their personal welfare and property and affairs. However it did not think that this was desirable. For example, a donor may want to include particular instructions about his or her healthcare on their personal welfare LPA form, but they would not wish this information to be seen by financial institutions which are following the property and affairs LPA. Following the consultation, regulations relating to lasting powers of attorney, enduring powers of attorney and the Public Guardian were placed before Parliament on 17 April 2007 and came into force on 1 October 2007.[3] They can be accessed through the Department for Constitutional Affairs (DCA) website.[4]

Who can make LPAs?

A person over 18 years can grant an LPA, but must have the requisite mental capacity at the time of its signature or execution.

How would capacity be defined?

The definition of mental capacity set out in Sections 2 and 3 of the MCA would be used to determine whether P had the necessary mental capacity to set up and execute a lasting power of attorney. Earlier case law on defining the requisite capacity, such as the case of Re K; Re F[5] where it was held that a person could have the necessary mental capacity to execute an enduring power of attorney even though he did not have the mental capacity to manage his own property and affairs, will probably be reconsidered in the light of the new statutory definition.

How are they drawn up?

Usually a person would seek legal advice in drawing up an LPA, to ensure that all the required formalities are complied with and that it is sufficiently clear what the donor intended. The statutory forms, which can only be completed from 1 October 2007, are in Schedules to the Regulations.

Scenario C2 considers the setting up of an LPA.

What could it cover?

General

An LPA could be general in the sense that it grants a power to the donee to make all welfare, property and affairs decisions on behalf of the donor, at the point at which the donor lacks mental capacity. The donee would be bound to act according to the principles of the MCA and in particular Section 1 (see Chapter 3) and Section 4 (see Chapter 5).

Specific

Alternatively the LPA could grant a specific power in relation to property or affairs or treatment and welfare. The donee would only have the powers granted in the instrument, and if the donee were to make decisions or take action on matters not included in the LPA, the donee would be acting *ultra vires*, i.e. outside the powers granted.

Who could the donee be?

The donor has the complete choice over whom he or she wishes to be appointed as a donee. The only legal requirements are that the donee should be over 18 years and have the requisite mental capacity. Alternatively for property and affairs decisions, the donee could be a trust corporation. There are special rules about bankrupts (see **Bankruptcy** on page 99).

Trust corporation

A trust corporation can be appointed as donee to make decisions on property and affairs. Section 64 of the MCA uses the definition given in Section 68(1) of the Trustee Act 1925 as the Public Trustee or a corporation appointed by the court in any particular case to be a trustee, or entitled by rules made under Section 4(3) of the Public Trustee Act 1906, to act as custodian trustee.

What if the donee did not know of the appointment?

It would not be possible for an LPA to be created with a specified person identified as a donee, but without the knowledge and consent of that person. Schedule 1 states that the instrument must include a statement by the donee (or if more than one, each one of them) that he or she has read the prescribed information and understands the duty imposed on a donee of a lasting power of attorney under Section 1 and Section 4 on the best interests.

What if the donee changes his or her mind?

The donee is entitled to disclaim the power of attorney and, if that person is the only nominated donee, the LPA will come to an end, unless there is a power in the LPA for another donee to be appointed. If the donee decides to change his or her mind, before the LPA comes into effect, the donor, if he or she still retains the necessary mental capacity, would have the opportunity of replacing the donee within the instrument. Para 20 and Schedule 6 of the Regulations[6] cover the disclaimer of appointment by a donee of a lasting power of attorney (drawn up by the Lord Chancellor under his powers given by Section 13(6)(a) of the MCA.)

The Regulations require the donee to complete the form (LPA 005) contained in Schedule 6 and send it to the donor, with a copy to the Public Guardian and to any other donee who, for the time being, is appointed under the power.

What conditions are required for a valid LPA?

The conditions for a valid LPA are set out in Section 10.

Firstly the donee must be **an individual who has reached 18 years**. This is the age of majority, and whilst for some purposes (such as the giving of consent under the Family Law Reform Act 1969) a young person of 16 and 17 years is recognised as having specific powers, for most legal situations a person is an adult at 18 years. Where the individual is over 18 years, then the powers under the LPA can cover both welfare decisions and property and affairs (see Chapter 12 on children). Scenario C1 considers the implications of this.

The donor must have the requisite mental capacity to sign the LPA

Mental capacity would be defined according to Sections 2 and 3 of the MCA.

If the LPA relates to P's property and affairs, **the donee must not be bankrupt**. This does not apply where the LPA relates to personal welfare.

Can more than one donee be appointed?

Section 10(4)–(7) covers the situation of two or more donees acting together.

The donees can act jointly or jointly and severally, or the instrument may appoint them to act jointly in respect of some matters and severally in respect of others.

'Jointly' means that the donees always act together in any decision and if one fails to meet the criteria in the Act, then a valid LPA will not be created.

'Severally' means that each donee can act independently.

'Jointly and severally' means that the donees can act together or independently.

If the LPA does not itself specify whether they are to act jointly or jointly and severally, the instrument is to be assumed to appoint them to act jointly.

It is possible for the instrument to grant certain powers to be exercised jointly and other powers to be exercised jointly and severally.

If donees are to act jointly, a failure as respects one of them to comply with the requirements of Section 10(1) or (2) or Part 1 or 2 of Schedule 1 prevents a lasting power of attorney from being created.

If they are to act jointly and severally, a failure as respects one of them to comply with the requirements of Section 10(1) or (2) or Part 1 or 2 of Schedule 1 prevents the appointment taking effect in his case, but does not prevent a lasting power of attorney from being created in the case of the other or others.

What happens if there are several donees who disagree?

In such a situation, it is likely that there would be an application to the Public Guardian or the Court of Protection to determine the dispute. Scenario C3 considers a dispute between donees.

What formalities must be followed?

The donor must make a statement to the effect that he has read the prescribed information, and intends the authority conferred by the instrument to include authority to make decisions on his behalf in circumstances where he no longer has capacity. The donor must also name a person(s) whom he wishes to be notified of any application for the registration of the instrument or state there are no such persons (Schedule 1 of the MCA).

Limitations on an LPA

The appointing of a replacement donee

An instrument used to create a lasting power of attorney cannot give the donee (or if more than one, any of them) power to appoint a substitute or successor.

However it may itself appoint a person to replace the donee (or, if more than one, any of them) on the occurrence of specified events.

These events are:

a.   the donee disclaiming his appointment in accordance with regulations[7] drawn up by the Lord Chancellor (S.13(6)(a));
b.   the death or bankruptcy of the donee (where the LPA relates to property or affairs an interim bankruptcy order merely suspends the LPA power as long as it lasts), or if the donee is a trust corporation, its being wound up (S.13(6)(b));
c.   the dissolution or annulment of marriage where donor and donee are married, unless the LPA made specific provisions that in such circumstances the donee's power would not cease (S.13(6)(c));
d.   the lack of capacity of the donee (S.13(6)(d)).

Where the donor is detained under the Mental Health Act 2007

The MCA expressly excludes the donee under an LPA having power to consent or refuse treatment for a mental disorder where the donor is detained under the Mental Health Act 2007 (Section 28 MCA and see Chapter 13). However if decisions relating to physical disorders are required (and therefore do not come within the aegis of the Mental Health Act 2007), then the donee under an LPA with powers relating to welfare decision would be able to make them on behalf of the mentally incapacitated donor.

Restraint of P

Qualifications on lasting powers of attorney

A donee is only authorised to restrain P if the three conditions laid down under Section 11 are satisfied.

The three conditions under Section 11 required to ensure that the restraint is limited are:

1. P lacks, or the donee reasonably believes that P lacks, capacity in relation to the matter in question.
2. The donee reasonably believes that it is necessary to do the act to prevent harm to P.
3. The act is a proportionate response to the likelihood of P's suffering harm and the seriousness of that harm.

These conditions are similar to those discussed in Chapter 5 on the principle of acting in the best interests of P. The donee of the LPA can only exercise the powers under the LPA in relation to care and treatment if P lacks the requisite mental capacity.

The definition of restraint by a donee is if he uses, or threatens to use, force to secure the doing of an act which P resists, or restricts P's liberty of movement, whether or not P resists.

The original provision in Section 11(6) that the donee does more than merely restrain P if he deprives P of his liberty within the meaning of Article 5(1) of the Human Rights Convention, is repealed by the Mental Health Act 2007, which amends the MCA to fill the Bournewood gap (see Chapters 3 and 13). Case law of the European Court of Human Rights (ECHR) distinguishes between a restriction of liberty and a deprivation of liberty. (This is further discussed in Chapter 3 and Box 3.1, page 23.)

An example of restriction of liberty would be a seat belt or restraining belt in a chair. A deprivation of liberty would be putting P in a locked room for which he did not have the key. A situation where a hoist is used which could be seen as a form of restraint is considered in Scenario C8. As a consequence of the amendments to the MCA made by the Mental Health Act 2007 to remedy the Bournewood gap, it would now be possible for a donee to restrict the liberty of P, but only if the conditions set down in the new proposed Sections 4A and 4B and Schedule A1 are met (see pages 24 and 25).

Decisions on personal welfare

In an LPA covering personal welfare decisions, the authority:

a. does not extend to making such decisions in circumstances other than those where P lacks, or the donee reasonably believes that P lacks, capacity;
b. is subject to Sections 24–26 (advance decisions to refuse treatment); and
c. extends to giving or refusing consent to the carrying out or continuation of a treatment by providing health care for P. (This does not authorise the giving or refusing of consent to the carrying out or continuation of life-sustaining treatment, unless the instrument contains express provision to that effect and is subject to any conditions or restrictions in the instrument – S.11(8).)

The Code of Practice gives the following as examples of the types of decisions which the donee of an LPA granting general powers in relation to personal welfare could make:[8]

- where the donor should live and who they should live with
- the donor's day-to-day care, including diet and dress
- who the donor may have contact with
- consenting to or refusing medical examination and treatment on the donor's behalf
- arrangements needed for the donor to be given medical, dental or optical treatment
- assessments for and provision of community care services
- whether the donor should take part in social activities, leisure activities, education or training
- the donor's personal correspondence and papers
- rights of access to personal information about the donor, or
- complaints about the donor's care or treatment.

What is the role of the LPA in advance decisions which relate to life and death issues?

There are strict provisions relating to the powers of a donee under an LPA where life and death decisions are involved. There was considerable concern in Parliament that a donee could be deciding in favour of a person being allowed to die, when there was no clear authorisation to that effect. Section 4(5) on the definition of the best interests of the donor states that:

> Where the determination relates to life-sustaining treatment he must not, in considering whether the treatment is in the best interests of the person concerned, be motivated by a desire to bring about his death.

Thus unless the donee of the LPA has explicit instructions from the donor about letting die or refusal of life saving treatment, the donee must act in the best interests of the donor and this cannot be motivated by a desire to bring about his death. This is further strengthened by Section 11, which states that the LPA authority does not authorise the giving or refusing of consent to the carrying out or continuation of life-sustaining treatment, unless the instrument contains express provision to that effect, and is subject to any conditions or restrictions in the instrument. The authority is also subject to the provisions relating to advance decisions set out in Sections 24–26 (see Chapter 9).

LPA and advance decision

If P sets up an advance decision, and then creates an LPA with instructions in the LPA which give powers to consent to or withhold consent to treatments specified in the advance decision, then the advance decision will cease to be effective. In other words, where there is a contradiction between the two instruments, i.e. the LPA and the advance decision, then the later instrument will be the effective one. To ensure that the advance decision remains effective, the LPA should explicitly refer to it and not be incompatible with its provisions. This is discussed in Scenario C5.

What is the significance if a patient in hospital has drawn up an LPA?

If the health professionals ascertain that a patient has drawn up an LPA in relation to personal welfare, it will not come into effect until and unless the patient lacks mental capacity. If mental incapacity is established, then the attorney or donee of the power, on being satisfied that the patient lacks capacity, can act according to the directions in the LPA. This may include giving consent or withholding consent to treatment (but if this is a life saving issue, the provisions discussed above apply). Health professionals should be entitled to have access to the LPA to ensure that the donee is acting within the powers granted by the donor. There could be a possible dispute between the donee of the LPA and the health or social services professionals. Such a situation is discussed in Scenario C8 in a dispute over manual handling. Scenario C6 considers a situation where a donee is considering whether the LPA enables her to refuse pain relief on the donor's behalf.

What is the significance for care homes if a resident has drawn up an LPA?

Similarly if a resident in a care home has drawn up an LPA which relates to his or her personal welfare, it will not come into effect until and unless the donor no longer has the requisite mental capacity, and the donee must be personally satisfied of that fact. Once the lack of mental capacity is established, then the donee can give consent to any care plans, or transfer of the resident to other accommodation, or take similar decisions, whilst being bound by the principles set out in Section 1 and whilst acting in the best interests of the donee according to the definition in Section 4. However, where there are specific instructions in the instrument of the LPA which are seen as not being in the best interests of the donor, these must be followed by the donee (see above provisions relating to life-sustaining treatment, page 92). In the event of a dispute over decisions by a donee under an LPA, an application could be made in the first instance to the Office of the Public Guardian, which has the responsibility of overseeing the proper execution of LPAs. It may subsequently be necessary to refer the matter to the Court of Protection.

LPA and the best interests of the patient

There is a statutory duty for the holder of an LPA covering personal welfare to act in the best interests of the donor. However this would be subject to the actual instructions within the instrument, as we have seen above in relation to the instruction to refuse life saving treatment. The holder of the power could not however insist that specific treatment was given (as opposed to a refusal) contrary to the best interests of the patient. This issue was considered in the case of *Burke* v. *GMC*,[9] which is considered in Chapter 9. In other words the holder of the LPA could refuse to give consent to treatment if that power was given in the LPA, even though health professionals considered that the treatment was necessary in the best interests of the patient. However, the holder of the LPA could not insist that health professionals provide treatment and care when such treatment was considered by the health professionals to be contrary to the best interests of the patient and against their professional discretion, even when the donor had stated in the LPA that he or she wished such treatment to be provided.

Gifts

When a lasting power of attorney exists in relation to property and affairs, the donee is not authorised to dispose of the donor's property by making a gift unless the following conditions are satisfied:

- gifts can be made on customary occasions to persons (including himself) who are related to or connected with the donor, or
- to any charity to whom the donor made or might have been expected to make gifts (S.12(2)).

These conditions only apply if the value of each such gift is not unreasonable having regard to all the circumstances and, in particular, the size of the donor's estate. Any conditions or restrictions in the instrument of the power of attorney would also have to be followed (S.12(4)).

'Customary occasion' is defined as:

- the occasion or anniversary of a birth, marriage or the formation of a civil partnership, or
- any other occasion on which presents are customarily given within families or among friends or associates.

The court may also authorise the making of gifts, which do not come within Section 12(2), under the powers granted by Section 23(4).

Scenarios C9 and C10 consider situations where gifts are made under the powers of an LPA.

How does the donee know when the LPA comes into effect?

LPA covering property and finance

This will come into effect at the time specified in the LPA. It can be whilst the donor still has the requisite mental capacity. It may be that it only comes into effect when the donor loses his mental capacity. The Office of the Public Guardian is laying down rules as to the bringing into effect of an LPA.

LPA covering personal welfare

This LPA will only come into effect when the donor loses mental capacity. Clearly the donee must maintain contact with the donor or his or her family to be sure at what point the LPA is now effective. The donee is advised to refer to guidance issued by the Office of the Public Guardian.

Scenario C4 is concerned with the execution of the two different forms of LPA.

What principles must be followed by the donee in making decisions?

The donee is obliged to follow any requirements drawn up in the LPA. However if the instructions in the LPA are of a very general nature e.g. 'to make all decisions in relation to my care and treatment', then the donee must follow the principles set out in Section 1 and act in the best interests of the donor as defined in Section 4.

In what circumstances can a donee act contrary to the best interests of the donor?

There may be situations where a specific requirement in the LPA is not seen by some to be in the donor's best interests, however the donee is obliged to follow the requirements laid down in the LPA.

How would action to control a donee commence and be followed through?

If there were a dispute over the interpretation of an LPA this could be referred to the Office of the Public Guardian (see Chapter 7).

Similarly, if there were fears that a donee was failing to act according to the LPA or was acting contrary to the statutory duties or duties at common law (see list of duties under the common law on page 97), any concerned person could apply to the Office of the Public Guardian.

The Code of Practice has suggested certain warning signs that a donee might be abusing his or her position. The list is clearly not intended to be exhaustive.[10] It is as follows:

- stopping relatives or friends contacting the donor – for example, the attorney may prevent contact or the donor may suddenly refuse visits or telephone calls from family and friends for no reason
- sudden unexplained changes in living arrangements (for example, someone moves in to care for a donor they've had little contact with)
- not allowing healthcare or social care staff to see the donor
- taking the donor out of hospital against medical advice, while the donor is having necessary medical treatment
- unpaid bills (for example, residential care or nursing home fees)
- an attorney opening a credit card account for the donor
- spending money on things that are not obviously related to the donor's needs
- the attorney spending money in an unusual or extravagant way
- transferring financial assets to another country.

Under Regulation 46 power is given to the Public Guardian to require information from donees of lasting powers of attorney in specified circumstances. These circumstances include where the donee may:

a. have behaved, or may be behaving, in a way that contravenes his authority or is not in the best interests of the donor of the power
b. be proposing to behave in a way that would contravene that authority or would not be in the donor's best interests, or
c. have failed to comply with the requirements of an order made, or directions given, by the court.

In such circumstances the Public Guardian may require the donee to provide specified information, or information of a specified description, or to produce specified documents or documents of a specified description. The Public Guardian can specify a reasonable time within which they must be produced and specify the place. The Public Guardian may require any information provided to be verified or any document to be authenticated.

Following a report to the Office of the Public Guardian (OPG), a Court of Protection visitor could be appointed to investigate any allegations against the donee of a lasting power of attorney. In serious situations, the OPG could refer the matter to the Court of Protection and also notify the police (see Chapters 7 and 11).

Who would represent P in checking up on the actions of the donee?

Where an LPA for personal welfare has come into effect, this would be at a time when P had lost, or was alleged to have lost, the requisite mental capacity. Any person concerned that the donee was not acting in P's best interests or according to the terms of the LPA, or the statutory duties of a donee, could contact the Office of the Public Guardian, which has the overall supervisory responsibility for donees (see Chapter 7). Scenario C.07 considers a situation where the exercise of the LPA is challenged.

Duties of donee or attorney

Some duties are specified under the Act:

- to act in accordance with the Act's principles
- to act or make decisions in the donor's best interests
- to have regard to the guidance in the Code of Practice
- to act within the scope of their authority.

Other duties would be specified under the common law:

- duty of care
- to carry out instructions
- not to delegate unless authorised to do so
- not to benefit themselves but to benefit the donor
- to act in good faith
- duty of confidentiality
- to comply with the directions of the Court of Protection
- not to disclaim without complying with the relevant Regulations
- (in relation to LPA for property and finance) to keep the donor's money and property separate from their own.

What happens if the donor changes his mind about setting up an LPA?

As long as the donor has the requisite mental capacity he or she can change his or her mind about the details in the LPA, or even as to whether there should be an LPA. Thus the name of the donee(s) could be changed as well as the details in the LPA by revoking the original LPA and setting up a new one (if required). Regulation 21[11] provides for the revocation by the donor of an LPA. It requires the donor to notify the Public Guardian that he has revoked the LPA and notify the donee(s) of the revocation. Where the Public Guardian receives a revocation notice from the donor, he must cancel the registration of the instrument creating the power, if he is satisfied that the donor has taken such steps as are necessary in law to revoke it. The Public Guardian may require the donor to provide such further information or produce such documents as the Public Guardian reasonably considers necessary to enable him to determine whether the steps necessary for revocation have been taken. Where the Public Guardian cancels the registration of the instrument he must notify the donor and the donee(s).

However once the donor loses capacity, the donor no longer has any power to revoke the LPA. The Court of Protection does however have the powers specified in Section 23, which include determining the meaning of the LPA and giving directions to the donee (see **Powers of the Court of Protection in relation to the validity of lasting powers of attorney** on page 100).

How long does an LPA last?

Once the LPA has come into effect it will last until the donor dies, or, if there are specific instructions, until these instructions have been carried out.

Regulation 22 provides for the revocation of a LPA on the death of the donor. It requires the Public Guardian to cancel the registration of an instrument as an LPA if he is satisfied that the power has been revoked as a result of the donor's death. Where the Public Guardian cancels the registration he must notify the donee(s).

How can an LPA be changed?

As long as the donor retains his or her mental capacity, then he or she can revoke a LPA. After it has been registered the donor would have to follow the rules relating to the revocation of a LPA and guidance issued by the Office of Public Guardian (see Regulation 21 above).

Once however the donor has lost capacity, it is not possible for the donor to change its provisions. The Court of Protection does however have the power under Section 23 to determine any question as to the meaning or effect of a lasting power of attorney or an instrument purporting to create one (see **Powers of the Court of Protection in relation to the validity of lasting powers of attorney** on page 100).

Revocation of lasting powers of attorney

The LPA can be revoked at any time when P has the capacity to do so (S.13(2) and Regulation 21). For the provisions relating to bankruptcy see below.

The following events terminate the donee's appointment and revokes the power:

- The death of the donor (Regulation 22).
- The disclaimer of the appointment by the donee in accordance with such requirements as may be prescribed for the purposes of this section in regulations made by the Lord Chancellor.
- The death or bankruptcy of the donee, or the winding-up or dissolution where the donee is a trust corporation (in a bankruptcy situation, only the power in relation to property and affairs is ended or, in an interim bankruptcy situation, suspended – S.13(6)(b) and (8) and (9)).
- The dissolution or annulment of a marriage or civil partnership between the donor and the donee ((S.13(6)(c) unless the instrument provided to the contrary – S.13(11)).
- The lack of capacity of the donee.

The following events terminate the donee's appointment but do not revoke the power:

- The donee is replaced under the terms of the instrument.
- The donee is one of two or more persons appointed to act as donees jointly and severally in respect of any matter and, after the event, there is at least one remaining donee.

Bankruptcy

Any reference to the bankruptcy of an individual includes a case where there is a bankruptcy restrictions order under the Insolvency Act 1986 in respect of that individual (S.64(3)).

If P becomes bankrupt, the power of attorney is revoked so far as it relates to P's property and affairs (S.13(3)). However if there are only interim bankruptcy restrictions the power of attorney in relation to P's property and affairs is suspended so long as the order has effect (S.13(4)). Under Section 13(9), where the donee is bankrupt because of an interim bankruptcy restriction order, then his power and appointment are suspended, so far as they relate to P's property and affairs, for so long as the order has effect.

The bankruptcy of a donee does not terminate his appointment, or revoke the power, in so far as his authority relates to P's personal welfare.

Bankruptcy restrictions orders include an interim bankruptcy restrictions order (MCA S.64(4)).

What happens if the donee is fraudulent?

Where the court is satisfied that fraud or undue pressure was used to induce P to execute an instrument for the purpose of creating a lasting power of attorney, or to create a lasting power of attorney, then the Court of Protection can declare that the instrument of the LPA is not to be registered (S.22(3) and (4)).

Where the fraud occurs after the LPA is registered and comes into effect, then the Court of Protection can, if P lacks capacity to do so, revoke the instrument or the lasting power of attorney. Clearly if P still has the requisite capacity he can revoke the LPA himself (see below).

What happens if the donee does not carry out what the donor would have wished?

An application can be made to the Office of the Public Guardian if there are fears that the donee of the power is not acting in accordance with the instructions therein, or, if there are no specific powers, not acting in the best interests of the donor. If the Public Guardian is unable to resolve the situation, then application can be made to the Court of Protection.

Protection of donee and others if no power is created or power revoked

Section 14 makes provision for the situation where, although an instrument has been registered as an LPA, in fact a valid LPA was not created. In such a situation, if the donee acts in purported exercise of the power, he does not incur any liability to P or any other person, because of the non-existence of the power. However to take advantage of these provisions, the donee must be unaware that a LPA was not created, or he must be unaware of circumstances which would have terminated his authority to act as a donee. In the circumstances where an LPA has not in fact been created, any transaction between the donee and another person is valid as if the power had been in existence unless that other person has knowledge of the non-existence.

For a purchaser there is a presumption in favour of the purchaser of the validity of the transaction, if the transaction was completed within 12 months of the date on which the instrument was registered or the other person makes a statutory declaration, before or within three months after the completion of the purchase, that he had no reason at the time of the transaction to doubt that the donee had authority to dispose of the property which was the subject of the transaction (S.14(4)). See Scenario C7.

Where two or more donees are appointed under a lasting power of attorney, Section 14 applies as if references to the donee were to all or any of them (S.14(6)).

Powers of the Court of Protection in relation to the validity of lasting powers of attorney (Sections 22 and 23)

Where P has executed or purported to execute an instrument with a view to creating a LPA, or an instrument has been registered as an LPA, then the court may determine any question relating to whether the requirements for the creation of a lasting power of attorney have been met, and any question relating to whether the power has been revoked or has otherwise come to an end.

The court has power to direct that an instrument purporting to create the lasting power of attorney is not to be registered or, if P lacks the capacity to do so, revoke the instrument or the lasting power of attorney in the following situations where the court is satisfied that:

- fraud or undue pressure was used to induce P to execute an instrument for the purpose of creating a lasting power of attorney or to create a lasting power of attorney, or
- the donee (or if more than one, any of them) of a lasting power of attorney has behaved or is behaving in a way that contravenes his authority or is not in P's best interests or proposes to behave in a way that would contravene his authority or would not be in P's best interests.

If there is more than one donee, the court may under Section 22(4)(b) revoke the instrument or the lasting power of attorney so far as it relates to any of them (S.22(5)).

The term donee includes an intended donee (S.22(6)).

These powers given to the Court of Protection are similar to those set out in Section 8 of the Enduring Powers of Attorney Act 1985, except that the administrative functions connected with registration will from October 2007 be performed by the Office of the Public Guardian.

Powers of the Court of Protection in relation to the operation of lasting powers of attorney

Section 23 gives the court the power to determine any questions as to the meaning or effect of an LPA or an instrument purporting to create one.

The court has the power:

a. to give directions with respect to decisions which the donee of a lasting power of attorney has authority to make and which P lacks capacity to make;
b. to give any consent or authorisation to act which the donee would have to obtain from P if P had capacity to give it (S.23(2)).

If P lacks capacity to do so, the court may:

a. give directions to the donee with respect to the rendering by him of reports or accounts and the production of records kept by him for that purpose;
b. require the donee to supply information or produce documents or things in his possession as donee;
c. give directions with respect to remuneration or expenses of the donee;
d. relieve the donee wholly or partly from any liability which he has or may have incurred on account of a breach of his duties as donee (S.23(3)).

The court may also authorise the making of gifts, which are not within Section 12(2). (The Explanatory Memorandum on the MCA suggests that this authorisation of such gifts could be used for tax planning purposes.)

Where two or more donees are appointed under a lasting power of attorney Section 23 applies as if references to the donee were to all or any of them (S.23(5)).

Application to the Court of Protection

The donor or donee or other interested person could apply to the Court of Protection for the use of its powers under Section 22 and Section 23. The Rules require that the applicant must ensure that those involved have a copy of the application form, so the donor must serve a copy on the donee(s), the donee(s) on the donor and if the applicant is not a donor or donee, on those parties respectively. The persons served with a copy of the application form in this way are known as a respondent to the proceedings (Rule 30).

All parties to the proceedings would of course be bound by the pre-action protocol and the Rules of the Court of Protection, which require the court to encourage co-operation between the parties and the settlement of the dispute without the need for court proceedings (see Chapter 7 and Scenario D2 on an application to the Court of Protection).

Registration

There were considerable concerns in the discussions of the Joint Committee[12] about the abuse of existing enduring powers of attorney, with estimates that abuse was possibly as high as 20%. The draft Bill therefore required an LPA to be executed and registered before it could be used. The Joint Committee stated (at para 144):

> We recommend that the Bill should make clear whether it is intended that personal welfare decisions, excluding those relating to medical treatment, may be taken when a donor retains capacity. Further, clarification of the extent and limitation of the powers, as well as adequate guidance and training for donees, are also strongly recommended.

The draft Bill was strengthened accordingly.

Problems were also envisaged by the Joint Committee because whilst the LPA must be registered when the power is granted, it does not become operational until the donor is actually incapable (unless the donor has specifically given this power in relation to finance and property), so how do those dealing with the donees know when the donor has become incapable? The Joint Committee stated (at para 157):

> We have concluded that the proposed system requiring the registration of LPAs before use will assist in monitoring the use of LPAs and detecting possible abuse. However, we recommend that donees should be placed under an obligation to notify both the donor and the Public Guardian that the donor is, or is becoming incapacitated, thereby putting this information on public record and opening it up to challenge. We further recommend that guidance should be provided to assist financial institutions to deal with the operational realities of LPAs.

An LPA must be registered with the OPG before it can be used. An unregistered LPA will not give the attorney any legal powers to make a decision for the donor. The donors can register the LPA while they are still mentally capable, or the attorney can apply to register the LPA at any time.[13]

The donor can identify persons who are entitled to receive notification of the application to register the LPA. Relatives will not automatically be notified of the application to register the LPA unless the donor has named them as being persons who should be given notice.

Objections to registration

The donor, where he or she is not the applicant to register, the attorney and persons named as entitled to be notified of the application to register, are all entitled to object to the LPA being registered. This is covered by Regulation 14,[14] which sets out time limits for making an objection to registration. Regulation 15 covers an application to the court over an objection to registration.

What do the registration provisions mean?

When the LPA is first drawn up

Unless an LPA has been registered with the OPG a valid LPA instrument has not been created. As a consequence no powers are given to the attorney once the donor lacks capacity (Sections 9(2)–(3)).

If the donor has failed to register the LPA , the donee can still apply for registration and must ensure that it has been effectively registered before attempting to exercise any of the powers under the LPA. The Code of Practice advises that if the LPA has been registered but not used for some time, the attorney should tell the OPG when they begin to act under it, so that the attorney can be sent relevant, up-to-date information about the rules covering LPAs.[15]

Schedule 1 provisions

Schedule 1 lays down the detailed requirements as to the making of instruments establishing LPAs. Additional requirements have been enacted by regulations made by the Lord Chancellor.[16] These regulations include the forms which are to be completed for registration. They can be down loaded from the DCA website or the Office of Public Sector Information website.[17]

The donor must make a statement to the effect that he has read the prescribed information and intends the authority conferred by the instrument to include authority to make decisions on his behalf in circumstances where he no longer has capacity. The donor must also name a person(s) whom he wishes to be notified of any application for the registration of the instrument or state there are no such persons.

The maximum number of persons the donor can name is five.[18] Where the donor states that there are no persons whom he wishes to be notified of any application for the registration of the instrument, then the instrument must include two LPA certificates (see below) and each certificate must be signed by a different person.[19]

The donee(s) must make a statement that he has read the prescribed information and understands the duties imposed upon a donee of an LPA under Section 1 (the principles) and Section 4 (best interests).

A prescribed person must provide a **lasting power of attorney certificate** that in his opinion at the time when the donor executes the instrument:

- the donor understands the purpose of the instrument and the scope of the authority conferred under it
- that no fraud or undue pressure is being used to induce the donor to create a LPA, and

- there is nothing else which would prevent a LPA from being created by the instrument.

Schedule 1 paragraph 3 sets out the effects of failure to comply with the prescribed form.

Under Regulation 8 the persons who are able to provide an LPA certificate are:

a. a person who has known the donor personally for at least two years, which ends immediately before the date on which the LPA certificate is signed, and
b. a person chosen by the donor who on account of his professional skills and expertise, reasonably considers that the donor is competent to make the judgments necessary to certify the matters set out in para 2(1)(e) of Schedule 1 to the MCA. (The following are cited as examples of such a person: a registered health care professional; a barrister, solicitor or advocate; a registered social worker, or an independent mental capacity advocate.)

Certain persons are disqualified from being able to give the LPA certificate, and these include:

- a family member of the donor
- a donee of the LPA or a donee of any other LPA executed by the donor
- a family member of the donee
- a director or employee of a trust corporation acting as a donee
- a business partner or employee of the donor or donee
- an owner, director, manager or employee of any care home in which the donor is living when the instrument is executed, or
- a family member of any of these persons.

Execution of the instrument

The 'execution' means the signing by the donor of the document which sets up the LPA. Regulation 9 sets out how the instrument is to be executed:

- The donor must read (or have read to him) all the prescribed information.
- As soon as reasonably practicable after reading the information, the donor must complete the provisions of Part A of the instrument and then sign Part A in the presence of a witness.
- The person (or persons if two are required) giving an LPA certificate must complete the LPA certificate at Part B of the instrument and sign it.
- The donee(s) must read or have read to him all the prescribed information and must complete the provisions of Part C of the instrument and sign in the presence of a witness.
- If the instrument is to be signed by a person at the direction of the donor or donee the signature must be done in the present of two witnesses.
- The donor may not witness any signature nor may the donee, apart from that of another donee.
- A person witnessing a signature must sign the instrument and give his full name and address.

Schedule 1 Part 2 of the MCA registration provisions

An application to the Public Guardian for registration of the instrument intending to create an LPA must comply with the requirements set out in Part 2 of Schedule 1 of the MCA and the regulations.[20]

Notice of the intention to apply for registration of an LPA must be on form LPA 001, found in Schedule 2 to the Regulations.[21] An application for registration must be on form LA 002 found in Schedule 3 to the Regulations. Form LPA 003A, on which the Public Guardian must notify the donees when he receives an application for registration, is found in Part 1 of Schedule 4 to the Regulations, and Form LPA 003B (found in Part 2 of Schedule 4 to the Regulations) is the form of notice to the donor when an application for registration is received by the Public Guardian.

Schedule 1 Part 3 of the MCA: cancellation of registration and notification of severance

This part sets out the circumstances in which the Office of the Public Guardian is obliged to cancel the registration of the LPA, and the circumstances in which the Court of Protection can order the OPG to cancel the registration.

Schedule 1 Part 4 of the MCA: records of alterations in registered powers

The Office of the Public Guardian must attach a note to the instrument of the LPA if the specified circumstances arise. In such a situation Regulation 18 applies,[22] and the OPG is required to give notice to the donor and the donee(s) requiring them to deliver the original of the instrument, any office copy and any certified copy. The Public Guardian will then attach the required note and return the document.

Non-registration

Where the Public Guardian is unable to register the instrument as a lasting power of attorney he must notify the person who applied for registration of that fact.

Fees in respect of the LPA and Court of Protection

The Consultation Paper on the fees for the Court of Protection and OPG[23] suggested that to register an LPA should cost £150, payable on application. Where an LPA has been drawn up to cover personal welfare as well as property and finance, both registrations will attract the fee, since there are separate registers for property and affairs and another for personal welfare LPAs. The fee for searching the Register should be £25. The fee of £25 also applies to a search of the Register to see if a deputy has been appointed. These are now set out in the Regulations.[24]

Conclusions

The extension of the powers of an attorney to cover personal welfare is to be welcomed, and it is likely that their use will become more popular and health and social services professionals will become familiar with their existence and operation. Extended powers of attorney will continue to be used, but no new EPAs can be created after October 2007. In time they will of necessity end as their creators die. Inevitably there will be disputes as to how the new provisions operate, and it is therefore likely that case law will develop over some of the issues raised in this chapter.

References

1   The Lasting Powers of Attorney, Enduring Powers of Attorney and Public Guardian Regulations 2007 (SI 2007/1253).
2   Office of the Public Guardian; Archway Tower, 2 Junction Road, London N19 5SZ; www.guardianship.gov.uk
3   The Lasting Powers of Attorney, Enduring Powers of Attorney and Public Guardian Regulations 2007 (SI 2007/1253).
4   www.dca.gov.uk/menincap/legis.htm
5   *Re K; Re F* [1988] 1 All ER 358.
6   The Lasting Powers of Attorney, Enduring Powers of Attorney and Public Guardian Regulations 2007 (SI 2007/1253).
7   *Ibid.*
8   Code of Practice for the Mental Capacity Act 2005. Department of Constitutional Affairs February 2007 para 7.21. TSO, London.
9   *R. (on the application of Burke)* v. *General Medical Council and Disability Rights Commission and the Official Solicitor to the Supreme Court* [2004] EWHC 1879; [2004] Lloyd's Rep Med 451.
10 Code of Practice for the Mental Capacity Act 2005. Department of Constitutional Affairs February 2007 para 7.70. TSO, London.
11 SI 2007/1253; see reference 1 above.
12 Joint Cttee. Chapter 9 paras 134–159.
13 Code of Practice for the Mental Capacity Act 2005. Department of Constitutional Affairs February 2007 para 7.14. TSO, London.
14 SI 2007/1253; see reference 1 above.
15 Code of Practice (see reference 8 above) para 7.16.
16 SI 2007/1253; see reference 1 above.
17 www.dca.gov.uk/menincap/legis.htm; www.opsi.gov.uk
18 SI 2007/1253 reg 6; see reference 1 above.
19 SI 2007/1253 reg 7; see reference 1 above.
20 SI 2007/1253 as amended by SI 2007 No 2161; see reference 1 above.

21 *Ibid.*
22 *Ibid.*
23 Court of Protection and Office of the Public Guardian Fees Consultation Paper CP23/06.
24 The Public Guardian (fees, etc.) Regulations Statutory Instrument 2007 No. 2051.

Scenarios C
Lasting Powers of Attorney

Introduction

The concept of the lasting power of attorney is one of the most important features of the Mental Capacity Act 2005. It permits a person, when they have the requisite mental capacity, to appoint another person to make decisions in relation to their personal welfare, as well as in relation to their property and finance. Under the existing power of attorney or the enduring powers of attorney, personal welfare decisions could not be delegated.

> **Scenario C1: Setting up a lasting power of attorney (LPA).**
>
> When Brian was 17 years old his mother, Ada, was diagnosed with a cancerous brain tumour. He had a brother and sister of 10 and 13 respectively. Ada was a widow and was concerned about how her family would cope when she died. She wished to set up a lasting power of attorney, so that she would be able to arrange for a person to make decisions for her, in the event of her becoming mentally incapacitated, including decisions not only about her property and affairs and but also her welfare. She wished Brian to be the donee of the LPA and to make the decisions for her. Is this legally possible?

Since the donee must be over 18 years at the time of the appointment, Brian will be unable to accept the appointment. Section 10(1)(a) stipulates that where the donee is an individual he or she must have reached 18 years. In addition Schedule 1 Para 2(d) requires the donee to state that he has read the prescribed information and understands the duties imposed upon the donee of a lasting power of attorney. As a consequence it would be impossible for Brian's mother to draw up an LPA appointing Brian at age 17 as a donee, which would come into effect when he is 18 years.

Could she appoint her sister until such time as Brian became 18 years?

Ada cannot in the instrument creating the lasting power of attorney appoint her sister as her donee and give powers for her sister to appoint Brian when he becomes 18 years. (Giving the power to a donee to appoint a substitute or successor is prevented by Section 10(8)(a).)

It is possible for the instrument creating the lasting power of attorney to appoint a person to replace the donee, on the occurrence of an event mentioned in Section 13(6)(a)–(d) (i.e. the disclaimer of the appointment by the donee, the death or bankruptcy of the donee, the dissolution of marriage or civil partnership between donee and donor, or the lack of capacity of the donee). However these exceptions do not cover the situation outlined here.

The simple answer therefore is that Brian cannot be appointed as a donee of an LPA (lasting power of attorney) until he is 18 years old.

Who could set up a lasting power of attorney?

Scenario C2: Requirements for setting up an LPA.

Christine, aged 17 years, was chronically ill with cystic fibrosis. She knew that unless she had a transplant she was unlikely to survive for very long, and she was almost reaching the stage of becoming too ill to cope with a transplant. Her parents were divorced and she lived with an older sister and her nieces and nephews. She was anxious that her sister, with whom she had a very close relationship, should make the decisions relating to her care and treatment, if she became too ill to make them herself. She explored whether she could arrange for her sister to be appointed to be the donee under a lasting power of attorney, to make decisions for her personal welfare.

The requirements for Christine to be able to establish a LPA are that:

- she must be at least 18 years at the time of the execution of the instrument setting up the LPA
- she must have the requisite mental capacity at the time of the execution
- the donee must be at least 18 years.

In Scenario C2 Christine could plan for the drawing up of the LPA and hope that she survives with the requisite mental capacity, so that when she becomes 18 she can execute the instrument and appoint her older sister as the donee. Until the time that she reaches adulthood, she could come under the provisions of the Children Act 1989. She could of course draw up a statement of her wishes which would constitute neither an LPA nor an advance decision (because for both of these she needs to be over 18 years). This statement should however influence those who are purporting to act in her best interests, since it may set out her wishes, feelings, beliefs and values, i.e. factors which should be taken into account in determining her best interests under Section 4 of the Act.

Dispute between donees

Scenario C3: Dispute between donees.

Mark drew up a lasting power of attorney appointing his son Matthew and his brother Harry to act as donees in decisions relating to his care and treatment. They both accepted the appointment. Mark subsequently suffered from dementia and was assessed as being unable to make decisions about his care and treatment. A dispute then arose between Matthew and Harry in relation to Mark's admission to a residential care home. Matthew considered that Mark should stay in the family home supported by carers. Harry was of the view that Mark should be admitted to a residential care home where he would have a better quality of life. He personally believed that Matthew was afraid that his inheritance would be lost in care home fees as the family home would have to be sold to pay the fees. How would such a dispute be resolved?

Clearly there would be evidence from social services and others as to what was seen to be in Mark's best interests. If the general view was that it was in Mark's best interests to be transferred to a residential care home, then if Matthew failed to agree to that, an application could be made initially to the Office of the Public Guardian and if necessary to the Court of Protection for the dispute to be resolved. The court may make a declaration as to what is in Mark's best interests. If Mark has not specified in the LPA whether the two are appointed to act jointly or severally, it will be presumed that a joint appointment is intended. This would mean that Matthew and Harry must act together.

Exercise of the LPA

Scenario C4: Exercise of the LPA.

Cynthia learnt by chance when she was 45 that she was in the early stages of Huntington's Chorea. An aunt had died from that condition and Cynthia was therefore familiar with the likely progress of the disease. She decided to give her daughter, Gwen, who was 23 years old, a lasting power of attorney over her personal welfare, since she felt that Gwen would know what Cynthia would want by way of care and treatment. She therefore drew up with the assistance of a solicitor, a lasting power of attorney to cover personal welfare. She notified Gwen of her intentions and Gwen agreed to become the holder of a lasting power of attorney. The solicitor asked her about decisions relating to property and finance and she asked her son Ben, who was 25, if he would take those kinds of decisions for her. He also agreed. Two separate documents were drawn up and appropriately signed by Cynthia, Gwen and Ben. Cynthia went on holiday abroad and asked Ben to take responsibility for selling her house. Whilst on holiday, she had a fall and Gwen was contacted about where Cynthia should be taken for treatment.

Following the consultation on the forms required for setting up an LPA, it was decided by the Government that there would be two different LPA forms: one to create a lasting power of attorney covering personal welfare decisions, the other covering property and finance. In Scenario C4 Ben and Gwen would have different documents appointing them as donees for their respective lasting powers of attorney. Both could be general, i.e. giving overall powers, or specific, i.e. giving instructions over a defined issue. Ben, for example, could have been given a specific power as attorney to arrange for the sale of Cynthia's house and to have the power to sign for the receipt of the payment and the reimbursement of any outstanding mortgage. The significant difference between the two kinds of LPA (i.e. personal welfare and property and finance) is that Gwen could only take up the lasting power of attorney when Cynthia has lost mental capacity to make her own personal welfare decisions.

On the facts of Scenario C4 Ben could act as Cynthia's attorney in relation to her property as soon as Cynthia makes that request. Ben would have to register the taking up of the power of attorney. Guidance from the Office of the Public Guardian explains how this is done. The fact that Cynthia still has her mental capacity is irrelevant.

In contrast, Gwen can only exercise her powers as a donee under the LPA when Cynthia loses her mental capacity to make decisions on her personal welfare. Gwen has been contacted by persons abroad about Cynthia's fall and treatment. She should immediately establish if Cynthia has the capacity to make her own decisions. If however she is unconscious, then Gwen could, depending upon the terms of the LPA governing personal welfare, register the fact of Cynthia's mental capacity and make personal welfare decisions on her behalf.

The LPA and advance decisions

Scenario C5: An LPA and an advance decision.

On the facts of Scenario C4 Cynthia realised from her aunt's history, that she was facing a future of suffering and pain, with possible indignities and loss of privacy. She therefore drew up an advance decision stating that in the event of her losing mental capacity as a result of Huntington's Chorea, she would not wish to be given resuscitation, ventilation, artificial feeding, antibiotics or other life saving treatments, but should be allowed to die. She also drew up and executed a lasting power of attorney covering personal welfare in which she appointed Gwen as her attorney. She then went on holiday abroad where she had a serious fall. She returned to England in an air ambulance and was admitted to a specialist hospital. Gwen visited and found her mother in a coma on a life support machine and being given artificial feeding. The consultant said that they had found the advance decision in Cynthia's handbag and asked Gwen if she thought that they should cease all life saving treatment.

Several questions arise for Gwen:

- Does Cynthia lack capacity?
- How do her powers under the LPA relate to the advance decision which Cynthia has drawn up?
- Do both the advance decision and the LPA apply to this situation or only one or neither?

The first issue over which Gwen must satisfy herself is Cynthia's lack of capacity. It is clear since she is in a coma, that there is a temporary loss of capacity, but Gwen would need to discover from the consultant the likelihood of Cynthia recovering consciousness and making her own decisions.

Gwen's powers under the LPA are subject to the advance decision to refuse treatment (S.11(7)(b)). However where the lasting power of attorney was created after the advance decision was made, and gives authority to the donee to give or refuse consent to the treatment to which the advance decision relates, then the advance decision is not valid (S.25(2)(b)). This is because the inconsistency would suggest that the donor of the LPA no longer saw the advance decision as valid since the LPA, which was drawn up afterwards, was incompatible with it.

If the advance decision was drawn up by Cynthia before the lasting power of attorney was executed, is that latter in conflict with the instructions in the advance direction?

Superficially it would appear that there is no incompatibility. However if the LPA referred to and confirmed the compatibility of the advance decision with the powers given in the LPA, there would be no conflict.

Applicability of the advance decision to the present situation?

However the question must be asked as to whether the advance decision is relevant and therefore applicable to the situation which has arisen. It refers to Cynthia becoming mentally incapacitated as a result of Huntington's Chorea. On the facts she has (possibly temporarily) lost her mental capacity because of the fall.

It could be concluded therefore that the advance decision does not apply to the situation which exists, i.e. the circumstances specified in the advance decision are absent (S.24(4)(b)).

Does the LPA apply?

It is assumed that Cynthia has drawn up an LPA appointing Gwen to make personal welfare decisions on her behalf on a general basis. Once it is established that Cynthia no longer has the requisite mental capacity, Gwen is bound by the Mental Capacity Act (MCA) to follow the principles set out in Section 1 and also to act in Cynthia's best interests according to the criteria set out in Section 4 and discussed in Chapter 5 of this book and Scenarios B.

As the donee of the lasting power of attorney, Gwen can make decisions about Cynthia's personal welfare, which includes the giving or refusing consent to the carrying out or continuation of a treatment by a person providing health care for P (S.11(7)(c)). Gwen could therefore, on Cynthia's behalf and acting in her best interests, give consent or refuse treatments suggested by the consultant for Cynthia. This power is however subject to a major qualification. Gwen would not be authorised to give or refuse consent to the carrying out of continuation of life-sustaining treatment unless the lasting power of attorney contains express provision to that effect. In addition Gwen is subject to any conditions or restrictions laid down in the instrument of the LPA.

On the facts of Scenario C5, Cynthia is on a life support machine. Even if the consultant recommended that this should be switched off, Gwen would not have the power to give consent to that, unless the LPA drawn up by Cynthia specifically mentioned the power to refuse life-sustaining treatment.

As we have noted above, the fact that the advance decision permitted the refusal of ventilation was irrelevant since the advance decision referred to Cynthia losing her mental capacity as a consequence of Huntington's Chorea.

Power in LPA to refuse life saving treatment

If the facts in Scenario C5 were different and the LPA drawn up for personal welfare by Cynthia did specifically give Gwen the power to refuse life-sustaining treatment, then she would be able to inform the consultant that she was refusing to give consent to Cynthia's continuation on a life support machine and the artificial feeding. The wording of the LPA must however be set out very clearly to cover this power, and there must be clear evidence that this actual situation would be covered by the powers granted in the LPA.

Refusing pain relief

Scenario C6: Refusal of pain relief.

Don, a Buddhist, had drawn up an LPA appointing his daughter Jane as the attorney. Subsequently he suffered from dementia and arthritis and was admitted to hospital. Jane had the power under the LPA to make decisions on treatment. The doctors stated that Don required a high level of pain killers to control the pain from the arthritis. Jane stated that as a Buddhist her father would not have agreed to any pain control and therefore he should not be given it. What is the law?

The Law Commission in its draft Mental Incapacity Bill in 1995 suggested that it should be impossible for a patient by means of an advance decision to refuse basic care, which would include direct oral nutrition and hydration and also pain relief. It would also follow that an attorney acting under an LPA relating to personal welfare could not refuse such basic care on the patient's behalf. The situation is not so clear under the 2005 Act (see Chapter 9) and the doctors may well wish an application to be made, initially to the Office of the Public Guardian and, if necessary, to the Court of Protection to determine whether pain relief could be validly withheld from Don in accordance with Jane's request.

Challenge to the donee of the power

> **Scenario C7: The donee's power is challenged.**
>
> David drew up a power of attorney whereby his son James would make all decisions relating to his property and finance. James undertook several transactions on his father's behalf, including the selling of some antique furniture. It subsequently comes to light that the LPA was never registered according to the provisions of Schedule 1. Since prices for antiques have subsequently risen steeply, James's sister considers that the furniture could now be sold for four times the amount which James received. She claims that the transaction was void because of the fact that an LPA was not created and the furniture should still be seen as belonging to her father. What is the legal situation of David and the purchaser?

In this situation, the fact that the LPA has not been registered means that no power of attorney has been created. What is the effect of this on the transactions which have taken place? The crucial question is the knowledge of David and the purchaser. If David is ignorant of the fact that the lasting power of attorney had not been created, then he is protected by Section 14(2) and he does not incur any liability to his father (i.e. the donor), or to any other person. In addition any transaction between David and another person is as valid as if the power had been in existence, unless at the time of the transaction that person has knowledge that the LPA was not created. Therefore if the purchaser of the furniture was unaware of the failure to register the LPA and the fact that an LPA had not been created, the transaction for the sale of the furniture will stand (S.14(3)). The purchaser's position is safeguarded and it is conclusively presumed in favour of the purchaser that the transaction was valid, if within three months of the completion of the purchase he signs a statutory declaration stating that:

> He had no reason at the time of the transaction to doubt that the donee had authority to dispose of the property which was the subject of the transaction (S.14(4)(b)).

The purchaser's position is also protected if the transaction was completed within 12 months of the date on which the instrument was registered (S.14(4)(a)).

Hypothetical dispute over LPA

An example, shown in Scenario C8, is given by Charles Hancock in an article[1] concerned with the problems which could arise for clinicians and managers over the introduction of LPAs under the MCA.

Scenario C8: LPAs and manual handling.

Patient A is a 67 year old woman suffering from complex physical handicaps and who has also developed senile dementia. She is normally cared for at home by her daughter Mrs F who has a lasting power of attorney for personal welfare. The patient is admitted to hospital for elective surgery. She is seen by the daughter when being transferred by hoist from the bed to a trolley to be taken to theatre. The daughter, who has strong views against the use of mechanical devices for moving and handling her mother, objects to the use of the hoist. The nurses refuse, stating that it is unsafe for both the patient and themselves to move the patient in another way. Mrs F then states that unless they follow her instructions precisely, they will face a civil action for battery and may be reported to the police. The ward sister tries to persuade Mrs F that it is the patient's best interests to be lifted in this matter. The hypothetical scenario continues with Mrs F subsequently presenting the ward staff with a note setting out her powers as the holder of a lasting power of attorney, her view that mechanical lifting and handling of the patient is not in the patient's best interests and may contravene Article 8 of the European Convention on Human Rights and that anyone who attempts to use mechanical devices may face a civil action. In addition any failure to provide personal care to the patient will result in a complaint of a contravention of Section 44 of the MCA (ill-treatment or neglect). Mrs F also asks the nursing staff to sign that they will not use mechanical devices in the care of her mother. The staff nurse refuses to sign the document and eventually, after discussions with hospital management and social services, an application is made to the Office of Public Guardian, who is responsible for dealing with complaints against the holders of lasting powers of attorney and court-appointed deputies.

The author of the article accepts that the overwhelming majority of people who will act as holders of lasting powers of attorney will do so in a sensible and co-operative manner with clinicians, managers and staff, in order to provide the best possible care. However he states that the scenario provides a realistic depiction of a simple way in which the issue of managing the care of those who lack capacity could go seriously wrong. He suggests that there needs to be an urgent dialogue between senior healthcare managers and the Public Guardian to ensure that there are robust and simple systems in place for such eventualities. He also recommends that there needs to be a system whereby staff can contact the Office of the Public Guardian in emergency situations, in order to request the suspension of the lasting power of attorney prior to any formal investigation.

Restraint

Scenario C8 raises the question of restraint. Could the use of a hoist be seen as a type of restraint in the care of the person lacking mental capacity?

Section 6(4) defines a person as using restraint if he:

(a)   uses, or threatens to use, force to secure the doing of an act which P resists, or
(b)   restricts P's liberty of movement, whether or not P resists.

Placing a person in a hoist would certainly appear to be a restriction of P's liberty of movement, whether or not P resists.

In what circumstances could the donee of the LPA covering personal welfare consent to restraint being used?

To use the hoist, which restricts P's liberty of movement and is therefore a restraint, could be justified under the MCA if:

- the patient/client lacks mental capacity
- it is reasonably believed to be necessary to prevent harm to the patient/client
- the restraint is a proportionate response to the likelihood of P's suffering harm and the seriousness of that harm.

It would appear that these conditions are satisfied in Scenario C8, since harm could befall the patient if she were to be manually handled.

Manual handling and human rights

The question of whether the use of manual handling was contrary to the rights of the patient was discussed in a case involving East Sussex County Council.[2] In this case two severely disabled women claimed that they had a human right not to be manually handled. The judge accepted that both A and B and also their carers had rights, under Article 8 of the European Convention on Human Rights, to dignity. He stated it was highly questionable to state that manual handling is dignified whereas mechanical handling is undignified, and said that:

> One must guard against jumping too readily to the conclusion that manual handling is necessarily more dignified than the use of equipment. . . . Hoisting is not inherently undignified, let alone inherently inhuman or degrading. I agree . . . that certain forms of manual lift, for example the drag lift, may in certain circumstances be less dignified than hoisting. Hoisting can facilitate dignity, comfort, safety and independence. It all depends on the context.

The judge went on to consider a framework for decision making, setting out the principles which should apply and considering the factors which should be taken into account in determining how to assess reasonable practicability.

Gifts

Scenario C9: Situation A – welcome gift.

Mavis was the donee of an LPA drawn up by her father, Amos, who had recently been admitted to a nursing home. Amos had been examined by a doctor who declared him to be lacking mental capacity. Amos had considerable assets including a stash of cash which Mavis was aware of. She therefore decided that she would make a gift of the cash to herself, since she believed that the powers of the LPA extended to her making gifts on behalf of her father. What is the law?

Mavis would be entitled to give herself the cash, provided that the provisions of Section 12 are satisfied. The following questions would have to be answered:

- Is Mavis related to the donor?
- Is it a customary occasion?
- Is the size of the gift reasonable in relation to all the circumstances and in particular Amos's estate?

Mavis would be wise to ensure that the gift related to an occasion such as her birthday, her marriage or some other particular occasion. Unless there was a specific requirement in the instrument to bestow a gift upon herself, she would also have to consider whether it was in her father's best interests for the gift to be made, and have regard to the principles in Section 1.

Acting contrary to the best interests of the donor

Scenario C10: Not in the best interests.

Harold drew up an LPA appointing his daughter Jean to be a donee in property decisions. She knew that he had always favoured giving money to an African charity and she intended to continue this tradition. However Harold had very little capital and only a small pension supplemented by social security for income. In spite of this, Jean decided that she would make a donation of £5000 from Harold's capital of £10 000 to the African charity. This gift was contested by Harold's son Michael as not being in Harold's best interests. Jean argued that that was not necessary since she was acting under an LPA.

If the donor had previously made regular or periodic donations to any charity, the attorney or donee would also be permitted to continue to make such donations from the donor's funds (S.12(2)(b)). However the gift to the charity is subject to the same conditions as a gift to relatives or to persons who are connected with the donor, i.e. the gift must be reasonable having regard to all the circumstances and particularly the size of the donor's estate. To donate half of Harold's estate to the charity would appear to be out of all proportion to the estate and therefore unreasonable. However if there were a specific requirement that Jean gave that amount to the charity in the LPA, then Jean would be acting in accordance with her instructions. Without such specific instructions Jean would have to comply with the provisions of Section 12, the principles set out in Section 1 and the definition of best interests as defined in Section 4.

References

1   Hancock, C. (2006) Power Games. *Health Management*, pp. 24–25.
2   *A and B* v. East *Sussex County Council (The Disability Rights Commission an interested party)* [2003] EWHC 167 (Admin).

7

Court of Protection, Court Appointed Deputies, the Office of the Public Guardian and Visitors

Introduction

The Court of Protection, whilst retaining the old title, is a new court with a much wider jurisdiction than its predecessor. It has the power to make decisions about both personal welfare and property and affairs for a person who lacks the requisite mental capacity, and can make declarations about advance decisions. It also has ultimate control over those appointed under a lasting power of attorney. Court-appointed deputies replace the previous system of receiverships and have extended powers to include welfare and health care matters, as well as financial and property affairs.

The significant new feature is that there is now a single integrated framework for making personal welfare decisions, health care decisions and financial decisions on behalf of those lacking the requisite mental capacity, as recommended by the Law Commission in 1995. The court can make both one-off orders and also appoint a deputy with continuing powers.

Court of Protection

Constitution of the Court of Protection

Part 2 of the Mental Capacity Act 2005 Sections 45–56 makes provision for a new Court of Protection. The provisions under Part 7 of the Mental Health Act 1983 are repealed.

The jurisdiction of the court covers England and Wales and it can sit at any place, on any day and at any time. It has a central office and registry located by the Lord Chancellor, who has the power to designate any district registry of the High Court and any county court office as an additional registry of the Court of Protection.

Judges are appointed by the Lord Chancellor or a person acting on his behalf. There are specified conditions of eligibility for the appointment of a judge to the Court of Protection, i.e.:

a.   the President of the Family Division
b.   the Vice-Chancellor
c.   a puisne judge of the High Court
d.   a circuit judge
e.   a district judge

The Lord Chancellor must appoint the President and Vice President of the court from one of categories a, b or c. From amongst the other categories the Lord Chancellor must appoint a Senior Judge of the Court of Protection, with administrative functions set by the Lord Chancellor.

General powers and effect of orders

The court has the same powers, rights, privileges and authority as the High Court (S.47(1)). This means that all the High Court powers in relation to witnesses, contempt of court and enforcement of its decisions apply to the Court of Protection.

The powers given by Section 204 of the Law of Property Act 1925, which lay down that the High Court orders are conclusive in favour of purchasers, apply to the Court of Protection. Office copies of the official documents of the court which are sealed with its official seal are admissible in all legal proceedings as evidence of the originals without any further proof.

Interim orders and directions

The Court of Protection has the power, pending the determination of an application to it, to make an order or give directions on any matter which is within its jurisdiction, if there is reason to believe that P lacks the capacity in relation to that matter and it is in the person's best interests to make the order, or give the directions without delay.

General powers of the Court of Protection

The Court of Protection is given powers under Section 15 of the Mental Capacity Act 2005 to make declarations, and under Section 16 to make decisions and appoint deputies. The power to make declarations covers the following:

a.   Whether a person has or lacks capacity to make a decision specified in the declaration.
b.   Whether a person has or lacks capacity to make decisions on such matters as are described in the declaration.

c.   The lawfulness or otherwise of any act (which includes an omission and course of conduct) done, or yet to be done, in relation to that person.

Examples of c. might include deciding whether the withholding or withdrawing of medical treatment is in the best interests of P.
 Scenario D1 illustrates how this section works.

Decisions of the Court of Protection

Where a person lacks capacity in relation to a matter or matters concerning his or her personal welfare or property and affairs, then the court may make an order which makes the decisions on P's behalf or may appoint a deputy to make the decision on P's behalf. The powers must be exercised in accordance with the principles set out in Section 1 of the Act (see Chapter 3 of this book) and in accordance with the best interests of P as defined in Section 4 (see Chapter 5 of this book).
 The powers of the court are extensive in that the court may make the order, give the directions or make the appointment on such terms as it considers are in P's best interests, even though no application is before the court for an order, directions or an appointment on those terms (S.16(6)).

Reports for the Court of Protection

Where proceedings are brought in respect of a person under Part 1 of the Mental Capacity Act (MCA), and the court is considering a question in relation to P, then the powers of the Court of Protection include the calling for reports from the Public Guardian (see below) or by a Court of Protection visitor (see below). The Court of Protection can also require a local authority or an National Health Service (NHS) body to arrange for a report to be made by one of its officers or employees or such other person as it thinks appropriate to make a report. The Court of Protection can specify matters which must be included in any such report and can also direct whether the report should be made in writing or by word of mouth.

Procedure for applications to the Court of Protection (S.50)

No permission is required for an application to the court for the exercise of any of its powers under the MCA by:

- a person who lacks, or is alleged to lack, capacity
- if such a person has not reached 18, by anyone with parental responsibility for him (parental responsibility has the same meaning as in the Children Act 1989 – see Chapter 12)
- by the donor or a donee of a lasting power of attorney to which the application relates

- by a deputy appointed by the court for a person to whom the application relates, or
- by a person named in an existing order of the court, if the application relates to the order.

The Mental Health Act 2007 has added a new Subsection 1A to Section 50 so that no permission is required for an application to the court under Section 21A (see Box 7.2) by the relevant person's representative.

Others not listed above will need to obtain permission to apply to the Court of Protection (see Scenario D2) subject to the Court of Protection Rules (see below) and declarations relating to private international law (see **Permission to apply to the Court of Protection** below and Chapter 3).

Rule 25 sets out the circumstances where, in addition to those listed above under Section 50(1), permission is not required. They include a situation where the application relates to a financial application in respect of a person who lacks capacity. The reasoning behind this exception is that most cases dealt with by the present Court of Protection are undisputed finance cases, where a quick decision is needed to ensure the financial security and well-being of a person who is losing capacity. Such cases include a situation where a third party such as a bank, building society or pension fund cannot accept a receipt or signature from anyone other than the person who lacks capacity. The commentary on the draft Rules suggests that to require a permission stage to access the Court of Protection would add unnecessary delay and complexity.[1]

Private international law

An interested person may apply to the court for a declaration as to whether a protective measure taken under the law of a country other than England and Wales is to be recognised in England and Wales, and no permission is required for an application to the court under this paragraph (Schedule 3, Para 20(2)).

Permission to apply to the Court of Protection

In considering whether permission for a person to apply is to be granted, the Court of Protection must have regard to:

- the applicant's connection with the person to whom the application relates
- the reasons for the application
- the benefit to the person to whom the application relates of a proposed order or direction, and
- whether the benefit can be achieved in any other way.

The Explanatory Memorandum suggests that the factors to which the court must have regard are designed to ensure that any proposed application will promote the interests of the person concerned, rather than causing unnecessary distress or difficulty for him.

Court of Protection Rules (S.51)

These can be made by the Lord Chancellor in relation to the practice and procedure of the court, and can cover the areas listed in Section 51(2). These include the areas shown in Box 7.1.

Box 7.1: Practice and procedure issues covered by the Court of Protection Rules.

- the manner and form in which proceedings are to be commenced
- the persons entitled to be notified of, and to be made parties to, the proceedings
- the allocation of any proceedings to a specified judge
- the exercise of the jurisdiction of the court by its officers or other staff
- to enable the court to appoint a suitable person to act in the name of or represent the person to whom the proceedings relate
- to enable an application to the court to be disposed of without a hearing
- to enable the court to proceed with a hearing in the absence of the person to whom they relate
- to enable proceedings or any part of them to be conducted in private, who should be admitted and who excluded
- what may be received as evidence and the manner in which it is to be presented
- the enforcement of orders made and direction given in the proceedings

---

Draft Rules were published in July 2006 for consultation, which ended on 6 October 2006. They were finalised and approved for implementation on 1 October 2007.

The Rules may make different provision for different geographical areas (S.51(4)).

The Rules can be accessed at the Department of Constitutional Affairs (DCA), Public Guardianship, Office of Public Sector Information (OPSI) or The Stationery Office websites. Court of Protection Rules Statutory Instrument 2007, No 1744.

Court of Protection practice directions (S.52)

The President of the Court of Protection with the agreement of the Lord Chancellor may give directions as to the practice and procedure of the court.

The Explanatory Memorandum makes it clear that these are directions about a court's practices and procedures issued for the assistance and guidance of litigants. They often support and add detail to the Rules of Court. Practice directions for the Court of Protection will have to be made by the President with the approval of the Lord Chancellor, or by another person (for example the Vice-President) with the approval of the President and the Lord Chancellor.

Section 52(3) enables the President of the Court of Protection to give directions which contain guidance as to law or making judicial decisions without the concurrence of the Lord Chancellor. Section 51(3) of the MCA states that the rules may, instead of providing for any matter, refer to provision made or to be made about that matter by the directions made under Section 52. The intention is to make rules accompanied by practice directions, on the model of the Civil Procedure Rules 1998.[2]

Rights of appeal (S.53)

An appeal from any decision of the Court of Protection lies to the Court of Appeal, but the Court of Protection Rules Part 20 enable appeals against decisions made by specified judges to be made to a higher judge of the Court of Protection. An appeal from a decision of a District Judge is heard by a Circuit Judge, and an appeal from the decision of a Circuit Judge is heard by a High Court Judge. An appeal from the decision of a High Court Judge would be heard by the Court of Appeal. The Court of Protection Rules provide that an appeal against the decision of the Court of Protection should not be made without permission and set out in Rule 172 who is able to grant permission to appeal. Rule 173 sets out the matters that the court will take into account when considering an application for permission to appeal. Rules 174–182 govern the process by which and time limits within which applications in respect of an appeal against a decision of the court must be made.

Under Section 53(4) no appeal may be made to the Court of Appeal from the decision of a judge hearing an appeal, unless the Court of Appeal considers that:

- the appeal would raise an important point of principle or practice, or
- there is some other compelling reason for the Court of Appeal to hear it.

This matches the '2nd appeal' test in the Civil Procedure Rules 1998, Rule 52.13.

Fees and costs

Rules laid down in Sections 54, 55 and 56 relate to the prescribing of fees and the awarding of costs by the Court of Protection. The Department of Constitutional Affairs published a second public consultation, this time on fees for the Court of Protection and the Office of the Public Guardian on 6 September 2006. The consultation closed on 29 November 2006. The fees are set out in SI. 2007 No 1745.

The Court of Protection Draft Rules suggested:

> . . . that fees should be paid where people are able to do so, but that access to justice should be protected for those who are not able to pay. Protection should be provided for clients of modest means as fees should not prevent access to justice.[3]

This is in keeping with the recommendations of the Joint Committee, which was concerned about the issue of costs in relation to accessibility. Costs should not act as a disincentive. The Joint Committee stated that:

We seek assurances that public funds will be made available to ensure that the Court of Protection is sufficiently accessible for those with limited assets. Furthermore, we seek clarification as to the types of cases for which legal aid will be provided to mentally incapacitated applicants and alternative remedies for those cases which will not qualify.

Application to the Court of Protection

The Rules of the Court of Protection govern the way in which applications can be made to the Court of Protection and the procedure which must be followed. The Rules of the Court of Protection require the applicant to bring proceedings by filing an application of notice and to comply with the pre-action protocols. The pre-action protocols specify:

a. the action which must be taken prior to an application being made to the court
b. any procedures that must be followed
c. time periods within which any actions must be taken or any procedures must be followed
d. the need to encourage co-operation between the parties
e. the promotion of an early exchange of information
f. the need to encourage the parties to settle any dispute, otherwise than by proceedings in a court
g. the need to support the efficient management of the court's proceedings.

(Scenario D2 illustrates a potential situation.)

Pre-action protocol

Parties must comply with the pre-action protocol and ensure that every reasonable action is taken to resolve the dispute prior to the application to the court being made. Failure to comply with this requirement could lead to costs being awarded against the party. The pre-action protocol covers the action which must be taken prior to making an application to the court, the procedures which must be followed, encouragement to the parties to co-operate, promotion of the early exchange of information and encouragement for the parties to settle any dispute without proceedings in court (Rule 9 applies the Civil Procedure Rules).

Overriding principle of the Court of Protection

The Court of Protection Rule 3 states that the overriding objective of the Rules of Court is to enable the court to deal with cases justly, having regard to principles contained in the Act. The Court of Protection is required to give effect to the overriding objective in its exercise of any power under the MCA or the Rules, and its interpretation of any Rule or provision of the MCA. Dealing with any case justly includes ensuring that it is dealt with expeditiously and fairly, dealing with the case in ways which are proportionate to the nature, importance and complexity of the issues. It must also ensure that the parties are on an equal footing (see Rule 3(3)(d)). Rule 5 requires the court to actively manage the cases, and Rule 5(2) lists the many ways in which the court should be involved in active management.

Attempting a reconciliation

The pre-action protocol and the Rules of Court require the parties to attempt to resolve the dispute prior to a court hearing. The Court of Protection as part of its duty of actively managing cases must encourage the parties to use an alternative dispute resolution procedure if the court considers that to be appropriate, and it must facilitate the use of such procedure. It must also help the parties settle the whole or part of the case.

Decisions which could only be made by the Court of Protection

There are certain kinds of serious decisions relating to medical treatment which have under common law been referred to the courts for a declaration as to their validity, and these cases will now be referred to the Court of Protection. They include the following:

- decisions about the proposed withholding or withdrawal of artificial nutrition and hydration (ANH) from patients in a permanent vegetative state (PVS)
- cases involving organ or bone marrow donation by a person who lacks capacity to consent
- cases involving the proposed non-therapeutic sterilisation of a person who lacks capacity to consent to this (e.g. for contraceptive purposes)
- all other cases where there is a doubt or dispute about whether a particular treatment will be in a person's best interests.
- termination of pregnancy in certain cases[4]
- any other cases where there are disputes and concerns over whether proposed treatment is in the best interests of the person lacking the requisite capacity.[5]

Powers of Court of Protection and the Bournewood provisions

As a consequence of the amendments to the Mental Capacity Act introduced to remedy the defects identified by the European Court of Human Rights in the Bournewood case, a new S21A was contained in the Mental Health Act 2007, defining the powers of the Court of Protection in relation to the new Schedule A1 and powers to restrict the liberty of persons in specified circumstances. Section 21A is shown in Box 7.2.

Box 7.2: New Section 21A added to the MCA by para 2 of Schedule 9 of the Mental Health Act 2007.

(1)   This section applies if either of the following has been given under Schedule A1:
    (a)   a standard authorisation
    (b)   an urgent authorisation.
(2)   Where a standard authorisation has been given, the court may determine any question relating to any of the following matters:
    (a)   whether any relevant person meets one of more of the qualifying requirements;
    (b)   the period during which the standard authorisation is to be in force
    (c)   the purpose for which the standard authorisation is given
    (d)   the conditions subject to which the standard authorisation is given.
(3)   If the court determines any question under subsection (2), the court may make an order:
    (a)   varying or terminating the standard authorisation, or
    (b)   directing the supervisory body to vary or terminate the standard authorisation.
(4)   Where an urgent authorisation has been given, the court may determine any question relating to any of the following matters:
    (a)   whether the urgent authorisation should have been given;
    (b)   the period during which the urgent authorisation is to be in force;
    (c)   the purpose for which the urgent authorisation is given.
(5)   Where the court determines any question under subsection (4), the court may make an order:
    (a)   varying or terminating the urgent authorisation, or
    (b)   directing the managing authority of the relevant hospital or care home to vary or terminate the urgent authorisation.
(6)   Where the court makes an order under subsection (3) or (5), the court may make an order about a person's liability for any act done in connection with the standard or urgent authorisation before its variation or termination.
(7)   An order under subsection (6) may, in particular, exclude a person from liability.

Court appointed deputy

The Court of Protection can make a single order or appoint a deputy in relation to a matter within its jurisdiction. Section 16 makes provisions for the Court of Protection to make decisions and for the appointment of deputies.

Single order or appointment of deputy?

The Joint Committee of the Houses of Parliament[6] were concerned to ensure that further guidance should be provided to assist the Court of Protection in deciding when a single order is more appropriate than the appointment of a deputy.

Section 16(4) therefore provides that when deciding whether it is in P's best interests to appoint a deputy, the court must have regard (in addition to the following the principles in Section 1 and the best interests of P as defined in Section 4) to the principles that:

- a decision by the court is to be preferred to the appointment of a deputy to make a decision, and
- the powers conferred on a deputy should be as limited in scope and duration as is reasonably practicable in the circumstances.

The court has the power to make further orders or give directions, and confer on a deputy such powers as it thinks necessary or expedient for giving effect to an order or appointment made by it. This power may prevent repeated applications to the Court of Protection itself, enabling the deputy to deal with questions as they arise. Scenario D3 illustrates the appointment of a deputy.

Control of a deputy by the Court of Protection

The court may vary or discharge an order made previously. Section 16(8) states:

> The court may revoke the appointment of a deputy or vary the powers conferred upon him if it is satisfied that the deputy
>
> a.   has behaved, or is behaving, in such a way that contravenes the authority conferred on him by the court or is not in P's best interests, or
> b.   proposes to behave in a way that would contravene that authority or would not be in P's best interests.

Scenario D6 illustrates the supervision of a deputy by the Court of Protection.

Deputy and personal welfare decisions

Whilst Section 5 enables the carers and professionals concerned with P's welfare to make decisions on P's care and treatment and take appropriate action on behalf of P (see Chapter 5), in cases of dispute the Court of Protection may appoint a deputy to resolve any issues on welfare and health.

Under Section 16 decisions can be made by the Court of Protection and the deputies can be given powers (with specified limitations) over matters of personal welfare which extend in particular to:

- deciding where P is to live (where a deputy makes a decision on this, it is subject to the restrictions on deputies – see **Restrictions on the powers of deputies** page 132)
- deciding what contact, if any, P is to have with any specified persons (the deputy has no power to make an order prohibiting a named person from having contact with P – see **Restrictions on the powers of deputies** page 132)
- giving or refusing consent to the carrying out or continuation of a treatment by a person providing health care for P.

A deputy cannot give a direction that a person responsible for P's health care should allow a different person to take over that responsibility: only the Court of Protection has that power (see **Restrictions on the powers of Deputies**, page 132).

The words 'extend in particular to' indicate that this list is not exhaustive and other powers could be added to those listed. In addition the list does not mean that these kinds of decisions have to be made by the Court of Protection or by deputies. They could, and generally will, be made by carers or professionals involved in the welfare of P.

Welfare powers and amendments introduced by the Mental Health Act 2007

The Mental Health Act section 50(3) introduced a new S.16A to be added to the Mental Capacity Act, as a consequence of the amendments introduced to fill the Bournewood gap (see Chapters 3 and 13).

Section 16A provides as follows below.

Section 16 powers: Mental Health Act patients etc

1. If a person is ineligible to be deprived of liberty by this Act, the court may not include in a welfare order provision which authorises the person to be deprived of his liberty
2. If:
    (a) a welfare order includes provision which authorises a person to be deprived of his liberty, and
    (b) that person becomes ineligible to be deprived of liberty by this Act, the provision ceases to have effect for as long as the person remains ineligible
3. Nothing in Subsection (2) affects the power of the court under Section 16(7) to vary or discharge the welfare order
4. For the purposes of this section:
    (a) Schedule 1A applies for determining whether or not P is ineligible to be deprived of liberty by this Act
    (b) 'Welfare order' means an order under section 16(2)(a)

Deputies and property and affairs

In connection with property and affairs, Section 18 makes provision for the decisions which can be made by the court, and the powers which can be given to deputies extend in particular to the matters shown in Box 7.3.

Box 7.3: Powers of deputy in relation to property and affairs.

- the control and management of P's property
- the sale, exchange, charging, gift or other disposition of P's property
- the acquisition of property in P's name or on P's behalf

- the carrying on, on P's behalf, of any profession, trade or business
- the taking of a decision which will have the effect of dissolving a partnership of which P is a member
- the carrying out of any contract entered into by P
- the discharge of P's debts and of any of P's obligations, whether legally enforceable or not
- the settlement of any of P's property, whether for P's benefit or for the benefit of others
- the execution for P of a will (unless P is under 18 years old) (subject to restriction on deputies)
- the exercise of any power (including a power to consent) vested in P whether beneficially or as trustee or otherwise
- the conduct of legal proceedings in P's name or on P's behalf

As in the list of powers in relation to personal welfare decisions, the list shown in Box 7.3 is not intended to be exhaustive, and other powers could be added as necessary. In addition the list does not mean that such decisions always have to go to the Court of Protection or be made by a deputy. They can be taken by carers and professionals. However, frequently in matters concerning property and affairs it may be necessary to have the formal authorisation of the Court of Protection or of a deputy.

Where deputies make such decisions on property and affairs they are subject to the restrictions laid down under Section 20 (see **Restrictions on the powers of deputies** page 132).

With the exception of the execution of a will (which cannot be made unless P is 18 years), the powers under Section 16 can be exercised, even though P has not reached 16, if the court considers that it is likely that P will still lack capacity to make decisions in respect of that matter when he or she reaches 18. Thus in the case of a young person with severe learning disabilities, a decision about his property and affairs can be made even though he is under 16 years, if it seems unlikely that he will have the necessary mental capacity at 18 years (see Chapter 12 on children).

However a will cannot be made for a person who has not reached 18 years (S.18 (2) and chapter 12).

Schedule 2

Schedule 2 provides supplementary provisions relating to property and affairs. These cover the making of a will and the effect of the execution of a will, the settlement of any property, variation of settlements, and the effects of disposing of any property.

Appointment of deputy

To be appointed as a deputy an individual must be 18 years or over. An individual of at least 18 years or a trust corporation can be appointed as a deputy in respect of powers relating to property and affairs. The deputy must give consent to the appointment. The holder of a specified office or position may be appointed as deputy. Two or more deputies could be appointed to act jointly or jointly and severally. ('Jointly' means that they act together in making decisions and exercising the powers; 'severally' means that they act as individuals separately.) Some powers could be specified to be taken by the deputies acting together, i.e. jointly, and others to be taken by the deputy acting separately. The court has the power to appoint a succession of deputies in certain circumstances and for a specified period. Scenario D4 illustrates the choice of a deputy.

The deputy as agent of P

The deputy is treated as P's agent in relation to anything done or decided by him within the scope of his appointment and in accordance with Part 1 of the MCA. This imports into the law of mental capacity the principles of agency law and the rules which apply to the agency/principal relationship in law.

Payment of deputies

Expenses

The deputy is entitled to be reimbursed out of P's property for his reasonable expenses in discharging his functions.

Remuneration

In addition, if the court so directs when appointing the deputy, the deputy can receive remuneration out of P's property for discharging his functions.

The court can give the deputy powers to take possession or control of all or any specified part of P's property, and to exercise all or any specified powers in respect of it, including such powers of investment as the court decides.

Security

A court may require a deputy to give to the Public Guardian such security as the court thinks fit for the due discharge of his functions.

Reports

A court may require a deputy to submit to the Public Guardian such reports at such times or at such intervals as the court may direct (S.19(9)). The Regulations make further provisions in relation to security and reports.[7] Under Regulation 38 a deputy can apply to the Public Guardian (see **Right of deputy to require review of decisions made by the Public Guardian** page 132) for an extension of the time within which the report must be submitted. The report must include any information required by the court and also contain or be accompanied by information and documents reasonably required by the Public Guardian. The Public Guardian may require the deputy (or where the deputy has died, his personal representative) to submit a final report on the discharge of his functions. If the Public Guardian is dissatisfied with any aspect of the final report he may apply to the court for an appropriate remedy (including the enforcement of security given by the deputy).[8]

Where the Public Guardian has concerns about the way in which the deputy is exercising his powers or any failure to exercise them, or there are concerns about the conduct of the deputy, the Public Guardian may require the deputy to provide specified information or documents.[9]

Right of deputy to require review of decisions made by the Public Guardian

The deputy may require the Public Guardian to reconsider any decision he has made in relation to the deputy under reg 42 of the Regulations. He has 14 days beginning with the date on which the notice of the decision is given to request the reconsideration.

Restrictions upon the powers of deputies

P must lack capacity

Under Section 20, a deputy does not have the power to make decisions on behalf of P in relation to a matter if he knows or has reasonable grounds for believing that P has capacity in relation to the matter.

The explanatory notes use the example of a person suffering from fluctuating mental capacity, and state that if P recovered his capacity, then the deputy could not carry on making decisions on his behalf.

No power to prohibit a person having contact with P

Nor does the deputy have power to prohibit a named person from having contact with P. This is a power which can only be exercised by the Court of Protection.

No power to replace a person responsible for P's health care

The deputy cannot direct a person responsible for P's health care to allow a different person to take over that responsibility. Again this is a power which can only be exercised by the court.

Restrictions on powers in relation to property

In relation to property, the deputy cannot be given powers in respect of the settlement of any of P's property (whether for P's benefit or of others), the execution for

P of a will, or the exercise of any power (including a power to consent) vested in P whether beneficially or as trustee or otherwise. These powers would be exercised by the court.

Cannot overrule a donee under an LPA

Nor may a deputy be given power to make a decision on behalf of P which is inconsistent with a decision made, within the scope of his authority and in accordance with the MCA, by the donee of a lasting power of attorney granted by P (or, if there is more than one donee, by any of them – S.20(4)).

Thus the deputy cannot go against what has been or is being decided by the donee(s) of a lasting power of attorney if the donee(s) is/are acting lawfully. If there is a dispute over the actions of a donee then the Court of Protection should use its powers under Sections 22 and 23 rather than appoint a deputy.

No power to refuse to consent to life-sustaining treatment

A deputy may not refuse consent to the carrying out or continuation of life sustaining treatment in relation to P (S.20(5)). (The words 'unless the court has conferred on the deputy express authority to that effect' and 'The court can only give express authority in exceptional circumstances' were contained in the Bill but omitted from the Act, so that the court cannot authorise the deputy to that effect. See discussion in Chapter 9 on advance decisions.)

The Joint Committee were strongly against giving powers to deputies to refuse life-sustaining treatment.[10] The Joint Committee strongly urged that the provisions allowing deputies to consent to treatment be restricted to exclude the withdrawal or refusal of life-sustaining treatment. The Joint Committee considered that unless there is a valid lasting power of attorney (LPA) or advance decision expressing the individual's wishes in relation to the subject, decisions relating to the carrying out or continuation of life-sustaining treatment should be referred to the Court of Protection for determination.[11]

Must follow Section 1 principles and Section 4 best interests

The deputy's authority is subject to the provisions of the MCA, and in particular the principles set out in Section 1 (see Chapter 3, Section 4 and the duty to act in the best interests of P, and Chapter 5). The Joint Committee was concerned that further guidance was required for deputies as to the standard of conduct they must maintain in the operation of their duties.[12]

Restriction on deputy in exercise of restraint of P

A deputy may not do any act intended to restrain P unless the four following conditions are satisfied:

1. that in doing the act the deputy is acting within the scope of an authority expressly conferred on him by the court

2. that P lacks, or the deputy reasonably believes that P lacks, capacity in relation to the matter in question
3. that the deputy reasonably believes that it is necessary to do the act in order to prevent harm to P
4. that the act is a proportionate response to:
    a. the likelihood of P's suffering harm, or[13]
    b. the seriousness of that harm

The definition of restraint for the purposes of this section is if the deputy uses, or threatens to use, force to secure the doing of an act which P resists, or restricts P's liberty of movement, whether or not P resists, or if the deputy authorises another person to take such action.

Section 20(13) stated that the deputy does more than merely restrain P if he deprives P of his liberty within the meaning of Article 5(1) of the European Convention on Human Rights. However like comparable provisions in the MCA (e.g. Section 6(5) (treatment) and Section 11(6) (donees)) this is to be repealed, as a consequence of the amendments to the MCA by the Mental Health Act 2007 required by the provisions to fill the Bournewood gap (see Chapters 3 and 13). An additional section to clarify the Court of Protection's powers in relation to welfare orders has been enacted (see Section 16A on page 129).

These restrictions on a deputy using restraint are the same as those imposed upon the donee of a lasting power of attorney (Section 11) and upon a carer or professional acting on behalf of P (Section 5). As in the other cases, depriving a person of his liberty within the meaning of Article 5 of the European Convention of Human Rights is more than restraint, and therefore not lawful for a carer, professional, donee of an LPA or deputy (see earlier discussion in Chapter 5 Scenario B10). This is however subject to the amendments to the MCA introduced by the Mental Health Act 2007, designed to fill the gap highlighted by the Bournewood case (see Chapter 13).

Duties of deputies

The Code of Practice identifies the following list as duties to be followed by the court-appointed deputy[14]. It notes that when agreeing to act as deputy, whether in relation to welfare or financial affairs, the deputy is taking on a role which carries power that he must use carefully and responsibly. The standard of conduct expected of deputies involves compliance with the following duties as an agent and with the statutory requirements:

- to comply with the principles of the Act
- to act in the best interests of the client
- to follow the Code of Practice
- to act within the scope of their authority given by the Court of Protection
- to act with due care and skill (duty of care)
- not to take advantage of their situation (fiduciary duty)
- to indemnify the person against liability to third parties caused by the deputy's negligence

- not to delegate duties unless authorised to do so
- to act in good faith
- to respect the person's confidentiality, and
- to comply with the directions of the Court of Protection.

Property and affairs deputies also have a duty to:

- keep accounts, and
- keep the person's money and property separate from own finances.

Scenario D5 illustrates the appointment of a deputy for a person in a care home.

A successor deputy

It is possible for the Court of Protection to appoint a successor to the deputy whom it appoints if the circumstances require. The Code of Practice uses the example of an elderly couple with a son with Down's syndrome who are appointed as joint deputies but are concerned what would happen when they die. In such a situation the Court of Protection could appoint other relatives to succeed them as deputies.[15]

Office of the Public Guardian

Public Guardian (S.57)

This officer, paid out of moneys provided by Parliament, is appointed by the Lord Chancellor with functions specified under Section 58 of the MCA. The Lord Chancellor may provide him with (or contract for the provision of) officers and staff. The functions may be performed by any of his officers. They are shown in Box 7.4.

Box 7.4: Functions which can be performed by the Office of the Public Guardian.

- establishing and maintaining a register of lasting powers of attorney
- establishing and maintaining a register of orders appointing deputies
- supervising deputies appointed by the court*
- directing a Court of Protection Visitor to visit:

  a donee of a lasting power of attorney
  a deputy appointed by the court, or
  the person granting the power of attorney.

To make a report to the Public Guardian on such matters as he may direct:

- receiving security which the court requires a person to give for the discharge of his functions
- receiving reports from donees of lasting powers of attorney and deputies appointed by the court

---

- reporting to the court on such matters relating to proceedings under the MCA as the court requires
- dealing with representations (including complaints) about the way in which a donee of a lasting power of attorney or a deputy appointed by the court is exercising his powers.*

*The two functions which are asterisked may be discharged in co-operation with any other person who has functions in relation to the care or treatment of P.

The Lord Chancellor may by regulations confer other functions on the Public Guardian and specify how he carries out his functions. These regulations can cover the security given by deputies appointed by the court, the fees which may be charged by the Public Guardian, how the fees are to be paid and the making of reports.

Regulations which came into force on 1 October 2007[16] cover the functions of the Public Guardian in establishing and maintaining the registers, applications for searches of the registers and the disclosure of additional information held by the Public Guardian. The Regulations also cover rules relating to security for the discharge of their functions (paras 33–7).

Statutory powers given to the Public Guardian include, at all reasonable times, the examination and taking of copies of:

- any health record
- any record health by a local authority and compiled in connection with a social services function, and
- any record held by a person registered under Part 2 of the Care Standards Act 2000 which relates to P.

The Public Guardian may interview P in private.

The Public Guardian is required under Section 60 to make an annual report to the Lord Chancellor about the discharge of his functions, and within one month of its receipt the Lord Chancellor must lay a copy of it before Parliament.

The Office of the Public Guardian has an important role to play in overseeing the registration of lasting powers of attorney. This was spelt out explicitly by Mr Burstow (a Liberal MP) in the House of Commons Select Committee:[17]

> That brings me to the role of the **Office of the Public Guardian**. In future, it will become aware of the vast majority of LPAs as they are registered, but the problem with that is that registration is no indication of the power being used, because one registers ahead of loss of capacity. How can we be certain that an LPA has been triggered and is being used appropriately? Under a later group of amendments, we will deal with safeguards relating to the individual who becomes the donee, checks on donees, and so on.

The new Public Guardian (Designate) was named as Richard Brook, who joined the Department of Constitutional Affairs in February 2006 as Chief Executive of the Public Guardianship Office and Public Guardian (designate). He will be responsible for the new Office of the Public Guardian (OPG) when launched in October 2007. As the Public Guardian, he will be responsible for regulating people appointed to make finance, health and welfare decisions for those who lack capacity. He defined his role as follows:

> Working in effective partnership with the judiciary, it will be our role to ensure that appropriate supervision regimes are in place which balance the autonomy of the individual with the most appropriate protection against abuse. We are currently considering how this regime can be effective yet as unobtrusive as possible. We will also have a role in providing the public with information about mental capacity issues and sign-posting people to the most appropriate form of help and assistance.[18]

Further information about the work of the Office of the Public Guardian and the forms used can be obtained from its website.[19]

Public Guardian Board

This Board established under Section 59 of the MCA has the duty of scrutinising and reviewing the way in which the Public Guardian discharges his functions and to make such recommendations to the Lord Chancellor about that matter as it thinks appropriate. The Lord Chancellor has a statutory duty to give due consideration to recommendations made by the Board in discharging its functions in relation to the appointment and function of the Public Guardian. The Lord Chancellor appoints the members of the Board, which must consist of at least one member who is a judge of the court and at least four members who are persons appearing to the Lord Chancellor to have appropriate knowledge or experience of the work of the Public Guardian. The Lord Chancellor has the power to make regulations covering the appointment and reappointment of the members, the selection of chairman, the term of office of chairman and members, their resignation, suspension or removal, the procedure and validation of proceedings. The Lord Chancellor also has the power to determine payments of expenses, allowances and remuneration to the members.

The Board must make an annual report to the Lord Chancellor about the discharge of its functions (S.59(9)).

Court of Protection visitors (S.61)

The Lord Chancellor can appoint a Court of Protection visitor to a panel of Special Visitors or a panel of General Visitors. (These Court of Protection visitors replace the current 'Lord Chancellor's Visitors' (see Section 102 of the Mental Health Act 1983).

Special Visitor

To be eligible for appointment as a Special Visitor a person must be a registered medical practitioner (or appear to the Lord Chancellor to have other suitable qualifications or training) and also appear to the Lord Chancellor to have special knowledge of and experience in cases of impairment of or disturbance in the functioning of the mind or brain.

General Visitor

In contrast a General Visitor need not have a medical qualification.

Duties of visitors

Visitors have the duty to carry out visits and produce reports, as directed by the court (Section 49(2)) or the Public Guardian (Section 58(1)(d)) in relation to those who lack capacity. Their functions and powers are similar to those of Lord Chancellor's Visitors appointed under Part 7 of the Mental Health Act 1983.

The Court of Protection visitor may be appointed for such term and subject to such conditions and may be paid such remuneration and allowances as the Lord Chancellor may determine.

Regulations set requirements for the notification of visits by the Public Guardian or the Court of Protection visitors[20].

Scenario D7 illustrates the appointment of a Visitor.

Powers of visitors

The Public Guardian (see above) or a Court of Protection visitor, in carrying out his functions, has the power at all reasonable times to examine and take copies of the following:

(a) any health record
(b) any record of, or held by, a local authority and compiled in connection with a social services function, and
(c) any record held by a person registered under Part 2 of the Care Standards Act 2000.

so far as the record relates to P.

The Public Guardian or the Court of Protection visitor may also interview P in private for the purpose of carrying out his functions.

If the Court of Protection visitor is a Special Visitor (i.e. a registered medical practitioner or someone with other suitable qualifications or training) and is making a visit in the course of complying with a requirement to make a report, he may, if the court so directs, carry out in private a medical, psychiatric or psychological examination of P's capacity and condition (S.49(9)).

When would a visitor be appointed?

The Code of Practice notes that:

> Court of Protection Visitors have an important part to play in investigating possible abuse. But their role is much wider than this. They can also check on the general wellbeing of the person who lacks capacity, and they can give support to attorneys and deputies who need help to carry out their duties.[21]

The Code of Practice describes a situation where a visitor is appointed, which is discussed in Scenario D7.

Advocacy and the Court of Protection

The Joint Committee was concerned that people lacking capacity might have considerable difficulties in accessing the Court of Protection, and recommended that consideration is given to the provision of independent advocacy services and other means of enabling people lacking capacity to participate as fully as possible in any hearing affecting their rights and entitlements[22] (this is discussed in Chapter 8).

People under 18 years

There is provision under Section 21 for the Lord Chancellor to make provision, in specified circumstances, for the transfer of proceedings relating to a person under 18, from the Court of Protection to a court with jurisdiction under the Children Act 1989 and vice versa (S.21) and Regulations were accordingly passed.[23] See Chapter 12 for further consideration on children and the Mental Capacity Act.

Code of Practice

The Joint Committee considered that further guidance is required for deputies as to the standard of conduct they must maintain in the operation of their duties. They also considered that guidance should also be issued to the Court of Protection to assist in the appointment of the most appropriate individual to act as a deputy. Paras 8.31–8.71 of the Code of Practice provide guidance on the appointment of deputies by the Court of Protection, their duties and responsibilities. The Code of Practice sets out the following analysis of the role of the Public Guardian in supervising deputies:[24]

[Para 8.70] The OPG is responsible for supervising and supporting deputies. But it must also protect people lacking capacity from possible abuse or exploitation. Anybody who suspects that a deputy is abusing their position should contact the OPG immediately. The OPG may instruct a Court of Protection Visitor to visit a deputy to investigate any matter of concern. It can also apply to the court to cancel a deputy's appointment.

The OPG will consider carefully any concerns or complaints against deputies [Para 8.71]. But if somebody suspects physical or sexual abuse or serious fraud, they should contact the police and/or social services immediately, as well as informing the OPG. Chapter 14 (of the Code of Practice) gives more information about the role of the OPG. It also discusses the protection of vulnerable people from abuse, ill treatment or wilful neglect and the responsibilities of various relevant agencies.

Court of Protection and lasting powers of attorney

The powers of the Court of Protection in relation to the validity and operation of lasting powers of attorney are set out in Sections 22 and 23, and are considered in Chapter 6.

Transitional provisions

As a result of the MCA, part 7 of the Mental Health Act 1983 is repealed, as is the Enduring Powers of Attorney Act 1985 (S.66(1)(a) and (b)). Schedule 5 of the MCA contains transitional provisions and savings in relation to Part 7 of the Mental Health Act (S.66(4)); see Chapter 17. The Court of Protection (Amendment) Rules 2005 (SI 2005, 667) made various amendments to the fees chargeable. They also enable the court to dispense with the service of a relevant application where the court considers it necessary to appoint an interim receiver.

Conclusions

The Court of Protection, its appointed deputies, the Office of the Public Guardian and its visitors and the Public Guardian Board have a key role to play in ensuring that the fundamental provisions of the new legislation are implemented, and that the rights of those lacking mental capacity are reasonably protected. It is hoped that in addition to the annual report required by the Public Guardian Board there will be regular monitoring of the work of the Court of Protection at an early stage, following implementation of the Act, to identify any weaknesses in the newly established institutions, systems and procedures. The implementation of the provisions relating to the new Court of Protection, the Office of the Public Guardian and lasting powers of attorney were delayed from April 2007 to October 2007 'in order to ensure adequate time to train the many civil servants and professionals affected by the Act and the very important changes that it brings'.[25]

References

1   Court of Protection Consultation Draft Rules CP 10/06 para 4.3.
2   Explanatory Memorandum on the Mental Capacity Act 2005, DCA para 138.
3   Court of Protection Consultation Draft Rules CP 10/06 para 4.16.
4   D v. *An NHS Trust (Medical Treatment: Consent: Termination)* [2004] 1 FLR 1110.
5   Code of Practice for the Mental Capacity Act 2005. Department of Constitutional Affairs February 2007 para 8.19–24. TSO, London.
6   House of Lords and House of Commons Joint Cttee on the Draft Mental Incapacity Bill, Session 2002-3, HL paper 189–1; HC 1083–1.
7   The Lasting Powers of Attorney, Enduring Powers of Attorney and Public Guardian Regulations 2007 (SI 2007/1253).
8   *Ibid.* reg 40.
9   *Ibid.* reg 41.

10 House of Lords and House of Commons Joint Committee on the Draft Mental Incapacity Bill, Session 2002-3, HL paper 189–1; HC 1083–1 paras 182–3.

11 *Ibid.* para. 184.

12 *Ibid.* para 180.

13 Code of Practice for the Mental Capacity Act 2005. Department of Constitutional Affairs February 2007 para 8.46 note 35 points out that the 'or' is a drafting error and it should be 'and' in keeping with Ss.6(3)(a) and 11(4)(b). Section 46 of the Mental Health Act 2007 amended Section 20(11) so that 'and' was substituted for 'or' (see Scenario D3).

14 Code of Practice for the Mental Capacity Act 2005. Department of Constitutional Affairs February 2007 para 8.56. TSO, London.

15 *Ibid.* para 8.44.

16 The Lasting Powers of Attorney, Enduring Powers of Attorney and Public Guardian Regulations 2007 (SI 2007/1253).

17 House of Commons Select Cttee 26 Oct 2004.

18 Mental Capacity update (2006). 7th edn. www.justice.gov.uk/whatwedo/mentalcapacity.htm/

19 www.guardianship.gov.uk

20 The Lasting Powers of Attorney, Enduring Powers of Attorney and Public Guardian Regulations 2007 (SI 2007/1253).

21 Code of Practice for the Mental Capacity Act 2005. Department of Constitutional Affairs February 2007 para 14.11. TSO, London.

22 Joint Committee para 170.

23 Mental Capacity Act 2005 (Transfer of Proceedings) order Statutory Instrument 2007 No 1899.

24 Code of Practice for the Mental Capacity Act 2005. Department of Constitutional Affairs February 2007 para 8.70. TSO, London.

25 Ministerial statement by Baroness Ashton of Upholland, Parliamentary Under-Secretary of State, DCA. House of Lords, 18 December 2006, Hansard.

Scenarios D
Court of Protection, Deputies
and Appointment of a Visitor

Court of Protection

The new Court of Protection has powers to make decisions on personal welfare in addition to decisions on property and finance, to which the former Court of Protection was restricted.

Scenario D1: Whose decision?

Henry, aged 84, was in hospital following a hip operation. A pre-discharge assessment was carried out by an occupational therapist who advised his wife, Monica, that it was highly likely that she would be unable to care for him at home and that it was preferable if they considered discharge to a care home. He would require a substantial input of nursing care which was not easily provided at home. Monica had not worked during her married life and was dependent upon Henry's occupational pension and state benefits. She feared that if he were to be admitted to a care home, and had to pay fees, she would have an inadequate income to live upon. She therefore opposed his admission to a care home and favoured his return back home. Henry was in the early stages of dementia. When lucid, he appeared to favour going to a care home, but his periods of lucidity were declining both in frequency and length. The hospital was concerned that Henry was blocking a bed and with the pressures of winter increasing, they wanted him discharged since he no longer needed hospital care. The social services was anxious to find accommodation for Henry since under the delayed discharges legislation it faced the possibility of a fine. Henry and Monica's two children were drawn into the dispute and whilst they sympathised with their mother's plight, they agreed that Henry would be too much for her to cope with and they raised the question of why Henry's accommodation should not be funded through the National Health Service (NHS), since his continuing care needs appear to meet the justification for top level fees being paid for his care. An independent mental capacity advocate was not appointed to represent Henry in the decision making, since it was considered that there were appropriate persons who could be consulted. In order to speed up the decision making, the social services department made an application to the Court of Protection for the issue of Henry's accommodation to be determined.

The first question which will have to be resolved is whether Henry has the requisite mental capacity to decide on the question of his future accommodation.

Evidence will be provided by social services and by Monica about Henry's capacity, and Henry should have the opportunity of trying to establish his capacity to make the decision (possibly with the assistance of the independent mental capacity advocate (IMCA) – see Chapter 8 – but this appointment will depend upon it being showed that there were no appropriate persons who could speak on behalf of Henry). If there is no agreement on Henry having the requisite capacity, then an application could be made to the Court of Protection for a court declaration on this point (see Chapter 4 and Scenarios A on the determination of capacity).

If the Court of Protection determines that Henry lacks the requisite capacity, it then has the option of the following measures:

- appointing a deputy with the power to decide on which accommodation is appropriate for Henry's needs
- making the decision on the basis of papers submitted
- holding a hearing to determine the issue.

In selecting which option is appropriate, the Court of Protection would be mindful of the statutory provisions that a decision of the court is to be preferred to the appointment of a deputy to make a decision (S.16(4)). Since there is a single issue to be determined in this case and therefore continuing supervision is not required, it is highly probable that the accommodation decision will be made either on the basis of the papers submitted to the court or after a short hearing of the court. In making its decision, the Court of Protection is bound to apply the principles set out in Section 1 of the Act (see Chapter 3) and also to use the criteria set down in Section 4 for deciding what is in the best interests of Henry (see Chapter 5 and Scenarios B). It would take into account the fact that Henry's condition, both mentally and physically, appears to be deteriorating and even if Monica could care for him initially, this would appear to be only for the short term.

Who should provide the accommodation?

The relatives have raised the question of why Henry's accommodation should not be funded through the NHS. Whoever becomes responsible for making decisions on behalf of Henry will have to ensure that Henry is represented in any application to the NHS Trust that it is the appropriate body to be providing his accommodation.

A recent case which considered the eligibility for NHS continuing care is discussed in Case D1 (see Continuing care on page 248).

Case D1: continuing care.[1]

G. applied for judicial review of a decision by an NHS trust that she did not qualify for continuing NHS healthcare. If the NHS provided care it would be free; if it were the social services, she would be means tested. The High Court held that an NHS trust should apply a primary health need test to determine whether accommodation should be provided by the NHS or social services. The criteria of the NHS trust for determining whether the patient had continuing care needs were fatally flawed, and it failed to give reasons why it considered that the patient's continuing care needs were neither complex nor intense. The court ordered the trust's decision to be set aside and remitted for fresh consideration.

What fees are payable?

The Court of Protection Fees Order[2] sets the fees to be charged. The fee for an application to the Court of Protection is £400; a hearing fee is £500; an appeal fee £400 and a copy of a document fee £5. There are exemptions from payment of those in receipt of specified benefits such as income support.

Who pays the fees?

The general rule set out in Rule 156 of the Court of Protection Rules[3] is that in proceedings relating to P's property and affairs, the fees shall be paid by P, or charged to his estate. In contrast in matters relating to personal welfare Rule 157 sets out the general rule that there will be no order as to the costs of the proceedings relating to personal welfare. Where proceedings relate to both property and affairs and personal welfare, there will be an apportionment of costs insofar as practicable (Rule 158). However under Rule 159 the court may depart from these principles if the circumstances so justify, taking into account the conduct of the parties, whether a party has succeeded on part of his case and the role of any public body involved. Conduct of the parties is defined in Rule 159 (2). Rule 9 of the Court of Protection Fees Order enables the Lord Chancellor to reduce or remit the fees payable where exceptional circumstances would involve undue hardship.

The underlying principle accepted by the DCA, which is not subject to the consultation, is that, for the first year of operation, the Court of Protection and the Office of the Public Guardian's (OPG) fees will be set at a level to recover approximately 80% of the costs of the two organisations. Fee exemptions and fee remissions will ensure that access to justice is protected for those unable to pay.

It may be that the costs to the public purse will be greater than that at present envisaged by the DCA since, once the new jurisdiction of the Court of Protection is extended to personal welfare issues, there will be many more cases where the person lacking (or alleged to be lacking) the requisite mental capacity who is either the applicant or the subject of the application does not have any significant financial resources. Such cases may become the majority of those heard by the Court of Protection. This would be very different from the former regime where only property and finance matters were the subject of its jurisdiction, and therefore by definition there would have been assets in the estate of the mentally incapacitated adult.

Making an application to the Court of Protection

On the facts of Scenario D1 how would the action be commenced? The situation is illustrated in Scenario D2.

Scenario D2: Making an application.

Social services under pressure to arrange for Henry's discharge to alternative accommodation was prepared to apply to the Court of Protection, but sought advice on how the application was to be made and what action was required of it.

Social services must comply with the pre-action protocol and make every effort to resolve the issue before it comes to court. Before it made its application to the Court, social services would have to ensure that all reasonable practicable steps had been taken to secure the agreement of the parties in the dispute. Only if these steps had been taken and failed, would social services be justified in seeking for permission to apply to the court. This is explained in Chapter 7.

Application to the Court of Protection

Social services is not one of the persons or organisations listed in Section 50(1) (i.e. the person lacking capacity, a deputy or donor or donee of a lasting power of attorney and the personal representative) who can make an application to the Court of Protection without seeking permission.

Social services would therefore have to seek the permission of the court to bring the application.

As applicant the social services department would begin the proceedings by filing an application notice on the approved form (unless there is an exception to this requirement) and comply with all the pre-action protocols.

The court would issue an application form. This must set out the information shown in Box D1 (paragraph 63 of the Court of Protection Rules (SI 2007 No 1744)).[4]

Box D1: Application form to commence Court of Protection proceedings.

- the matter which the applicant wants the court to decide
- the order which the applicant is seeking
- whether the applicant is acting in a representative capacity and if so, what that capacity is
- if the names of the applicant; P; any person with an interest; any person the applicant intends to notify
- any other relevant information and material (a practice direction will set this out).

The application form will be accompanied by any written evidence on which the applicant intends to rely and any other documents referred to in the application form. This may include written evidence that P is a person who lacks capacity to make the decision(s) in relation to the matter to which the application relates.

On receipt of the application the court will consider:

- whether to grant permission (if that is required)
- whether it could be linked with another application relating to P.

Informing P

Once the application form has been issued the applicant, the social services department must provide Henry with the information shown in Box D2 in a way that is appropriate to his circumstances (using simple language, visual aids or other means). (Paragraph 42 and 46 of the CP Rules SI 2007 No 1744).

Box D2: Informing P about an application to the Court of Protection.

- that an application relating to P has been issued
- who the applicant is
- that the application raised the question of whether P lacks capacity in relation to the matter or matters
- what will happen if the court makes any order or direction that has been applied for
- that P may seek advice and assistance, and
- where the application contains a proposal for an appointment of a person to make decisions on P's behalf in relation to the matter or matters to which the application relates, who that person is (if different from the applicant).

Henry must be provided with this information personally (Rule 46(2)) and it must be accompanied by a form for acknowledging service (Rule 47).

The social services department is also required under Rule 70 to serve a copy of the form on any person who is named as a respondent in the application, unless they have already been served with the form under another rule. Other persons specified in the practice direction must be notified of the application. These are listed in Box D3.

Box D3: Notice of the application form.

Must be given to:

- if P is under 18 years, his parent or guardian or a person with parental responsibility
- any person who has authority to act as an attorney or deputy in relation to a matter to which the application relates
- relatives of P (but where the applicant is a relative of P this need only be sent to those relatives who have the same or nearer degree of relationship to P than the applicant)
- any other person that the applicant reasonably considers has an interest in matters relating to P's best interest.

Any person served with the notice of the application must file an acknowledgement of service within 21 days, beginning with the date on which the document is served (Rule 72(2)). If that person opposes the application or seeks a different order, then his acknowledgement of service must be accompanied by written evidence on which the person intends to rely. Where P is notified under Rule 42 or one of the persons listed in Box D3 opposes the application or seeks a different order, the acknowledgement of service would be accompanied by an application for joinder as a party (Rule 75).

Failure by any of the persons, who have been served notice, to file an acknowledgement of service within the time limit means that they are bound by any order made or directions given as if he or she was a party to the proceedings.

Consideration of applications

Once the time allowed for the filing of an acknowledgment of service has passed, a court officer will give notice of the date on which the application is to be considered by the court. The notice will be given to P, each person who has filed an acknowledgment of service and any other person the court may direct.

Dispensing with a hearing

The court may deal with an application without a hearing if the parties agree that the court should dispose of the application without a hearing or if the court does not consider that a hearing would be appropriate. The court would have regard to the factors listed in Box D4 in deciding whether a hearing was necessary.

Box D4: Dispensing with a hearing (Rule 84(3)). Factors to be considered.

- the nature of the proceedings and the order sought
- whether the order sought is, or is likely to be, opposed by a person who appears to the court to have an interest in matters relating to P's best interests
- whether the case is likely to involve a substantial dispute of fact
- the complexity of facts and laws
- any wider public interest in the proceedings
- the circumstances of P and of any party with an interest
- any other matter specified in the relevant practice direction.
- whether the parties agree that the court should dispose of the application without a hearing

---

Would a hearing be likely in Henry's situation in Scenarios D1 and D2?

Let us assume that the social services department has requested an order declaring that Henry lacks the mental capacity to make his own decision on accommodation, and that it requires him to be discharged from hospital and transferred to a named care home.

It could be assumed that the IMCA (if one has been appointed) will have assisted Henry in returning an acknowledgement of service together with a joinder notice. Henry's wife and possibly the two children should have received notice under Rule 70 as relatives of Henry, and they could have responded with an acknowledgement of service together with a joinder notice.

The court will be faced with disputed evidence over whether Henry lacks capacity and to which accommodation Henry is discharged. Whilst the issues appear simple, the court may propose to hold a hearing because of the substantial dispute over the facts and the fact that an order is required as to whether Henry has the requisite mental capacity.

Public hearing

Once the court decides that a hearing is necessary and the decision cannot be made on the basis of the written information submitted, then the general rule is that the hearing should be in private (Rule 90(1)). However there are exceptions recognised under Rule 92 where a hearing could be held in public.

Rule 90(2) states that a private hearing is a hearing which only the following persons are entitled to attend:

- the parties
- P (whether or not a party)
- any person acting as a litigation friend
- any legal representative of a person specified above
- any court officer.

Rule 91 gives the Court general powers to authorise publication of information about proceedings and impose restrictions in identifying parties.

P and attendance at court

Henry should be able to attend at court and be heard on the question of whether an order should be made (whether or not he is a party to the proceedings). However the court can proceed with a hearing in his absence unless it considers that it would be inappropriate to do so.

P and his representation

At any stage, the court may give a direction as it sees fit for the appointment of a litigation friend to conduct proceedings on behalf of P or any other person with sufficient interest, if P or the other person lacks capacity to conduct the proceedings him/herself. A person may act as a litigation friend if he can fairly and competently conduct proceedings on behalf of P, and he has no interest adverse to that of P. The person who wishes to act as a litigation friend must file a certificate of suitability stating that he satisfies the above conditions, and serve the certificate of suitability on any person who is P's attorney or deputy and every person who is party to the proceedings. If the person wishing to be a litigation friend is a court-appointed deputy for P then he must serve a copy of the court order which appointed him (Rule 142(4)). This Rule does not apply to the Official Solicitor.

The court can under Rule 143 appoint the Official Solicitor or some other person to act as P's litigation friend. The court has considerable powers under Rule 144 to direct that a person cannot act as a litigation friend, or to terminate the appointment or appoint a new litigation friend in substitution for an existing one.

If P regains capacity, then if a litigation friend has been appointed for him this person will continue with his appointment until it is brought to an end by order of the court (Rule 148).

Deputies

In certain circumstances the Court of Protection will decide that it is preferable if a deputy were to be appointed, rather than the Court of Protection itself making the decision. The legal powers and restrictions upon a deputy are considered in Chapter 7. In Scenario D3 we take a situation where a deputy is appointed.

Scenario D3: The appointment of a deputy.

Ralph was severely injured in a road accident. After many months in hospital he was discharged home but required 24-hour nursing care. Under a compensation settlement agreed with the court, he received £2 million which was in trust to be administered on his behalf. A dispute arose between the trustees, which included Ralph's father and one brother, as to whether some of these funds should be used to build a new property or whether an extension on his parents' existing home should be built for him. He has two older brothers who are opposed to the idea of an extension, since they consider that their share in the parental home would be forfeited were Ralph to have an extension there, and they consider that Ralph should have his own accommodation. Ralph himself had serious head injuries and appears unable to understand information given to him or to communicate. In addition ongoing decisions relating to Ralph's contact with an uncle whom the father and brothers consider has an upsetting effect upon Ralph, and decisions relating to the treatment which Ralph should be receiving in the future need to be made.

The Court of Protection decides to appoint a family friend (Bob) as deputy for Ralph. Bob, since he does not seem to be involved in the family dispute, could be trusted to act in Ralph's best interests and such an appointment is acceptable to him.

Bob must consent to the appointment and be at least 18 years.

Bob could make the following decisions:

- he could decide where Ralph is to live
- he could specify how much contact Ralph's uncle is to have with Ralph but he would not be able to prohibit the uncle having any contact at all
- he could agree the treatment regime which Ralph is to have with the General Practitioner and visiting nurses but he could not refuse consent to the carrying out or continuation of life-sustaining treatment
- he must make all these decisions in the best interests of Ralph and follow the principles set down in Section 1 of the MCA
- he cannot carry out an act which is intended to restrain Ralph unless:
    a. he is acting within the scope of an authority expressly given him by the Court of Protection
    b. he believes Ralph to lack mental capacity to make these decisions
    c. he believes it necessary to do the act in order to prevent harm to Ralph and
    d. the act is a proportionate response to the likelihood of Ralph's suffering harm or[5] (and) the seriousness of that harm
- he will be treated as Ralph's agent in relation to anything done or decided by him within the scope of his appointment
- he will be entitled to be reimbursed out of Ralph's property for his reasonable expenses in discharging these functions
- he will be entitled to remuneration out of Ralph's property for his work if the court of Protection had made the appropriate direction when he was appointed
- he may be required to give a security to the Public Guardian, as directed by the court, for the due discharge of his functions, and
- he may be required by the Court of Protection to submit such reports to the Public Guardian at such times or at such intervals as directed by the court.

Who can be appointed as deputy?

Scenario D4 considers the issue as to who is the appropriate person to be appointed as deputy.

> ## Scenario D4: Who should be the deputy?
>
> Beryl has motor neurone disease and has been moved to a residential home. She is unable to speak, but carers are able to communicate with her through signs and pictures. There are many decisions relating to her care and treatment and accommodation which require to be determined. Social services recommends that an application should be made to the Court of Protection for a deputy to be appointed. Who is likely to be the chosen person?

The Court of Protection would, if it decided that a deputy was the most suitable means of acting in Beryl's best interests, consider all possible persons. If Beryl has no close friend or relative who was able to act on her behalf, it is likely that it would appoint someone who is an office-holder or in a specified position, such as a director of social services or other person to be the deputy.

The deputy must be over 18 years and consent to being appointed as deputy. The Code of Practice recommends that:

> Paid care workers (for example, care home managers) should not agree to act as a deputy because of the possible conflict of interest – unless there are exceptional circumstances (for example, if the care worker is the only close relative of the person who lacks capacity). But the court can appoint someone who is an office-holder or in a specified position (for example, the Director of Adult Services of the relevant local authority). In this situation, the court will need to be satisfied that there is no conflict of interest before making such an appointment (see paragraphs 8.58–8.60).[6]

It would be possible in Scenario D4 for the Court of Protection to appoint two deputies: one with the power to make care and treatment decisions, the other with responsibilities in relation to property and affairs.

Scenario D5 considers the situation where the manager of a home is informed that a deputy has been appointed for one of the residents.

> ## Scenario D5: Deputy appointed for resident.
>
> Joyce is the manager of a care home. She is a registered nurse and has considerable experience in the residential care sector. Freda is admitted to the home from her family home. Freda has suffered a severe stroke which has left her unable to speak and with limited mobility. She is unable to communicate her decisions and the Court of Protection has appointed a deputy to take decisions on her behalf. Following her admission Freda suffers a cardiac arrest and Joyce is uncertain what action should be taken.

As soon as Joyce becomes aware that a deputy has been appointed on behalf of a resident she needs to investigate to establish the following facts:

- What powers have been given to the deputy?
- How long do these powers last?
- How can contact be made with the deputy?
- What information must be given to the deputy?
- In what circumstances must the deputy be contacted?

In Scenario D5 it is possible that the Court of Protection has only given the deputy powers in relation to Freda's financial affairs and the deputy has no duties in relation to Freda's care and treatment. Nevertheless it is in the best interests of Freda that Joyce should have regular contact with the deputy, since it may be that further funding of outings and extras to the basic care Freda receives could improve her quality of life. In the circumstances of the heart attack, Joyce has a duty of care to ensure that Freda receives immediate medical attention and an ambulance should be called.

Supervision of a deputy

In Scenario D6 we consider issues relating to the supervision of a deputy.

Scenario D6: Supervision of a deputy.

Jack was appointed by the Court of Protection as a deputy with responsibilities for the property and affairs of his brother, Amos, who had been injured at birth as the result of negligence by the midwife. He had received compensation from the NHS trust and Jack had specific powers to take financial decisions in the best interests of Amos.

Mandy, the sister of Jack and Amos, suspected that Jack was not acting in Amos's best interests, but was funding his own family from Amos's money. She wished to challenge his actions.

The first step Mandy should take would probably be to see if her concerns could be resolved by direct contact with Jack. Jack should have prepared accounts showing how Amos's property had been used. If these inquiries fail to meet her concerns, then she could ask the OPG to investigate whether Jack was acting appropriately. As the supervising authority for court-appointed deputies, the OPG has a responsibility to hear complaints. The Public Guardian can direct a Court of Protection visitor to visit a deputy to investigate any matter of concern (see Scenario D7). If Mandy's fears prove to be based on sound evidence, then Jack could be removed as deputy. In addition a report could be made to the police that Jack is guilty of a criminal offence of theft or fraud.

Appointment of a visitor

In the Code of Practice guidance is given on the anticipated role of the OPG, and the following situation set out in Scenario D7 is provided.[7]

Scenario D7: The appointment of a General Visitor.

Mrs Quinn made a lasting power of attorney (LPA) appointing her nephew, Ian, as her financial attorney. She recently lost capacity to make her own financial decisions, and Ian has registered the LPA. He has taken control of Mrs Quinn's financial affairs. But Mrs Quinn's niece suspects that Ian is using Mrs Quinn's money to pay off his own debts. She contacts the OPG, which sends a General Visitor to visit Mrs Quinn and Ian. The visitor's report will assess the facts. It might suggest the case go to court to consider whether Ian has behaved in a way which:

- goes against his authority under the LPA,

or

- is not in Mrs Quinn's best interests.

The Public Guardian will decide whether the court should be involved in the matter. The court will then decide if it requires further evidence. If it thinks that Ian is abusing his position, the court may cancel the LPA.

References

1 *R. (on the application of Grogan)* v. *Bexley NHS Care Trust* [2006] EWHC 44; (2006) 9 CCL Rep 188.
2 Court of Protection Fees Order Statutory Instrument SI 2007 No 1745.
3 Court of Protection Rules Statutory Instrument SI 2007 no 1744.
4 Court of Protection Rules Statutory Instrument SI 2007 no 1744 para 63.
5 Code of Practice for the Mental Capacity Act 2005. Department of Constitutional Affairs February 2007 para 8.46 note 35 points out that the 'or' is a drafting error and it should be 'and', in keeping with Ss. 6(3)(a) and 11(4)(b). Section 46 of the Mental Health Act 2007 amended S. 20(11) so that 'and' was substituted for 'or'.
6 Code of Practice for the Mental Capacity Act 2005. Department of Constitutional Affairs February 2007 para 8.41. TSO, London.
7 *Ibid.* para 14.10.

8 Independent Mental Capacity Advocates

Background to the provision on independent advocates

There was considerable concern during the parliamentary debates on the Bill and the discussions of the Joint Committee that adults who lacked mental capacity did not in the earlier drafts have a right of access to an independent mental capacity advocate or advocacy service. As a consequence of these concerns significant provisions were made in Sections 35–40 for an Independent Mental Capacity Advocacy service (IMCA).

In July 2005 the Department of Health (DH) issued a consultation paper on the new IMCA service.[1] The consultation period ended on 30 September 2005. Consultation covered the following main areas:

- the operation of the IMCA service
- the main functions the IMCA will carry out
- the definition of 'serious medical treatment' – one of the triggers for involving an IMCA
- whether to extend the service to cover other groups of people or different circumstances.

The DH published the results of its consultation on the IMCA service on 19 April 2006. The report includes the Government's response on the implementation and operation of the service.[2] (Separate consultation took place in Wales – see Chapter 16.)

The principle of advocacy

The philosophy behind the appointment of an advocate, which is given statutory force, is that a person to whom a proposed act or decision relates should, so far as practicable, be represented and supported by a person who is independent of any person who will be responsible for the act or decision (S.35(4)).

When should an advocate be appointed?

There are three provisions for the involvement of independent mental capacity advocates contained in the Mental Capacity Act (MCA). They are in relation to the provision of:

- serious medical treatment by National Health Service (NHS) body (S.37)
- accommodation by NHS body (S.38), and
- accommodation by a local authority (S.39).

In addition, using the powers given in the MCA, the Secretary of State and the Welsh Assembly may make regulations as to the functions of independent mental capacity advocates. Regulations made under these provisions[3] for England (for Wales see Chapter 16) extend the appointment of an IMCA to the following circumstances:

- where there is a review of the accommodation arrangements (reg 3), or
- where an NHS body or local authority (LA) proposes to take protective measures in relation to a person who lacks the requisite mental capacity (reg 4).

There are conditions specified for each of these situations which are considered in detail below.

Who can be an advocate?

Following the consultation on the IMCA services the Government in its response document stated that:

> Regulations should set out minimum standards for individual advocates – in particular, that they should all be subject to Criminal Records Bureau (CRB) checks on employment and receive appropriate training. In addition, the organisations who will be commissioned to provide the service will also have to meet appropriate standards as part of the commissioning/contract arrangements.

It also proposed that there should be a national training qualification developed, which includes specific pathways for both the IMCA and for Mental Health advocates.

The IMCA services will therefore be obliged to ensure that potential independent advocates have the requisite training to be able to support the person who lacks the requisite mental capacity.

In its response to the consultation, the Government stated that it agreed that advocates providing the IMCA service should receive appropriate training covering the key competencies, skills and knowledge required, including the law, diversity issues and communication skills. It intended to put such a requirement into the regulations.

The Government agreed that training for IMCAs should be linked where appropriate to independent mental health advocates training. Officials are working with stakeholders on the feasibility of developing a national advocacy qualification, to be accredited by the Qualifications and Curriculum Authority (QCA) and provided by an awarding body such as the Open College Network (OCN). The intention is that this qualification should be modular, with basic units covering key competencies, and additional units or pathways separately covering IMCA and independent mental health advocates requirements. Other pathways could be added in the future. This would enable advocates to build up their qualification by undertaking different pathways. The intention is for the DH to commission the training materials and to have the training course approved by the QCA by April 2007. Colleges and other bodies could apply to provide the training on a regional basis, with the aim of maximising flexibility of delivery as far as possible.

General Regulations[4] stipulate that:

No person may be appointed to act as an IMCA for the purposes of Sections 37–39 or under the regulations made under Section 41, unless:

a. he is for the time being approved by a local authority on the grounds that he satisfies the appointment requirements, or
b. he belongs to a class of persons which is for the time being approved by a local authority on the grounds that all persons in that class satisfy the appointment requirements.

The appointment requirements are defined as:

a. he has appropriate experience or training or an appropriate combination of experience and training
b. he is a person of integrity and good character, and
c. he is able to act independently of any person who instructs him.[5]

Before deciding if a person is of integrity and good character, an enhanced criminal record certificate issued under Sections 113A or B of the Police Act 1997 as amended by Section 163 of the Serious Organised Crime and Police Act 2005 is required.

IMCAs were named as a group that is subject to mandatory checking under the new vetting and barring system in the Safeguarding Vulnerable Groups Act 2006.

Powers of the independent mental capacity advocate (S.35(6))

In order to enable him to carry out his functions, an independent mental capacity advocate may:

a. interview in private the person whom he has been instructed to represent, and
b. at all reasonable times, examine and take copies of:
    - any health record
    - any record of, or held by a local authority and compiled in connection with a social services function, and
    - any record held by a person registered under Part 2 of the Care Standards Act 2000,

which the person holding the record considers may be relevant to the independent mental capacity advocate's investigation.

These statutory provisions followed significant criticisms by the Joint Committee,[6] which noted the absence of provision in the Bill to clarify rights of access to information about the mentally incapacitated persons by advocates.

What are the duties and functions of the independent mental capacity advocate?

In addition the MCA gives powers to the appropriate authorities to draw up regulations[7] which may require the advocate to take specified steps towards the purposes shown in Box 8.1.

Box 8.1: Purposes of the IMCA (S.36(2) MCA).

a.   providing support to the person whom he has been instructed to represent (P) so that P may participate as fully as possible in any relevant decision
b.   obtaining and evaluating relevant information
c.   ascertaining what P's wishes and feelings would be likely to be, and the beliefs and values that would be likely to influence P, if he had capacity
d.   ascertaining what alternative courses of action are available in relation to P
e.   obtaining a further medical opinion where treatment is proposed and the advocate thinks that one should be obtained.

The regulations have also made provision as to circumstances in which the advocate may challenge, or provide assistance for the purpose of challenging, any relevant decision (see below).

The regulations which came into force on 1 April 2007 specify the following functions for the IMCA in England (for Wales see Chapter 16):

The general duty of the IMCA, when instructed by an authorised person to represent a person 'P', is that he **must determine in all the circumstances how best to represent and support P.**

In particular, the IMCA must:

a.   verify that the instructions were issued by an authorised person;
b.   to the extent that it is practicable and appropriate to do so
  • interview P, and
  • examine the records relevant to P to which the IMCA has access under Section 35(6) of the Act;
c.   to the extent that it is practicable and appropriate to do so, consult
  • persons engaged in providing care or treatment for P in a professional capacity or for remuneration, and
  • other persons who may be in a position to comment on P's wishes, feelings, beliefs or values; and

d.   take all practicable steps to obtain such other information about P, or the act or decision that is proposed in relation to P, as the IMCA considers necessary.[8]

The IMCA must evaluate all the information he has obtained for the purpose of:

a.   ascertaining the extent of the support provided to P to enable him to participate in making any decision about the matter in relation to which the IMCA has been instructed;
b.   ascertaining what P's wishes and feelings would be likely to be, and the beliefs and values that would be likely to influence P, if he had capacity in relation to the proposed act or decision;
c.   ascertaining what alternative courses of action are available in relation to P;
d.   where medical treatment is proposed for P, ascertaining whether he would be likely to benefit from a further medical opinion.[9]

The IMCA is required to prepare a report for the authorised person who instructed him (reg 6(6)) and may include in the report such submissions as he considers appropriate in relation to P and the act or decision which is proposed in relation to him (reg 6(7)).

It should be noted that the IMCA does not actually make the decision. His or her role is to support P by ascertaining what P's wishes and feelings, beliefs and values would likely have been, had P had the requisite capacity. The IMCA collates all the relevant information and passes it on to the authority responsible for making the decision. The IMCA can also obtain a second medical opinion where he or she considers it necessary. The regulations also enable the IMCA to challenge any decision which has been made, according to the power granted in Section 36(3) (see **Disputes between IMCA and others** page 173).

How is an advocate held to account, if he has failed to fulfil these duties?

The IMCA service would be responsible for ensuring that the individual advocate performs his or her duties in accordance with the statutory provisions, and ensures that P's wishes and feelings, beliefs and values are made known to the appropriate authorities.

Who monitors what the advocate is doing?

The IMCA service would carry out a monitoring role and would report to its commissioners on the overall effectiveness and functioning of the service.

What about payment to the advocate?

The individual advocate would be paid by the IMCA service, which in turn would look to the appropriate NHS body or local authority to fund the service. Government funds are being allocated to the statutory bodies for this purpose.

Who can challenge the appointment of an advocate, e.g. if there is a split in the family?

In the event of a dispute over the appointment of an IMCA, the complainant would be encouraged to discuss his or her concerns with the appropriate body. It may be that a family member considers that an advocate should not have been appointed, or that the wrong person, who is not independent, has been appointed. Eventually such concerns which relate to whether the decision making will be in the best interests of the person lacking the requisite mental capacity, would be resolved by the Court of Protection.

Can an advocate access the patient's records?

As noted above the advocate has a statutory power, at all reasonable times, to examine and take copies of: any health record; any record of, or held by a local authority and compiled in connection with a social services function, and any record held by a person registered under Part 2 of the Care Standards Act 2000. However the person holding the record must consider that the record may be relevant to the independent mental capacity advocate's investigation. If the holder of the record is of the view that the record in question is not relevant, access can be refused.

Is an advocate under a duty of confidentiality?

The advocate has a duty to ensure that information he or she obtains about P is only made known to a person or authority, which, because of the decision which has to be made, has a legal right to that information. To pass on that information to a person who is not so eligible would be a breach of confidentiality and also an offence under data protection legislation.

What training will an advocate have?

The IMCA service will arrange for training to be made available for the advocates.

The DH working with the Social Care Institute for Excellence (SCIE) has commissioned Action for Advocacy (A4A)[10] to develop induction training materials for people who are appointed to act as IMCAs in England and Wales. The training pack was ready before the implementation of the IMCA service in April 2007.[11]

The Department for Constitutional Affairs (DCA) has commissioned the Making Decisions Alliance (MDA)[12] and the National Care Association (NCA)[13] to write two information booklets on the Mental Capacity Act. One is for people who may lack capacity and the other for family and unpaid carers. They are available from the DCA website.

When could an advocate be appointed in spite of family and friends being available?

When decisions are being made about serious medical treatment, the NHS body has a duty to arrange for the appointment of an IMCA, only if it is satisfied that there is no person, other than one engaged in providing care or treatment for P in a professional capacity or for remuneration, whom it would be appropriate to consult in determining what would be in P's best interests (S.37(1)(b)). Thus if a family member or close friend of P is able to speak on behalf of P, then the duty to appoint an IMCA does not arise.

The wording here is important: 'whom it would be appropriate to consult' would hopefully rule out those family members or friends who have decided views on the outcome and would not ascertain P's own wishes, feelings, beliefs and values. Hopefully resource constraints will not affect the decision on when it would be 'appropriate' to have an IMCA in such circumstances. Similar requirements exist in relation to the appointment of an advocate when accommodation decisions are being made by an NHS body or a local authority. Section 38(1)(b) states that '. . . if it is satisfied that there is no person, other than one engaged in providing care or treatment for P in a professional capacity or for remuneration, whom it would be appropriate for it to consult in determining what would be in P's best interests.' There is similar wording for Section 39(1)(b) and the arrangements by a local authority for accommodation.

Who else could be consulted before an IMCA is appointed?

There is a statutory duty on the decision maker under Section 4(7), when determining what is in P's best interests, to take into account, if it is practicable and appropriate to consult them, the views of:

(a) anyone named by the person as someone to be consulted on the matter in question or on matters of that kind
(b) anyone engaged in caring for the person or interested in his welfare, as to what would be in the person's best interests and, in particular:
   - the person's past and present wishes and feelings (and, in particular, any relevant written statement made by him when he had capacity)
   - the beliefs and values that would be likely to influence his decision if he had capacity, and
   - the other factors that he would be likely to consider if he were able to do so.

Exceptions to the appointment of an IMCA

The authorities are not required to arrange for the appointment of an IMCA where there is:

(a) a person nominated by P (in whatever manner) as a person to be consulted in matters affecting his interests

(b)   a donee of a lasting power of attorney created by P
(c)   a deputy appointed by the court for P, or
(d)   a donee of an enduring power of attorney (within the meaning of Schedule 4) created by P.

IMCA and court appointed deputy

It is clear from the statutory provisions that if a deputy has been appointed for P, then an IMCA cannot be appointed. The deputy makes decisions on behalf of P within the powers granted by the Court of Protection. However it is clear that where decisions relating to serious treatment, NHS and LA accommodation are to be made, then the deputy will be consulted by the decision maker and an IMCA will not be appointed. Similar provisions would apply where a lasting power of attorney has been appointed by P.

How can an advocate challenge decisions made in the light of information he has provided which seems to have been ignored?

There is a statutory duty for the NHS body or the LA to take into account the report of the IMCA. If the question of serious medical treatment arises, then the NHS body must, in providing or securing the provision of treatment for P, take into account any information given, or submissions made, by the independent mental capacity advocate (S.37(5)). Where the NHS is involved in providing accommodation, then under Section 38(5), the NHS body must, in deciding what arrangements to make for P, take into account any information given, or submissions made, by the independent mental capacity advocate. Likewise the local authority must, under Section 39(6), in deciding what arrangements to make for P take into account any information given, or submissions made, by the independent mental capacity advocate.

The authorities only have to 'take into account' the information or submissions of the IMCA. It may be difficult for the IMCA to provide evidence that they failed in this duty, even when the decision made is completely contrary to his or her report. However the Regulations provide that where an IMCA has been instructed to represent a person and a decision affecting P is made (including a decision as to his capacity) then the IMCA has the same rights to challenge the decision as he would have if he were a person (other than an IMCA) engaged in caring for P or interested in his welfare.[14] This is illustrated in Scenario E6 and see page 173.

Can an advocate delegate responsibility?

The appointment of the IMCA would be a personal one, and any change of IMCA would be subject to the decision of the IMCA service. It is highly unlikely that they would permit any delegation of the IMCA's duties.

What problems might an advocate face?

Perhaps the biggest problem that an advocate might face will be the time constraints within which the information has to be obtained and the report prepared. Resource issues means that only a limited time is available for this work to be done. The IMCA may be fortunate if paid carers have a long-standing knowledge of and relationship with P. They would then be able to pass on to the IMCA much information about P's wishes, feelings etc. However where there is a swift turnover of staff and they do not know P so well, then more time would have to be taken by the IMCA to obtain this information. Because of communication difficulties and the fact that a considerable time is taken for systems of communication to develop, the IMCA might not find it possible to obtain the information and write the report within the expected time. Some conditions, for example strokes, might leave a person with profound communication problems and for an IMCA to determine whether or not they have capacity, and also if they are deemed to lack capacity, what would their wishes and feelings be, could take a considerable time. It must be remembered that principle 2 in Section 1 states that:

> A person is not to be treated as unable to make a decision unless all practicable steps to help him to do so have been taken without success.

This principle must be followed by the IMCA and so all practicable steps must be taken by the IMCA to enable P to make his or her own decisions. Research into the advocacy role of the learning disability nurse has shown the complexity of the advocacy role.[15] It showed that clients with learning disabilities considered that the relationship between themselves and any possible advocate was of the utmost importance and that these relationships should preferably be long term, enabling the development of mutual trust and understanding which they considered vital to the successful advocacy partnership.[16] This will clearly not be a feature of the one-off statutory provision of independent mental capacity advocates.

The problem of obtaining sufficient information in the time available is illustrated in Scenario E8.

What happens if an advocate wishes to have an input into decisions on which the responsible authority decides that there is no need to seek IMCA advice?

This is considered in Scenario E9.

It is likely that this situation will arise frequently, since at present the situations specified by the MCA and the subsequent regulations cover only a tiny proportion of those occasions where the person lacking the requisite mental capacity may need independent advocacy. There are of course many advocacy arrangements in place run by voluntary groups, charities, statutory and other organisations, and it may be possible for a person to receive such help, even though it is outside of the provisions of the MCA. (See list of websites for some of these organisations.) In the future of course, as resources permit, the remit of the IMCA may be extended further by new regulations.

Scenarios E5 and E9 illustrate situations which could arise when the IMCA who has been commissioned to represent a person incapable of making the requisite decision in a specific area, considers that he should be represented in other types of decisions, where the authority is not yet obliged to appoint an IMCA.

What if P disagrees with the IMCA?

It is difficult to see this arising, since the main role of the IMCA is to report to the appropriate authority what P's wishes, feelings, values and beliefs would likely to have been had P had the capacity to make his or her own decisions. The IMCA represents P, and therefore his or her own personal opinion as to what should happen to P is irrelevant. If a dispute arises between P and the IMCA over what is in P's best interests, it is likely that the IMCA is not representing P appropriately and a complaint could be made to the service which contracted the IMCA. However a dispute could arise over whether in fact P lacks capacity. In this situation, it is open to P to apply to the Court of Protection for a declaration that he or she has the requisite capacity to make his or her own decisions.

What about documentation by advocate?

The IMCA is required to prepare a report for the authorised person who instructed him.[17] It will therefore be essential for the IMCA to keep records on his discussions with P and with other people and the contents of his submission and report to the relevant authorities. The IMCA services will probably provide guidance on the documentation to be kept.

Statutory situations where an IMCA must be appointed

Providing serious medical treatment (S.37)

Scenario E2 illustrates the appointment of an IMCA under this Section.

Serious medical treatment is defined (S.37(6)) as treatment which involves providing, withholding or withdrawing treatment of a kind prescribed by regulations to be drawn up by the Secretary of State or National Assembly for Wales. Following the consultation on the IMCA service, the Government stated that the definition of serious medical treatment in the regulations should not list specific treatments, but the regulations should set out the characteristics of the decision to be reached. As a consequence reg 4[18] defines serious medical treatment as follows:

Treatment which involves providing, withdrawing or withholding treatment in circumstances where:

a. in a case where single treatment is being proposed, there is a fine balance between its benefits to the patient and the burdens and risks it is likely to entail for him,

b. in a case where there is a choice of treatments, a decision as to which one to use is finely balanced, or

c. what is proposed would be likely to involve serious consequences for the patient.

The instruction of an independent mental capacity advocate must be made in the following circumstances:

- if serious medical treatment is being considered for P and P lacks capacity to consent to the treatment, and
- there is no person, other than the person providing treatment in a professional capacity or for remuneration, whom it would be appropriate to consult to determine what would be in P's best interests.

If these conditions exist then, under Section 37(3) before treatment is provided, the NHS body must instruct an independent mental capacity advocate to represent P.

The NHS body has been defined in reg 3 of the regulations[19] drawn up by the Secretary of State or the National Assembly for Wales (S.37(7)) as:

- a Strategic Health Authority
- an NHS Foundation Trust
- a Primary Care Trust
- an NHS Trust, or
- a Care Trust.

Even though the regulations do not list the kinds of treatments which would come under the definition of serious medical treatment, the Code of Practice does give an illustrative list as follows:

- chemotherapy and surgery for cancer
- electro-convulsive therapy
- therapeutic sterilisation
- major surgery (such as open-heart surgery or brain/neuro-surgery)
- major amputations (for example, loss of an arm or leg)
- treatments which will result in permanent loss of hearing or sight
- withholding or stopping artificial nutrition and hydration, and
- termination of pregnancy.

But it warns that it depends on the actual circumstances and consequences as to whether these come within the definition in any particular case, and they are illustrative examples only. The Code of Practice points out that there are also many more treatments which will be defined as serious medical treatments under the Act's regulations.[20]

The NHS body has a statutory duty (S.37(5)) to take into account any information given, or submissions made, by the independent mental capacity advocate, in providing or securing the provision of treatment for P. See Scenario E2 for a situation involving an IMCA for serious medical treatment decisions.

Urgent serious medical treatment

In an emergency situation where treatment needs to be provided as a matter of urgency, it may be provided even though the NHS body has not been able to comply with the requirement to instruct an independent mental capacity advocate to represent P (S.37(4)).

Section 37 does not apply if P's treatment is regulated by Part 4 of the Mental Health Act 2007 (S.37(2)) (see Chapter 13).

Extremely serious medical treatments and other decisions

Some treatments such as a non-therapeutic sterilisation, ending artificial feeding of a PVS patient and other decisions must be made by a declaration of the Court of Protection. However an independent mental capacity advocate should still be appointed under the provisions of Section 37 (see Code of Practice para 10.48 and Chapter 8 of the Code of Practice).

Arranging accommodation by NHS body (S.38)

An NHS body (as defined above) must instruct an independent mental capacity advocate to represent P if it is proposing to make arrangements

a. for the provision of accommodation in a hospital or care home for a person P who lacks capacity to agree to the arrangements, or
b. for a change in P's accommodation to another hospital or care home

and the NHS body is satisfied that there is no person, other than one engaged in providing care or treatment for P in a professional capacity or for remuneration, whom it would be appropriate for it to consult in determining what would be in P's best interests (S.38(1)).

An amendment to the Mental Capacity Act made by the Mental Health Act 2007 (Para 4(2) of Schedule 8) makes it clear that a person appointed under Part 10 of Schedule A1 to be P's representative is not, by virtue of that appointment, engaged in providing care or treatment for P in a professional capacity or for remuneration.

Before making the arrangements, the NHS body must instruct an independent mental capacity advocate to represent P unless it is satisfied that:

a. the accommodation is likely to be provided for a continuous period which is less than the applicable period, or
b. the arrangements need to be made as a matter of urgency.

If the NHS body

a. did not instruct an independent mental capacity advocate to represent P before making the arrangements because it was satisfied that these subsections applied, but
b. subsequently has reason to believe that the accommodation is likely to be provided for a continuous period
    *   beginning with the day on which accommodation was first provided in accordance with the arrangements, and
    *   ending on or after the expiry of the applicable period

it must instruct an independent mental capacity advocate to represent P.

This requirement ensures that persons placed in accommodation for less than the prescribed periods will come under the provisions of Section 38 if their stay is extended beyond the prescribed period.

Where an independent mental capacity advocate is instructed, the NHS body must take into account any information given, or submission made, in deciding what arrangements to make for P (S.38(5)).

'Applicable period' means 28 days in relation to accommodation in a hospital and eight weeks in relation to accommodation in a care home (S.38(9)).

This statutory requirement for the NHS body to instruct an independent mental capacity advocate does not apply if P is accommodated as a result of an obligation imposed on him under the Mental Health Act (S.38(2)) (see Chapter 13). A new Subsection 2A to Section 38 has been added to the Mental Capacity Act by the Mental Health Act 2007 (Para 4(2) of Schedule 9) and Section 2A states:

This section [i.e. Section 38] does not apply if:

(a) an independent mental capacity advocate must be appointed under Section 39A or 39C (whether or not by the NHS body) to represent P and

(b) the hospital or care home in which P is to be accommodated under the arrangements referred to in this section is the relevant hospital or care home under the authorisation referred to in that section.

The definition of 'NHS body' for the purpose of Section 38 is the same as that for Section 37 (see **Providing Serious Medical Treatment (S.37)** page 164).

Arranging accommodation by a local authority body (S.39)

Scenarios E1 and E4 illustrates the effect of this provision.

Advice from an independent mental capacity advocate must be sought by a local authority if it is proposing to make arrangements:

a. for the provision of residential accommodation for a person P who lacks capacity to agree to the arrangements, or

b. for a change in P's residential accommodation

and the local authority is satisfied that there is no person, other than one engaged in providing care or treatment for P in a professional capacity or for remuneration, whom it would be appropriate for them to consult about P's best interests (S.39(1)).

The section only applies if the accommodation is to be provided in accordance with:

a. Section 21 or 29 of the National Assistance Act 1948, or

b. Section 117 of the Mental Health Act.

as the result of a decision taken by the local authority under Section 47 of the NHS and Community Care Act 1990 (S.39(2)).

This statutory requirement for the local authority to instruct an independent mental capacity advocate does not apply if P is accommodated as a result of an obligation imposed on him under the Mental Health Act (S.39(3)).

Amendments to the MCA are made by the Mental Health Act 2007 which adds two new Sections to Section 39, i.e. 39A and 39B (see below). In addition a new Subsection 3A states that Section 39 does not apply if:

(a)   an independent mental capacity advocate must be appointed under section 39A or 39C (whether or not by the local authority) to represent P, and

(b)   the place in which P is to be accommodated under the arrangements referred to in this section is the relevant hospital or care home under the authorisation referred to in that section.

It is therefore implied in this exception to the duty under Section 39 that Section 117 accommodation under the Mental Health Act (MHA) 1983 is not accommodation as a result of an obligation imposed on him under the MHA (see Chapter 13 on mental capacity and mental health and Scenario E6). Sections 39A, 39B and 39C can be found in Chapter 13.

Before making the arrangements, the local authority must instruct an independent mental capacity advocate to represent P unless they are satisfied that:

a.   the accommodation is likely to be provided for a continuous period of less than eight weeks, or

b.   the arrangements need to be made as a matter of urgency (S.39(4)).

If an independent mental capacity advocate was not instructed because one of these subsections was thought to apply, but subsequently the local authority has reason to believe that the accommodation is likely to be provided for a continuous period that will end eight weeks or more after the day on which accommodation was first provided, then the local authority must instruct an independent mental capacity advocate to represent P (S.39(5)). This provision ensures that those persons are covered by Section 39 if the initial period of the accommodation is outside the specified period but is later extended.

The local authority must take into account any information given, or submission made, by the independent mental capacity advocate in deciding what arrangements to make for P (S.39(6)).

Sections 39A and 39C added by Mental Health Act

Where a person has lost his or her liberty under the provisions of Schedule A1 as added to the Mental Capacity Act by the Mental Health Act 2007, then an IMCA must be appointed in accordance with Sections 39A or 39C. These Sections are shown in Box 13.1 on page 299. Part 11 of Schedule A1 of the MCA (as added by the Mental Health Act 2007 Schedule 7) sets out the functions of 39A and 39C IMCAs.

Review of accommodation arrangements by NHS body or LA ('care reviews')

Where a review is proposed or in progress for accommodation provided for P for a continuous period of 12 weeks or more, then the NHS body or LA **may** instruct an IMCA to represent P if it is satisfied that it would be of particular benefit to P to be so represented. This does not apply if there is an appropriate person who could be consulted.[21] This, unlike the duties under Sections 37, 38 and 39, is a discretionary duty, and the Code of Practice has given guidance on when the power to appoint an IMCA should be used in care reviews.[22] The power only applies where the person lacks the requisite mental capacity. The power does not apply where accommodation is provided under an obligation imposed by the Mental Health Act 1983 (see Chapter 13 and Scenario E6).

Adult protection cases

Where an NHS body or LA are proposing or have taken protection measures in relation to a person P who lacks capacity to agree to one or more of the measures, then the NHS body or LA **may** instruct an IMCA to represent P if it is satisfied that it would be of particular benefit to P to be so represented. The Code of Practice gives guidance on when this discretionary power may be used.[23] The regulations do not require the person in an adult protection situation to have no friends or family to consult. The protective measures must be proposed or taken as a result of an allegation that P is being abused or neglected or is abusing another person. Protective measures includes measures to minimise the risk that any abuse or neglect of P, or abuse by P, will continue.[24] Scenario E3 illustrates the appointment of an IMCA when protective measures are being taken.

Guidance on adult protection and care reviews

Guidance has been provided by the DH on the regulations relating to adult protection and care reviews.[25] In care reviews, it suggests that the LA or NHS body should draw up a policy statement outlining the criteria to be applied when deciding for each eligible individual having an accommodation review whether there would be a benefit from having the safeguard of an IMCA. This policy statement should be made widely available, so that all relevant staff in the local authority or NHS body are aware of the criteria to be applied, thus ensuring consistency in decisionmaking in these cases.

For both care reviews and adult protection cases the guidance emphasises that where the qualifying criteria are met, it would be unlawful for the LA or NHS body not to consider the exercise of their power to instruct IMCAs for accommodation reviews and adult protection.

The guidance quotes statements made by adult protection co-ordinators and IMCAs in the pilot schemes to assist in the development of the policies. It could be questioned whether it might not have been more helpful for the DH itself to have provided a national policy statement to ensure consistency across the country.

The Independent Mental Capacity Advocacy services

Independent mental capacity advocates

The Secretary of State (for England) and the National Assembly for Wales (for Wales) (i.e. the appropriate authority – S.35(7)) must make such arrangements as it considers reasonable to enable persons (independent mental capacity advocates) to be available to represent and support persons to whom acts or decisions proposed under Sections 37, 38 and 39 (S.35(1)) relate and those specified in the regulations.

Regulations on independent mental capacity advocates[26]

Part of these regulations came into force on 1 November 2006 to enable the Secretary of State to make arrangements under Section 35 to enable persons known as independent mental capacity advocates to be available to represent and support persons to whom acts or decisions proposed under Sections 37, 38 and 39 relate. The remaining regulations came into force on 1 April 2007.

The appropriate authority may make regulations as to the appointment of independent mental capacity advocates (S.35(2)).

These regulations may, in particular, provide:

a.   that a person may act as an independent mental capacity advocate only in such circumstances, or only subject to such conditions as may be prescribed
b.   for the appointment of a person as an independent mental capacity advocate to be subject to approval in accordance with the regulations.

In making arrangements for independent mental capacity advocates to be available, the appropriate authority must have regard to the principle that a person to whom a proposed act or decision relates should, so far as is practicable, be represented and supported by a person who is independent of any person who will be responsible for the act or decision (S.35(4)).

This is a significant statutory provision. It prevents health or local authorities saving funds by using their own staff as IMCAs. The IMCA must be independent of any person who will be responsible for the act or decision which is to be made.

These arrangements may include provision for payments to be made to or in relation to, persons carrying out functions in accordance with the arrangements (S.35(5)).

How is it commissioned?

Following the consultation, the Government decided that the IMCA services are to be commissioned locally, with Local Social Services Authorities (LSSAs) having financial responsibility within joint commissioning arrangements with Primary Care Trusts (PCTs).[27]

How is it funded?

The DH has estimated that the cost of funding the IMCA service[28] in England will be £6.5m per annum and is making this new resource available through the annual local authority settlement using a population-based formula. The DH has issued guidance that identifies some of the issues for local authorities to consider when deciding how to commission the new IMCA service. The DH has published a best practice tool to assist organisations in testing their readiness to comply with the requirements of the Act, and to assist local implementation initiatives.[29]

The appropriate authorities (i.e. Secretary of State for England and National Assembly for Wales) have the responsibility of laying down the arrangements, which may include provision for payments to be made to, or in relation to, persons carrying out functions in accordance with the arrangements.

How is it managed?

The Government in its response to the consultation stated that independent advocacy organisations who will be commissioned to provide the IMCA services should also have to meet appropriate organisational standards as part of the commissioning or contract arrangements. The Government will work with independent advocacy organisations, commissioners and other stakeholders in developing these standards.

How is its independence secured?

Following the consultation, the Government stated that:

> The Government believes that the independence of the IMCA can be achieved through national standards that will apply to all organisations offering an IMCA service and through the contracting process. Guidance on commissioning will be available to those responsible at local level. Guidance will recommend that engagement protocols should set out how to address situations where a conflict of interest may arise, whether organisational, financial or personal.
>
> There are two key areas where independence is essential:
>
> - the IMCA must not have any professional or paid involvement with the provision of care or treatment for any vulnerable person for whom they may be appointed to act, and
> - they must be completely independent of the person responsible for making the decision or doing the act in question.

These features and further guidance on the IMCA role are covered in Chapter 10 of the Code of Practice.

How is it held accountable?

Following the consultation the Government stated that monitoring arrangements should be managed via local contracts/commissioning, but it would also produce an annual report on the IMCA service for the first three years.

It also stated that:

> The Government believes that all contracts or engagement protocols between the commissioner and IMCA service provider should include agreed complaints procedures. Complaints about the individual advocate providing the IMCA service should be directed in the first instance to the independent advocacy organisation employing the IMCA. All IMCA services should have a

clear and accessible complaints procedure. They should be required to report complaints about them to their commissioning body.

The Government will also consider whether the requirement to have agreed complaints procedures in place should be part of the national standards for independent advocacy organisations.

The Government believes that compliance with standards should primarily be part of contract monitoring, validated by performance assessment and service inspection evidence gathered by commissioners and by the Commission for Social Care Inspection (CSCI) and/or the Healthcare Commission. We will discuss this with the regulatory bodies.

What if it fails to provide advocates?

A situation might arise where an NHS organisation or LA was making a decision for a person lacking the requisite mental capacity which was covered by the IMCA and where there was no appropriate person who could be consulted and yet an IMCA was not appointed. In such a case there would be a breach of the statutory duty under Sections 37, 38 or 39 as appropriate (see above). If the situation were covered by the urgent provisions of Ss. 38(3)(b) and 39(4)(b), then the respective authority has a duty to arrange for an IMCA to be appointed if the accommodation is required for more than the specified time. In the event of a breach of the statutory duty to appoint an IMCA, a complaint could be raised and attempts made to remedy the situation. If this could not be resolved, and the complaint was not dealt with satisfactorily, then a judicial review of the failure to appoint an IMCA could be sought. (See Chapter 2 on judicial review.)

Who sets the standards?

The commissioning authorities will be responsible for ensuring that the IMCA organisations who arrange for the appointment of individual IMCAs will have to follow the standards which are to be developed nationally, and which will be incorporated into the individual contracts between the commissioning body and the IMCA service provider.

Who enforces the standards?

These standards will be enforced by the commissioning authorities, who are ultimately responsible to the Secretary of State.

Who monitors?

Ultimately of course the Government is responsible for the overall standards of the IMCA services, and has stated in its response to the consultation on the IMCA service that:

We will evaluate the IMCA service after the first year of implementation to determine if we have sufficiently addressed the advocacy needs of the unbefriended.

Does it have to provide an annual report?

The IMCA organisations commissioned by each local authority will have to provide an annual report on its activities to the commissioning authority. In addition
the Government has promised to provide an annual report on the overall situation relating to IMCAs. This report would be submitted to Parliament.

The responsible authorities

The appropriate authorities, i.e. the Secretary of State for England and the
National Assembly for Wales, have the responsibility of ensuring that IMCA services are available and of laying down the more detailed functions and remit of
the IMCAs.

Exceptions to the duty to instruct an independent mental capacity advocate (S.40)

The duty to instruct an independent mental capacity advocate (under Sections
37(3), 38(3), 39(4) and (5) and *39A(3) and 39C(3)* (italicised words added by Mental
Health Act 2007 Schedule 8) does not apply if there is:

a. a person nominated by P (in whatever manner) as a person to be consulted in
    matters affecting his interests
b. a donee of a lasting power of attorney created by P
c. a deputy appointed by the court for P or
d. a donee of an enduring power of attorney (within the meaning of Schedule 4)
    which has been created by P, or if
e. the decision relates to treatment or accommodation provided under the
    Mental Health Act 1983.

The Mental Health Act 2007 has added a new Subsection 40(2):

> A person appointed under Part 10 of Schedule A1 to be P's representative is not,
> by virtue of that appointment, a person nominated by P as a person to be con-
> sulted in matters affecting his interests.

Disputes between IMCA and others

Section 36(3) states that the regulations may make provision as to the circumstances in which the advocate may challenge, or provide assistance for the purpose of challenging, any relevant decision. This is provided for in Regulation 7 of
the general regulations for England.[30] See Scenario E7.

In its response to the consultation on IMCA services, the Government stated that:

> The Government intends to use regulations made under s36(3) to set out the circumstances in which the advocate may challenge or assist in challenging the decision maker. Whilst the IMCA should aim to reach consensus and exhaust every avenue in reaching decisions before challenging decisions, there will be situations where disputes arise about the decision reached or the process followed. In such cases, the intention is that the IMCA should use existing complaints mechanisms to resolve cases locally as far as possible. However, in particularly serious cases or where there is no other way of resolving the matter, the IMCA may as a last resort seek to refer the matter to the Court of Protection – following the process as set out in paragraph 21 below.

Informal dispute resolution

Chapter 10 of the Code of Practice[31] suggests possible informal ways of resolving disputes at an early stage which could include:

- In relation to disagreements about health care or treatment:
  - involving the Patient Advice and Liaison Service (PALS) (in England) or the Community Health Council (in Wales)
  - using the NHS Complaints Procedure
  - referring the matter to the local continuing care review panel
- In relation to disagreements about social care:
  - if the person is in a care home, using the care home's own complaints procedure
  - using the local authority complaints procedure.

In particularly serious cases where there is no other way of resolving the matter, an IMCA may seek permission to refer the matter to the Court of Protection.

Formal dispute resolution

The Code of Practice[32] gives the following advice for pursuing disputes formally:

> The first step in making a formal challenge is to approach the Official Solicitor (OS) with the facts of the case. The OS can decide to apply to the court as a litigation friend (acting on behalf of the person the IMCA is representing). If the OS decides not to apply himself, the IMCA can ask for permission to apply to the Court of Protection. The OS can still be asked to act as a litigation friend for the person who lacks capacity.
>
> In extremely serious cases, the IMCA might want to consider an application for judicial review in the High Court. This might happen if the IMCA thinks there are very serious consequences to a decision that has been made by a public authority. There are time limits for making an application, and the IMCA would have to instruct solicitors – and may be liable for the costs of

the case going to court. So IMCAs should get legal advice before choosing this approach. The IMCA can also ask the OS to consider making the claim.

Codes of Practice (see also Chapter 17)

Much of the detail about the way in which independent mental capacity advocates will operate is not contained in the regulations but is set out in the Code of Practice. This was a specific recommendation of the Joint Committee,[33] which said on the subject of the role and status of advocates:

> We recommend that the Codes of Practice produced under the Bill provide guidance on the appropriate use of advocacy services, in particular suggesting priority situations when it may be essential for an incapacitated person to have access to an advocate. (306)

The Joint Committee also recommended when in considering the standards and quality of advocacy services:

> All organisations commissioning or providing advocacy services to incapacitated adults should have satisfactory procedures in place to ensure that the standards and quality of independent advocacy services are monitored and maintained. (308)

The importance of the Code of Practice was emphasised in the House of Lords by Baroness Ashton of Upholland[34] who also noted that:

> Not everyone would want to feel obliged to have an advocate. There are real issues too about how families interact and the support that family members can provide for individuals. We should not presume that everyone wishes to have an advocate any more than we should insist that people have to use their relatives. I am not taken with the idea of making that a requirement.

Changes to the role of the independent mental capacity advocate (S41)

The Secretary of State and the Welsh Assembly Government have the power to make regulations which:

a. expand the role of the independent mental capacity advocate in relation to persons who lack capacity, and
b. adjust the obligations to make arrangements imposed by Section 35 (see above).

As noted above, regulations have already been made which prescribe different circumstances from those set out in Sections 37, 38 and 39, in which an independent mental capacity advocate must, or circumstances in which one may, be instructed by a person of a prescribed description to represent a person who lacks capacity, and include provisions similar to any made by Sections 37, 38 and 39. Further regulations may be made in due course.

Implementation

Pilot schemes were set up for the implementation of the IMCA service, and these are further considered in Chapter 17.

Care reviews

There was considerable discussion on whether the IMCA service should extend to care reviews and in its response to the Consultation, the Government stated that:

> The Government will need to review the involvement of IMCAs in care reviews as part of its reassessment of planning assumptions and in light of the mixed response to this consultation question. It wants to avoid creating an administrative burden, but to ensure that IMCAs can be part of the care review process where appropriate. Therefore it intends that this will be a discretionary function of the IMCA – that LAs and NHS bodies will have the discretion about when to involve the IMCA in a care review.
>
> The Government will consider providing in regulations that where an emergency medical treatment decision is taken without involving the IMCA, the IMCA may be involved in reviewing any ongoing decision – again as one of the discretionary functions of the IMCA. We think that the Code of Practice should set out the normal time limits for this.
>
> The Government believes that section 37 of the Act as it stands requires the involvement of an IMCA where there is ongoing treatment following an initial decision to provide treatment on an emergency basis. We will clarify this in the Code of Practice.

Extending the service

Following the consultation, the Government stated that:

> The Government recognises that many stakeholders support extending the IMCA service to other groups of people and situations. The consultation also clearly demonstrated the diverse nature of views – none of the six identified options received unqualified support.
>
> The Government's main priority is to introduce safeguards to protect the rights of individuals who do not have family or friends to advocate on their behalf. We are mindful of concerns about introducing a good quality service for this group before looking to extend it further. Therefore the Government will revisit the planning assumptions along the lines of option ii – to provide a more intensive service for those who have no family or friends.

However, it is clear that there may be other situations beyond those listed in the Act where a person who lacks capacity may be particularly vulnerable. The Government wants commissioners to have the flexibility to extend the IMCA service within the resources available to other groups and situations. Therefore, it intends to specify in regulations other circumstances in which LAs and NHS bodies may provide the IMCA service on a discretionary basis. This may, for example, include involving the IMCA in a care review; or in other situations where the person is particularly vulnerable. LAs will be required to take a strategic view in assessing local priorities and to publish the additional areas where IMCAs will be used.

We will evaluate the IMCA service after the first year of implementation to determine if we have sufficiently addressed the advocacy needs of the unbefriended. If we have, it would then be possible to consider using regulation-making powers to extend access to other groups or situations if resources allow it.

Non-statutory advocacy

It must be recognised that across the country there are many groups; voluntary, charitable, not for profit and other organisations which provide an independent advocacy service for those needing support and advice. How will these differ from those who are appointed under the provisions of the MCA to act on behalf of those lacking the requisite mental capacity in the situations defined in the Act and by the regulations, i.e. serious medical treatment decisions, accommodation arrangements by NHS organisations and LAs, and where the NHS bodies or LAs intend to take protective measures in relation to a person lacking the requisite mental capacity?

The main differences are:

- There is a statutory duty in these specified situations for an IMCA to be appointed unless there is an appropriate person who can be consulted.
- There are regulations prescribing what the IMCA is to do and what rights and powers they have (e.g. in relation to access to records).
- There is a statutory duty upon the NHS organisations or LAs to take into account any information given, or submissions made, by the independent mental capacity advocate.
- The IMCA has a statutory right to challenge any relevant decision.

It may well be that as a consequence of these statutory powers regulating the appointment and use of IMCAs under the Act, these provisions will influence the use of advocates in other situations not specified in the statute, that the non-statutory advocates will be given similar responsibilities and that the NHS organisations and the LAs will take into account their reports and submissions. However in the meantime they may find it difficult without clear statutory authorisation to obtain the same powers and rights that the statutory IMCA has (i.e. interview in private the person whom he has been instructed to represent, and examine and take copies of the relevant records).

Conclusions

The resource implications of an advocacy service have led to a more limited provision than many organisations and individuals would have wished for. Even before the IMCA was established, regulations in England[35] provided for an extension to the service envisaged in the MCA. (For Wales see Chapter 16.) The Government has made it clear that the service will be monitored after the first year, and a further extension of the service will be considered if the advocacy needs of the unbefriended have been insufficiently addressed.

References

1   Department of Health (2005) *New Independent Mental Capacity Advocate*. Consultation 269342. DH, London.
2   http://www.dh.gov.uk/Consultations/ResponsesToConsultations/fs/en
3   The Mental Capacity Act 2005 (Independent Mental Capacity Advocates)(Expansion of Role) Regulations 2006 (SI 2006/2883).
4   The Mental Capacity Act 2005 (Independent Mental Capacity Advocates)(General) Regulations 2006 (SI 2006/1832) reg 5(1).
5   *Ibid*. reg 5(2).
6   House of Lords and House of Commons Joint Committee on the Draft Mental Incapacity Bill Session 2002–2003; HL Paper 891–1; HC 1083–1, Chapter 18.
7   The Mental Capacity Act 2005 (Independent Mental Capacity Advocates)(General) Regulations 2006 (SI 2006/1832) reg 6.
8   *Ibid*. reg 6(4).
9   *Ibid*. reg 6(5).
10 www.actionforadvocacy.org
11 (2006) Mental Capacity Act Update. 9th edn. www.justice.gov.uk/whatwedo/mentalcapacity.htm/
12 www.makingdecisions.org.uk
13 www.nca.gb.com
14 The Mental Capacity Act 2005 (Independent Mental Capacity Advocates) (General) Regulations 2006 (SI 2006/1832) reg 7.
15 Llewellyn, P. (2005) An investigation into the advocacy role of the learning disability nurse. PhD thesis. University of Glamorgan.
16 *Ibid*. p 287.
17 The Mental Capacity Act 2005 (Independent Mental Capacity Advocates)(General) Regulations 2006 (SI 2006/1832) reg 6(6).
18 The Mental Capacity Act 2005 (Independent Mental Capacity Advocates)(General) Regulations 2006 (SI 2006/1832).
19 *Ibid*.
20 Code of Practice for the Mental Capacity Act 2005. Department of Constitutional Affairs February 2007 para 10.45. TSO, London.
21 The Mental Capacity Act 2005 (Independent Mental Capacity Advocates)(Expansion of Role) Regulations 2006 (SI 2006/2883) reg 3 and 5.
22 Code of Practice for the Mental Capacity Act 2005. Department of Constitutional Affairs February 2007 para 10.62–65. TSO, London.
23 *Ibid*. para 10.66–68.

24   The Mental Capacity Act 2005 (Independent Mental Capacity Advocates)(Expansion of Role) Regulations 2006 (SI 2006/2883) reg 4 and 5.

25   Department of Health (2006). *Adult Protection, Care Reviews and IMCAs. Guidance on interpreting the Regulations extending the IMCA Role.*

26   The Mental Capacity Act 2005 (Independent Mental Capacity Advocates)(General) Regulations 2006 (SI 2006/1832).

27   See http://www.dh.gov.uk/Consultations/ResponsesToConsultations/fs/en; or from DH Publications Orderline, PO Box 777, London SE1 6XH.

28   Mental Capacity Act Update edn 9 September 2006. www.justice.gov.uk/whatwedo/mentalcapacity.htm/

29   www.dh.gov.uk/PublicationsAndStatistics/Bulletins/ChiefExecutiveBulletin/

30   The Mental Capacity Act 2005 (Independent Mental Capacity Advocates)(General) Regulations 2006 (SI 2006/1832).

31   Code of Practice for the Mental Capacity Act 2005. Department of Constitutional Affairs February 2007. TSO, London.

32   *Ibid.* para 10.38 and 10.39.

33   House of Lords and House of Commons Joint Committee on the Draft Mental Incapacity Bill Session 2002–2003 HL Paper 189–1; HC 1083–1.

34   House of Lords, 25 Jan 05, Honsard columns 1299–1252.

35   The Mental Capacity Act 2005 (Independent Mental Capacity Advocates)(Expansion of Role) Regulations 2006 (SI 2006/2883).

Scenarios E
Independent Mental
Capacity Advocates

These Scenarios should be read in conjunction with Chapter 8 which sets out the law relating to the appointment of an independent mental capacity advocate (IMCA).

Arrangements for local authority (LA) accommodation

> **Scenario E1: Arrangements for LA accommodation.**
>
> Justin had been injured in a road accident and was in a coma for several months. He recovered consciousness but was severely paralysed with brain damage. He was transferred to a home for young people with disabilities. He has now been offered a transfer to sheltered accommodation owned by a charity which tries to create work in its industrial therapy unit for the residents. There is a dispute between the manager of his present residential home where he appears to be reasonably happy, and his social worker who considers that he would benefit from the move.

Should an independent mental capacity advocate be appointed for Justin?

The first question to be answered is:

'Does Justin have the mental capacity to make the decision for himself?'

The provisions of Section 2 apply (see Chapter 4 and Scenarios A). If the answer to that question is 'Yes', then Justin is entitled to make the decision.

If however the answer is 'No', then the consideration of the appointment of an IMCA should proceed.

It must be established whether these are the kind of circumstances envisaged by the Act, where an IMCA would be appointed and whether there are any exceptions.

The decision to be made is about arrangements for accommodation being made by the LA. Section 39 covers the situation where the local authority is to make arrangements for the provision of residential accommodation for a person who lacks capacity to agree to a change in the arrangements for his residential accommodation.

Is there an alternative?

The duty to appoint an IMCA does not apply if there is another person, not including a person engaged in providing care or treatment for P in a professional capacity or for remuneration, whom it would be appropriate for them to consult in determining what would be in P's best interests. Does Justin have a friend, relative or some other person who could be consulted over the move? He may have struck up a close relationship with a member of staff, but this person is excluded from the possibility of being formally consulted under the section. If a deputy has been appointed by the Court of Protection or Justin has appointed an attorney under a lasting power, then the appointment of an IMCA is not required. If there is no other person, other than the paid carers, whom the LA could consult, then the duty to provide an IMCA would apply unless any of the exceptions apply (see below).

Is it the right kind of accommodation?

The duty of the LA to arrange for the appointment of an IMCA only applies to the provision of certain kinds of accommodation. This includes accommodation provided following an assessment by the LA under Section 47 of the National Health Service and Community Care Act 1990 (duty of the LA to carry out a community care assessment). In Justin's case his accommodation would be provided under Section 29 of the National Assistance Act 1948 (under this section the LA may make arrangements for promoting the welfare of persons over 18 who are blind, deaf, dumb, or who suffer from mental disorder, and other persons who are substantially and permanently handicapped by illness, injury or congenital deformity or such other disabilities).

Do any of the exceptions apply?

The LA does not have to instruct an IMCA to represent Justin if it is satisfied that either the accommodation is likely to be provided for a continuous period of less than eight weeks, or that the arrangements need to be made as a matter of urgency. Neither of these exceptions would appear to apply to Justin's case.

Who should be the advocate?

There should be, in each area, an IMCA service which will provide advocates when required by the local authority or health services organisation. The IMCA service will select a person to represent Justin. The LA must follow the basic principle that the appropriate person to whom a proposed act or decision relates should, so far as practicable, be represented and supported by a person who is independent of any person who will be responsible for the act or decision. This means that the LA could not appoint one of its own staff or a person connected with either the residential accommodation in which Justin is currently living, nor a person connected with the proposed accommodation.

Under the Regulations[1] a person would not be able to act as an IMCA unless he is approved by a local authority as satisfying the appointment requirements, or he belongs to a class of persons which is approved by a local authority on the grounds that all persons in that class satisfy the appointment requirements.

Under these appointment requirements the proposed advocate must have the appropriate experience or training, or an appropriate combination of experience and training. He must be a person of integrity and good character; and he must be able to act independently of any person who instructs him. Before deciding if a person is of integrity and good character, an enhanced criminal record certificate issued under Ss.113A or B of the Police Act 1997 as amended by Section 163 of the Serious Organised Crime and Police Act 2005 is required.

What will Paul do as the advocate?

Paul is nominated as the IMCA for Justin. He has received the appropriate training, is on the panel of approved IMCAs held by the local authority, and he has received clearance from the criminal records search. His specific function is to represent and support persons who lack capacity. He visits Justin and tries to explain to him all the options. He would possibly take Justin to visit the proposed accommodation. He would speak to the paid carers, Justin's fellow residents and any others with whom Justin has had contact in the past and present, including any family and friends.

What powers does the IMCA have?

Paul may interview Justin in private and may, at all reasonable times, examine and take copies of any health record, any record of, or held by, a local authority and compiled in connection with a social services function, and any record held by a person registered under Part 2 of the Care Standards Act 2000, if the person holding the record considers it may be relevant to the IMCA's investigation. There may a dispute over what is considered to be relevant and it would be difficult for Paul, without seeing a document which has been withheld, to maintain that it should be disclosed to him as being relevant to his role as IMCA.

What considerations should Paul take into account?

Paul is bound to observe the principles set out in Section 1 of the Mental Capacity Act 2005. He should also determine what are Justin's best interests in accordance with the criteria for best interests as set down in Sections 3 and 4 (see Scenarios B). This means that he should be:

a.   providing support to Justin, so that Justin may participate as fully as possible in any relevant decision
b.   obtaining and evaluating relevant information
c.   ascertaining what Justin's wishes and feelings would be likely to be, and the beliefs and values that would be likely to influence Justin, if he had capacity to make that particular decision
d.   ascertaining what alternative courses of action are available in relation to Justin.

In taking these steps Paul would be able to investigate Justin's history prior to the road traffic accident, and find out from persons who once knew Justin about his beliefs and values, his wishes and feelings. He might, for example, find out that Justin always hated change and, once he was settled, preferred to stay.

What is the effect of Paul's report?

The local authority must, in deciding what arrangements to make for Justin, take into account any information given, or submissions made, by the IMCA, i.e. Paul. This does not mean that it has to follow the opinion or view of the IMCA, but it would have to show in its documentation that it had taken account of the submissions and information provided by the IMCA. If it decides not to follow the conclusion of the IMCA, it would have to show in its records the reasons why it decided on a different course of action. For example it might be that the IMCA, having talked to Justin and the paid carers, decided that it was preferable for Justin to remain in the present accommodation, since he was settled, apparently very happy and would miss his fellow residents. On the other hand, the LA may place greater weight on the long term benefits he would receive by being in a rehabilitative environment, with the future prospects of obtaining paid work and becoming independent, and therefore recommend the transfer.

Paul's remuneration

Paul is entitled to be paid according to the rates agreed by the local IMCA service.

Urgent transfer to new accommodation – no IMCA

What would be the situation in Scenario E1 if a decision on the new accommodation that was being considered for Justin had to be made within a week as other clients were considering moving there? In such a situation, the LA could make the decision that a transfer was in Justin's best interests, and because of the urgency. In this case the LA would not be required to appoint an IMCA to represent and support Justin. However in this case if subsequently the LA has reason to believe that the accommodation will continue for over eight weeks from the date of transfer, then it must instruct an IMCA to represent Justin.

If Paul were to be appointed in this situation, he would have a very different task. Justin would be in the new accommodation and Paul would have to ascertain whether it was in Justin's best interests to remain where he now was or whether it was preferable for him to return to his previous accommodation, assuming of course that that accommodation is still available.

Serious medical treatment

The second area where there are statutory requirements for the instruction of IMCAs to be considered is where serious medical treatment decisions have to be made on behalf of an adult who lacks the mental capacity to make that particular decision (S.37 Mental Capacity Act (MCA)). This is illustrated in Scenario E2.

Scenario E2: Serious medical treatment and the IMCA.

Brian has Down's syndrome and his eyesight is becoming weaker. He has very little sight in his right eye and the pressure from glaucoma is reducing his sight in the other eye. There is also a cataract in the same eye. It is recommended by his ophthalmic surgeon that he should have an operation to remove the cataract and reduce the pressure. He warns the carers that there is a risk, even if all reasonable care were taken, that he could lose the sight in his left eye and would for all intents and purposes have almost no sight. His carers are concerned about the risks involved, and feel that it may be preferable to retain the sight he now has and not risk the operation until there is no alternative.

Should an advocate be appointed?

This situation would come under Section 37 of the MCA, since a health service body is proposing to provide, or secure the provision of, serious medical treatment for Brian, who lacks capacity to consent to the treatment. The health service body must be satisfied that there is no person, other than one engaged in providing care or treatment for P in a professional capacity or for remuneration, whom it would be appropriate to consult in determining what would be in Brian's best interests. If therefore Brian's parents were still alive or there were other family members or friends who could be consulted over what are in Brian's best interests, there would be no duty on the heath service organisation to instruct an IMCA.

When must the IMCA be appointed?

The National Health Service (NHS) trust is required to instruct an IMCA to represent Brian before the treatment is provided. If however the treatment must be provided as a matter of urgency then different provisions apply (see **Urgent medical treatments**, page 186).

Serious medical treatment

Does the eye operation proposed for Brian come within the definition of serious medical treatment? The MCA itself did not propose a definition but suggested that it should be left to the Regulations[2]. Regulation 4 defines serious medical treatment as:

> Treatment which involves providing, withdrawing or withholding treatment in circumstances where:
>
> a. in a case where single treatment is being proposed, there is a fine balance between its benefits to the patient and the burdens and risks it is likely to entail for him
> b. in a case where there is a choice of treatments, a decision as to which one to use is finely balanced, or
> c. what is proposed would be likely to involve serious consequences for the patient.

It would seem in Brian's case that a. and c. are both satisfied. There is a fine balance between the benefits, burdens and risk of the eye operation and the possibility of total blindness, which would involve serious consequences for him.

Who would be appointed as the IMCA?

The same provisions on the suitability of the person to be appointed as the IMCA apply here as they did in Scenario E1 on the transfer of a person to new accommodation. These include the requisite training, independence and also the criminal records clearance.

What actions must the IMCA take?

An IMCA appointed to represent and support a person who lacks the requisite mental capacity has the same powers and duties as one appointed in connection with accommodation arrangements (S.38 and 39) (see Chapter 8 and Scenario E1). However, in addition the IMCA is able to obtain a further medical opinion where treatment is proposed and the advocate thinks that one should be obtained.

What is the effect of the IMCA appointment?

As in Scenario E1 the IMCA does not actually make the decision. For example, Brian's advocate might state that it appeared to be in Brian's best interests for the operation not to proceed, until there is evidence that his sight has deteriorated to the point that there is no alternative. However the consultant surgeon might disagree with that view. The NHS body must take into account any information given, or submissions made, by the IMCA. It is not obliged to accept the view of the IMCA. Its documentation, however, should show the basis for its decision making and the reason why the IMCA's views were not followed. The IMCA has the power to challenge the decision of the statutory authority (see Scenario E7 below).

Best interests and reasonable medical opinion

In the past, in the absence of statutory provision, decisions on behalf of mentally incapacitated adults have been made on the basis of the common law (i.e. judge made decisions or case law), and in particular the decision of the House of Lords in *Re F*.[3] This stated that, where decisions had to be made on behalf of an adult who lacked the capacity to make his or her own decisions, then it should be in his or her best interests according to the reasonable professional practice of those involved in his or her care. (See Chapter 5 on best interests.)

The wider criteria in Sections 3 and 4 enable many other factors to be taken into account than medical ones, and it is possible that the NHS organisation might decide differently from the consultant's view.

Who would make the decision within the NHS Trust?

Prior to the implementation of the MCA, decisions on serious medical treatment for those lacking the capacity to make their own decisions were left to the clinical practitioner who would carry out the treatment. The requirement at common law was for these decisions to be made in the best interests of the mentally incapable patient, according to the reasonable standard of the medical practitioner (i.e. the Bolam Test).

In contrast, following the implementation of the MCA the definition of best interests is much wider and would go beyond just the clinical best interests. The patient services officer, or some other person delegated with the responsibility of carrying out the duties of the health service organisation under the MCA, will have the task of taking into account not only the clinician's opinion but also the information provided by the IMCA or other representative of the patient. The non-medical considerations should be more clearly enunciated and have a bigger impact upon the determination of best interests. The significance of this change remains to be seen.

Urgent medical treatment

Where urgent medical treatment is required, such as immediate life saving treatment, then there is no requirement to appoint an IMCA (S.37(4)). The Code of Practice recommends that this decision must be recorded with the reason for the non-referral to an IMCA. Responsible bodies will, however, still need to instruct an IMCA for any serious treatment that follows the emergency treatment.[4]

Extension of IMCA role

Two further situations where there should be consideration of the appointment of an IMCA were set out in regulations.[5] These include the review of arrangements as to accommodation and the taking of protective measures for an adult who lacks capacity. Scenario E3 illustrates the latter.

Scenario E3: Protective measures.

A prosecution has been brought by the Crown Prosecution Service against the parents of Tom, who has severe learning disabilities. It is claimed that the parents abused Tom by failing to provide adequate care for him, by misappropriating his benefits and not using them to provide proper and sufficient food and clothing for him. The social services are considering taking protective measures for Tom. Is an IMCA required?

Under regulations 4 and 5[6] in a situation where an adult lacking mental capacity is either the cause or the victim of abuse, and an NHS body or a local authority proposes to take or have taken protective measures in respect of that person, then an IMCA can be instructed if the NHS body or LA is satisfied that it would be of particular benefit for the person to be so represented. There is no requirement to ascertain if there is an appropriate person to represent P. An IMCA could therefore be instructed to represent Tom. Where an IMCA is instructed, then the NHS body or the LA must take into account any information provided or submissions made by the IMCA in making decisions about the protective measures. The definition of 'protective measures' includes measures to minimise the risk that any abuse or neglect of P, or abuse by P will continue. This regulation does not apply if Regulation 3 (dealing with review of arrangements as to accommodation), Section 37 (serious medical treatment), Section 38 (arrangements for accommodation by NHS body) or Section 39 (arrangements for accommodation by LA) apply.

An appropriate adult for consultation

Scenario E4 illustrates a possible problem with a restricted view of the present MCA and regulations.

Scenario E4: Appropriate for consultation?

Paula, 21 years old, lives with her father, her mother having died several years before. She has severe learning disabilities, and social services are considering moving her from the family home to live in a small community home with four other young people with disabilities. Her father is opposed to the move. The social services are concerned that the father may be sexually abusing Paula. The police investigated similar allegations in relation to an older sister, but the CPS abandoned the prosecution for lack of evidence. Could Paula have an IMCA?

Under Section 39 social services, in determining the accommodation needs for Paula, has a duty to arrange for an IMCA to be appointed, if Paula lacks the capacity to agree to the arrangements and is satisfied that there is no person, other than one engaged in providing care or treatment for Paula in a professional capacity or for remuneration, whom it would be appropriate for it to consult in determining what would be in Paula's best interests.

Once it is determined that Paula lacks the requisite mental capacity, then the next question is, does the father constitute 'an appropriate' person for social services to consult in determining what is in Paula's best interests? From the social services perspective, it may consider that the father would not be an appropriate person because of the allegations about his conduct. It might therefore recommend that an IMCA is appointed. If the father were to protest, he would have to provide evidence that he was appropriate to be consulted and able to advise as to what was in Paula's best interests. Clearly any IMCA appointed would have to include in his or her report the father's evidence as to what he thought was in Paula's best interests. In the event that local agreement could not be obtained, an approach could be made to the Official Solicitor giving the facts of the case. It may then be necessary for an application to be made to the Court of Protection, with Paula being represented by the Official Solicitor (see Chapter 8).

Scope of the IMCA's remit

Scenario E5 illustrates a situation which could arise when the IMCA, who has been commissioned to represent a person incapable of making the requisite decision in a specific area, considers that they should be represented in other types of decision, where the authority is not yet obliged to appoint an IMCA.

Scenario E5: Representation in another area?

In the situation discussed in E4, Jonathan is appointed as an IMCA to represent Paula on the proposed change in her accommodation. He obtains evidence from her father, her older sister and Paula herself on whether the transfer to the new home would be in her best interests. Whilst preparing his report he discovers that moneys which Paula is entitled to receive from a family trust fund and from social services are being used by Paula's father, who appears to have a gambling problem. He is advised by the LA social worker that his remit is only to concern himself with questions on accommodation and anything else is outside his remit.

Jonathan would seek advice from the IMCA service which has employed him and which has the contract to provide IMCAs on behalf of the LA and the NHS body. Depending upon the contract and the commissioning authority, the IMCA service could probably give Jonathan the authorisation to report on other aspects of her care. What is being alleged is a criminal offence, and action should be taken by the LA to ensure that it is reported to the police and appropriately investigated.

Accommodation for those with mental health problems

Scenario E6 illustrates a situation where a detained patient is being discharged and accommodation under Section 117 is being sought.

> **Scenario E6: Section 117 of the MHA and accommodation. Which legislation applies?**
>
> Barbara has been detained in a psychiatric hospital under Section 3 of the Mental Health Act 1983. She is shortly to be discharged, and a meeting to consider after-care to be provided under Section 117 is being convened. It is decided that she does not require after-care under supervision. Thomas, her occupational therapist, considers that she is incapable of making decisions on accommodation and that she should be represented under the Mental Capacity Act 2005. The consultant psychiatrist maintains that the MCA does not apply, because she comes under the provisions of the Mental Health Act 1983.

It is correct that Section 39(3) states that Section 39 (i.e. the duty to arrange for an IMCA where the LA is arranging accommodation), does not apply if P is accommodated as a result of an obligation imposed on him under the Mental Health Act. Is accommodation under Section 117 an obligation imposed under the Mental Health Act? Section 39(2) specifies that the duty under Section 39 only applies if the accommodation is to be provided in accordance with either Section 21 or 29 of the National Assistance Act 1948, or under Section 117 of the Mental Health Act, as the result of a decision taken by the local authority under Section 47 of the National Health Service and Community Care Act 1990. Therefore the effect of Section 39(2) and Section 39(3) is that accommodation provided under Section 117 of the MHA, following a community care assessment under Section 47 of the

NHS and Community Care Act, is not accommodation being provided under an obligation imposed by the Mental Health Act 1983.

Therefore if a person who has been detained under the Mental Health Act 1983 is discharged from hospital and comes under the requirements for after-care set out in Section 117 of the Mental Health Act 1983, if that person has no close relatives, friends or any other person to protect their interests, then the LA will have a duty to consult with an IMCA over any accommodation which is being planned. The situation would be different if Barbara was granted leave under S17 and was obliged to stay in specified accommodation.

It follows that the consultant psychiatrist is wrong in saying that an IMCA does not have to be appointed under the MCA. If Barbara is unable to make her own decisions about accommodation, and if there is no unpaid appropriate adult who could be consulted about her best interests, then an IMCA should be appointed. Thomas cannot act as her advocate since he is providing care and treatment for her in a professional capacity and for remuneration.

Right of IMCA to challenge the decisions

The regulations provide that an IMCA may challenge a decision. This is illustrated by Scenario E7.

Scenario E7: Challenging the decision.

Paul is nominated to act as the IMCA for Sheila, who is 22 years old and has Down's syndrome. She has lived with her family all her life and attends a day centre where she met Jimmy, who also has Down's syndrome. They became friendly and wanted to move into the same community home together. Her parents have opposed the move but the manager of the day centre disagreed with their refusal. He suggested that an IMCA should be appointed for Sheila and Paul was appointed. After interviewing Sheila and talking to her parents and others who had been involved in her care, Paul wrote a report which put firmly his conclusion that Sheila wished to move out of the family home and that it appeared to be in her best interests to do so. He noted however that her parents were opposed to the move. He was surprised to learn subsequently that the local authority had decided that it was in Sheila's best interests to remain with her parents. He suspected that the driving force behind the decision was not Sheila's best interests but the resource issues. The local authority was not subsidising Sheila's care at present since she was being cared for by the parents (apart from the day centre). However were she to be moved to a community home there would be significant cost implications. Paul wished to challenge the decision. How should this proceed?

Regulation 7 enables Paul, the IMCA, to challenge the decision. The following conditions are required:

- Paul must have been instructed to represent Sheila
- a decision affecting Sheila has made.

Paul then has the same rights to challenge the decision as he would have if he were a person (other than an IMCA) engaged in caring for P or interested in his welfare.[7]

The means of challenge would be first to take up the question of the decision through the local authority's complaints and representations procedures. Then, if that fails, and Paul still considers that the wrong decision has been made for Sheila, he could go to the Official Solicitor (OS). The OS would then decide if a case should be brought, in which case he would consider acting as Litigation Friend. The Court of Protection would then make a decision on what was in Sheila's best interests.

It might be questioned whether in practice such a situation would arise, since in all likelihood the local authority might decide that there was no requirement for an IMCA, since Sheila lived with her parents who could be consulted on her behalf and therefore Paul would not have been appointed.

A question of time

Scenario E8: Time constraints.

Andy was asked to act as the IMCA on behalf of Sophie, who lived in a community home for those with challenging behaviour. Discussions were taking place over the transfer of Sophie to another home, where the social worker felt that Sophie would have closer ties with other residents. The home manager opposed such a transfer on the grounds that Sophie had been in his home for over ten years, and any move would be contrary to her best interests. Sophie, who had severe learning disabilities, had no one who could be consulted on her behalf. She was unable to speak but was however able to communicate by signs and facial expressions. Unfortunately a care assistant who had worked for many years with Sophie and had developed a close rapport with her, had recently left the home. The high turnover of staff meant that there was no one who could give any considered views on what was in Sophie's best interests. Andy realised that if he was to be able to get a full picture of Sophie's best interests in terms of accommodation and prepare a considered report, he would require much longer than the half day allowed for the interview, the record research and the preparation of the report. What is the situation?

It is hoped that the conditions and terms of service of the appointment of IMCAs will take into account the fact that there will be occasions where an IMCA will need longer than the average assumed time to prepare his or her submissions. Andy may be able to trace and talk to the care assistant to find more about Sophie's best interests. Hopefully the monitoring of the IMCA following its first year of full implementation will consider the existence and implications of any such time constraints.

An issue of discrimination

Scenario E9: Treated differently.

Rodney lives in a community home for those with challenging behaviour with three other residents. The local day centre has recently changed its policy and no longer accepts Rodney and his co-residents, but expects the home to provide its own activities. The home has a van which it can use for excursions, but the van is rarely used since visits to local cafes, sports centres and pubs have resulted in the service users being abused and ridiculed. It is not always possible for the staff to arrange individual outings since the staffing is such that two people could not be spared to take one person on a trip. As a consequence the residents find that they rarely leave the home and their quality of life is diminished.

Scenario E9 paints a situation where someone should be standing up for the rights of the residents and challenging the discrimination to which they are subjected on their trips outside the home. A case could be made for representation to the Equality and Human Rights Commission for action to be taken on their behalf. Perhaps too, those responsible for the change of policy at the day centre could be persuaded to permit the residents to attend. If the paid staff or other interested persons fail to take up any of these issues there are at present no statutory provisions for an IMCA to be appointed, and the Scenario illustrates the fact that there may be many situations and many persons who, because of the present narrow definition of the situations identified by statute requiring the appointment of an IMCA, are not receiving the representation and support which they need. From December 2006 public bodies have a new disability equality duty to fulfil (see page 31). It remains to be seen how far this improves the circumstances of those lacking the requisite mental capacity.

Checklist for the appointment of an IMCA

1. Is P lacking the requisite mental capacity?
2. If the answer to 1 is 'no', then P can make his or her own decisions.
3. If the answer to 1 is 'yes', then question 4 below must be asked.
4. Does the decision relate to serious medical treatment, accommodation arranged by an NHS body or LA, a review of such accommodation or an adult protection issue?
5. If the answer to 4 is 'yes', does it come within the discretion of the NHS body or LA to arrange for the appointment of an IMCA?
6. If the answer to 4 is 'no', then an IMCA cannot be appointed under the MCA provisions.

7. If the answer to 4 is 'yes', is there an appropriate unpaid adult who can be consulted over P's best interests?
8. If the answer to 7 is 'yes', then an IMCA would not be appointed.
9. If the answer to 7 is 'no', then an IMCA can be appointed, provided that a deputy or lasting power of attorney has not been appointed.

References

1 The Mental Capacity Act 2005 (Independent Mental Capacity Advocates)(General) Regulations 2006 (SI 2006/1832).
2 *Ibid.*
3 *F* v. *West Berkshire Health Authority* [1989] 2 All ER 545; [1990] 2 AC 1.
4 Code of Practice for the Mental Capacity Act 2005. Department of Constitutional Affairs February 2007 para 10.46. TSO, London.
5 The Mental Capacity Act 2005 (Independent Mental Capacity Advocates)(Expansion of Role) Regulations 2006 (SI 2006/2883).
6 *Ibid.*
7 The Mental Capacity Act 2005 (Independent Mental Capacity Advocates)(General) Regulations 2006 (SI 2006/1832) reg 7.

9 Advance Decisions

Introduction

The most hotly debated and contentious provisions of the Mental Capacity Bill were those relating to advance decisions and the fear that the provisions were legalising euthanasia. The Bill allowed for a person nominated by the patient to be able to make decisions on behalf of the patient (at a time when the patient lacked the requisite mental capacity), and it has been argued by opponents that if this power were not limited, it could lead to the death of a patient by food, water and other necessities being withdrawn. In addition it was argued that there was no provision to cover the possibility that a person who had drawn up a living will had changed his or her mind. An amendment proposed by Iain Duncan Smith was defeated but the Government promised that, when the Bill was discussed in the House of Lords in January 2005, changes would take place to make it explicit that the Bill did not allow decisions to be made which are aimed at killing the patient.

The Government response on safeguards on withdrawal of life-sustaining treatment led to changes to the Bill to make

> it absolutely clear that no person, whether doctor, attorney, deputy or court, can, when making a best interests determination, have the motive of causing death, regardless of what would be in his best interests [Para.41]

As a consequence Subsection 5 was added to Section 4:

> (5) Where the determination relates to life-sustaining treatment he must not, in considering whether the treatment is in the best interests of the person concerned, be motivated by a desire to bring about his death.

Further safeguards were introduced to tip the legislation in favour of preserving life. Tough tests of validity and applicability have been set that must be satisfied if an advance decision is to be binding.

Eventually the final amendments made provision for many of these concerns and gave statutory recognition to the situation, which had already been recognised at common law in the Tony Bland case,[1] that a person when mentally capacitated could make advance decisions refusing treatment in a specified set of circumstances at a later time when he or she lacked capacity. In the case of *HE* v. *NHS Trust A and AE*[2] the High Court held that the anticipatory refusal of a patient to have blood at a subsequent time when he no longer had mental capacity was valid at common law (i.e. judge made/case law) and binding on health professionals. This common law principle has now been given statutory recognition in the Mental Capacity Act 2005 .

Advance decision to refuse treatment: general

Definition

An 'advance decision' means a decision made by a person, who is over 18 years and has the capacity to make the decision, that if at a later time and in such circumstances as he may specify, a specified treatment is proposed to be carried out or continued by a person providing health care for him, and at that time he lacks the capacity to consent to the carrying out or continuation of the treatment, then the specified treatment is not to be carried out or continued.

An advance decision has also been known as a living will, or advance refusal or advance direction. The Law Commission in its Report in 1995[3] used the term advance refusal rather than advance decision. It considered that the document would constitute a refusal for the commencement or continuation of treatment, but the possibility of an advance decision requiring treatment to be given has been considered in a recent case, *Burke* v. *GMC* (see **Burke decision**, page 205).

Who can draw up an advance decision?

Age of person

The person preparing the advance decision must be over 18 years. This is because there have been situations where the refusal of a person under 18 years has been overruled by the court on the grounds that it was life saving treatment and in the best interests of the young person, and therefore their refusal could be overruled. This occurred in the case of *Re W*[4] a girl of 16 years suffering from anorexia nervosa, who was refusing treatment. The Court of Appeal held that it was in her best interests to receive life saving treatment and her refusal could therefore be overruled (see Chapter 12 on children). As a result of Section 40 of the Mental Health Act 2007 a parent can no longer overrule the refusal of young person of 16 and 17 years with the requisite mental capacity to be admitted to a psychiatric hospital. This reduction in parental powers may eventually lead to the recognition of the right of autonomy of the mentally capacitated 16- and 17-year-old.

The present situation contrasts with the situation for a mentally capacitated person over 18 years, as can be seen from the case of *Re B*,[5] an adult patient, who was tetraplegic but who had the requisite mental capacity, and who was therefore able to refuse ventilation. The case is considered in detail in Chapter 2.

How is it to be drawn up?

Layman's language

The decision may be regarded as specifying a treatment or circumstances, even though expressed in layman's terms (S.24(2)).

The fact that the patient is not required to use the jargon of the health professional is important, but this could present some difficulties in determining exactly what the patient wants covered by the advance decision. Clearly help by a health professional in drawing up the advance decision would greatly assist in identifying what is covered by the advance refusal.

What are the legal formalities?

There are very few formalities which are required to constitute a valid advance decision. A written document is only required if the advance decision is intended to cover situations where life-sustaining treatment is being refused (see **Conditions for an advance decision to cover life-sustaining treatment to be valid**, page 199). The statutory provisions are minimal, but the Code of Practice suggests recommended procedures:[6]

> A written document can be evidence of an advance decision. It is helpful to tell others that the document exists and where it is. A person may want to carry it with them in case of emergency, or carry a card, bracelet or other indication that they have made an advance decision and explaining where it is kept.

The Code of Practice para 9.19 says there is no set form for written advance decisions, because contents will vary depending on a person's wishes and situation. But it is helpful to include the information shown in Box 9.1.

Box 9.1: Information which the Code of Practice recommends should be included in an advance decision.

- full details of the person making the advance decision, including date of birth, home address and any distinguishing features (in case healthcare professionals need to identify an unconscious person, for example)
- the name and address of the person's GP and whether they have a copy of the document
- a statement that the document should be used if the person ever lacks capacity to make treatment decisions
- a clear statement of the decision, the treatment to be refused and the circumstances in which the decision will apply
- the date the document was written (or reviewed)

- the person's signature (or the signature of someone the person has asked to sign on their behalf and in their presence)
- the signature of the person witnessing the signature, if there is one (or a statement directing somebody to sign on the person's behalf).

More formalities are required if the advance decision is to cover life-sustaining treatments (see **Conditions for an advance decision to cover life-sustaining treatment to be valid**, page 199).

The Law Commission in 1995 was concerned not to insist that specific formalities were followed:

> To disregard valid decisions on that account would be contrary to our aims of policy. Matters of form and execution are essentially questions of evidence in any particular case.

The important point for the health professional is that the patient's wishes should be clear, and it should be understood to which treatments the patient is referring and the circumstances envisaged for the instruction to apply.

This contrasts very starkly with the strict formalities required for an ordinary will which comes into operation after the patient's death.

Oral advance decisions

Instructions by word of mouth may be given in advance by a mentally competent patient relating to a future refusal. There is no legal requirement that these should be made in writing, unless they are intended to refer to life-sustaining treatments. The Code of Practice[7] suggests that where a patient has given instructions by word of mouth, the health professional should document this and certain information should be recorded in the patient's notes, which will produce a written record that could prevent confusion about the decision in the future. The record should include:

- a note that the decision should apply if the person lacks capacity to make treatment decisions in the future
- a clear note of the decision, the treatment to be refused and the circumstances in which the decision will apply
- details of someone who was present when the oral advance decision was recorded and the role in which they were present (for example, healthcare professional or family member), and
- whether they heard the decision, took part in it or are just aware that it exists.

The situation is illustrated in Scenario F4.

How can it be changed? Withdrawal or alteration of an advance decision

P may withdraw or alter an advance decision at any time when he or she has capacity to do so (S.24(3)). It is not necessary for the withdrawal or a partial withdrawal to be in writing (S.24(4)). Nor need an alteration of an advance decision be in writing unless it is applicable to life-sustaining treatment (S.24(5) – see **Conditions for an advance decision to cover life-sustaining treatment to be valid**, page 199).

In a case heard prior to the implementation of the Mental Capacity Act (MCA), the Family Division decided that a woman of 24, mentally incapable of giving consent to treatment, could be given a blood transfusion, in spite of the existence of an advance decision created at a time when she was a Jehovah's Witness, since there was evidence that she had rejected her faith as a Jehovah's Witness and intended to marry a Muslim. It emphasised the importance of the hospital referring any case of uncertainty about the validity of an advance decision to the court for a declaration.[8] The case is further discussed in Case F1 and see Scenario F11.

Validity and applicability of advance decisions

An advance decision must be valid and applicable to the treatment proposed at a particular time in order to give rise to liability on the part of a defendant (S.25(1)). For example P in an advance decision may refuse a blood transfusion, but ventilation and artificial feeding may still be administered.

An advance decision is not valid if P:

a.   has withdrawn the decision at a time when he had capacity to do so
b.   has, under a lasting power of attorney which was created after the advance decision was made, conferred authority on the donee (or, if more than one, any of them) to give or refuse consent to the treatment to which the advance decision relates, or
c.   has done anything else clearly inconsistent with the advance decision remaining his fixed decision (S25(2)).

One of the crucial concerns for any health professional or carer who finds that a now mentally incapacitated patient has drawn up a living will is knowing whether or not it is valid (see Scenario F1). Although treatment can continue to keep the patient alive, whilst the validity of the advance decision is determined by the Court of Protection, the health professional would not wish to have to go to court every time an advance decision is produced. The important requisite in law is that the advance decision should reflect the patient's wishes, so that at the time it comes into play it is absolutely clear what the now mentally incapacitated patient would wish to happen to him or her.

The Act states that any action clearly incompatible with the advance decision taken by the patient after it has been drawn up, would negate the applicability of the advance decision. So appointing a lasting power of attorney with powers to consent or refuse treatments, which are covered by the advance decision, after the advance decision was drawn up, would indicate that the person no longer wished to keep to the advance decision, which would therefore be treated as withdrawn.

Other actions may also imply an intent on the patient's part to withdraw the advance decision. For example see Scenario F2.

Capacity of P

P must have the necessary mental capacity to create a valid advance decision and to withdraw or alter it. The advance decision does not come into effect until P lacks mental capacity. As long as P is capable of giving or refusing consent, the advance decision remains ineffective.

An advance decision is not applicable to the treatment in question if at the material time P has capacity to give or refuse consent to it (S.25(3)).

Relevance of the advance decision

An advance decision is not applicable to the treatment in question if:

a. that treatment is not the treatment specified in the advance decision
b. any circumstances specified in the advance decision are absent, or
c. there are reasonable grounds for believing that circumstances exist which P did not anticipate at the time of the advance decision, and which would have affected his decision had he anticipated them (S25(4)).

See Scenarios F1, 2 and 3 on the relevance and applicability of an advance decision.

Life-sustaining treatment

Special provisions apply to advance decisions and life-sustaining treatment. An advance decision is not applicable to life-sustaining treatment unless P specified in the decision that it was to apply to such treatment (S.25(5)) and that the decision or statement complies with Section 25(6).

What are life-sustaining treatments?

These are defined in Section 4(10) as

> treatment which in the view of a person providing health care for the person concerned is necessary to sustain life.

Nutrition, hydration and ventilation obviously come into the definition, but at some point even such day-to-day treatments and care as nail cutting, dental care or bodily cleansing could, if neglected for too long, become life-threatening. True elective surgery, such as a face lift, would not usually become life-threatening.

The Explanatory Memorandum suggests (Para 89)[9] that 'life' includes the life of an unborn baby, but there is nothing in the Act itself to give that interpretation and a court decision to interpret this must be awaited.

If the Explanatory Memorandum is correct there are significant implications for the pregnant woman (see pages 204 and 213).

Conditions for an advance decision to cover life-sustaining treatment to be valid

It must be clear in the advance decision that P intends the refusal to apply to treatments, even though his or her life would be at risk. In addition Subsection 5 of Section 25 states that subsection 6 must be complied with:

The decision or statement complies with subsection (6) only if:

a. it is in writing
b. it is signed by P or by another person in P's presence and by P's direction
c. the signature is made or acknowledged by P in the presence of a witness
d. the witness signs it, or acknowledges his signature, in P's presence.

The stipulations of Subsections 5 and 6 are strict and were designed to meet the concerns of those who felt that a person could inadvertently, through an advance decision, fail to receive the appropriate treatment, because they had not realised that it could be a life-threatening situation.

These formalities also apply to any alteration of an advance decision which requires life-sustaining treatment to be withheld or withdrawn. An alteration must be in writing, signed by P or by another person in Ps presence and by P's direction, and P's signature acknowledged in the presence of a witness who signs it or acknowledges his signature in P's presence. See Scenario F4.

In writing

In a memorandum submitted to the Joint Committee on Human Rights in response to their letter of 18 November 2004, the Joint Committee of the Houses of Parliament questioned why advance directives did not carry the additional safeguard of having to be made in writing.

In the light of this comment and also in the light of comments by the Joint Scrutiny Committee, the Government amended the Bill to say that advance decisions relating to the withdrawal of life-sustaining treatment should be put in writing and should be witnessed (the Government response can be downloaded from the Department of Constitutional Affairs website).[10]

The Code of Practice and future guidance will stress the importance of making advance decisions as clear as possible. It must be clear that the patient knows what he or she is doing and is aware of the implications. Otherwise a doctor may not be satisfied that an advance decision (1) exists, (2) is valid and (3) is applicable.

Specifying treatments in an advance decision

If a person has not specified that the refusal is to apply where artificial nutrition and hydration (ANH) is necessary to sustain life, then ANH (if in the person's best interests) will have to be given. It is not necessary for a patient to spell out all treatment options which he is refusing. However it is essential that the patient makes it clear that the refusal applied to treatments necessary to sustain life. This requirement could be easily met where a person is suffering from a specific disease such as motor neurone disease, and draws up an advance decision which makes it clear that if the disease progresses and they cease to have the mental capacity to make a decision on treatment, then certain forms of specified treatment (e.g. resuscitation, ventilation and artificial feeding) should not be given.

However where the patient has not made it clear what treatments he is refusing and in what circumstances the refusal would apply, a health professional caring for that person would, with that uncertainty, have no alternative but to provide treatments in the best interests of the patient. An application could be made to the Court of Protection for a declaration on the validity of the advance decision to the patient's particular circumstances and treatment (see Scenario F10).

In such circumstances where P has not satisfied the strict conditions for the validity of the advance refusal of life-sustaining treatment, the National Council for Palliative Care has suggested that the refusal should be called an 'advance statement' as opposed to an advance decision, and should be taken note of when the best interests of P are being determined, as evidence of P's past wishes and feelings.[11]

Lasting powers of attorney and advance decisions

Where P has created a lasting power of attorney after an advance decision was made, which conferred authority on the donee (or, if more than one, any of them) to give or refuse consent to the treatment to which the advance decision relates, then the advance decision is invalid. However any other lasting power of attorney does not prevent the advance decision from being regarded as valid and applicable (S.25(7)).

It is only in these circumstances that the advance decision is overruled. Where a lasting power of attorney does not refer to treatments or refers to different treatments, it can exist side by side with the advance decision (S.25(7)).

Effect of a valid advance decision

If P has made an advance decision which is valid and applicable to a treatment, then the decision has effect as if he had made it, and had had the capacity to make it, at the time when the question arises whether the treatment should be carried out or continued (S.26(1)).

Therefore anyone who believed that a valid advance decision exists which covers the treatment in question, yet ignored the provisions of that refusal and carried on giving the treatment, could be liable for the tort of trespass to the person in the civil courts and also, in some circumstances, the criminal offences of assault and battery (see Chapter 11).

A person does not incur liability for carrying out or continuing the treatment unless, at the time, he is satisfied that an advance decision exists which is valid and applicable to the treatment (S.26(2)).

Where a health professional gave life-sustaining treatment to a mentally inca-pacitated patient in ignorance that there was a valid advance decision, he or she would not be liable in the tort of trespass or be criminally liable.

This is illustrated in Scenario F5.

Reasonable belief on the validity of an advance decision

A person does not incur liability for the consequences of withholding or with-drawing a treatment from P if, at the time, he reasonably believes that an advance decision exists which is valid and applicable to the treatment (S.26(3)).

Court declaration on the validity of an advance decision

The court may make a declaration as to whether an advance decision:

a. exists
b. is valid
c. is applicable to a treatment (S.26(4)).

It should be noted that if the Court of Protection concludes that the advance deci-sion is valid and applicable, it does not have the power to overrule it.

Nothing in an apparent advance decision stops a person:

a. providing life-sustaining treatment, or
b. doing any act he reasonably believes to be necessary to prevent a serious deterioration in P's condition.

while a decision as respects any relevant issue is sought from the court (S.26(5)).

This could of course give rise to problems, as illustrated in Scenario F7 when the treatment being refused is the very treatment required to keep the patient alive, whilst the validity of the advance decision is being considered.

Application to the Court of Protection

The Code of Practice considers the situations where an application to the Court of Protection may be necessary.[12]

> The Court of Protection can make a decision where there is genuine doubt or disagreement about an advance decision's existence, validity or applicability. But the court does not have the power to overturn a valid and applicable advance decision.
>
> 9.68 The court has a range of powers (sections 16–17) to resolve disputes con-cerning the personal care and medical treatment of a person who lacks capacity (see chapter 8 of the Code of Practice). It can decide whether:
>
> ● a person has capacity to accept or refuse treatment at the time it is proposed
> ● an advance decision to refuse treatment is valid

- an advance decision is applicable to the proposed treatment in the current circumstances.

9.69 While the court decides, healthcare professionals can provide life-sustaining treatment or treatment to stop a serious deterioration in their condition. The court has emergency procedures which operate 24 hours a day to deal with urgent cases quickly.

Examples of the concerns which might arise over the validity of an advance decision include:

- a disagreement between relatives and healthcare professionals about whether verbal comments were really an advance decision
- evidence about the person's state of mind raises questions about their capacity at the time they made the decision (see Code of Practice paras 9.7–9.9)
- evidence of important changes in the person's behaviour before they lost capacity that might suggest a change of mind.

In cases where serious doubt remains and cannot be resolved in any other way, it will be possible to seek a declaration from the court.[13]
The possibility of a dispute over an advance decision is considered in Scenario F6.

What can P refuse?

The Law Commission had recommended in its 1995 report[14] that a person drawing up an advance decision should not be able to opt out of basic care. Basic care was defined as 'care to maintain bodily cleanliness and to alleviate severe pain, and the provision of direct oral nutrition and hydration'. There is no such provision in the MCA, and therefore in theory P could refuse any kinds of treatment, including pain relief, by means of an advance decision. However the effect of Section 25(5) is that life-sustaining treatment cannot be withheld or withdrawn unless P specified in writing that the advance decision was to apply, even if life is at risk and all the procedural requirements of Section 25(6) are satisfied.
Refusal to have pain relief is considered in Scenario F.8.

Refusal of care

Section 5 refers to the provision of care and treatment and an advance decision can only cover treatment, so it follows that an advance decision cannot include care. This is the view taken by the Code of Practice,[15] which suggests that Section 5 is intended to cover basic care and would prevent a patient refusing basic care in an advance decision.

[Para 9.28] An advance decision cannot refuse actions that are needed to keep a person comfortable (sometimes called basic or essential care). Examples include warmth, shelter, actions to keep a person clean and the offer of food and water by mouth. Section 5 of the Act allows healthcare professionals to carry out these actions in the best interests of a person who lacks capacity to consent (see chapter 6).

There is in the Act no definition of care, and Section 64 on interpretation suggests that 'treatment' includes a diagnostic or other procedure. There is therefore room for doubt as to what would come within the definition of 'care' and could not therefore be excluded by an advance decision, and what will come under the definition of 'treatment' and could therefore be excluded. Section 5(4) states that:

> Nothing in this section affects the operation of sections 24–26 (advance decisions to refuse treatment)

Eventually case law will determine the extent to which, if any, an individual can, when he or she has the requisite mental capacity, refuse specific types of care at a future time, when the capacity is lost. Scenario F8 illustrates the dilemma.

Conscientious objection

Could a health professional ignore an advance decision on the grounds that he or she has a conscientious objection to withholding or withdrawing life-sustaining treatment? There is no such provision in the MCA. The Law Commission in its report in 1995 considered that it was inappropriate to include such a provision. Treating a patient despite a refusal of consent will constitute the civil wrong of trespass to the person and may constitute a crime.[16] Just as it would be a civil wrong of trespass to the person and even a criminal wrong of assault for a health professional to insist on providing treatment against the wishes of a mentally capacitated person, so it would be a civil wrong or an offence to ignore an advance decision made by a mentally capacitated person which applied to the treatment in question and complied with the statutory requirements. In the words of the Law Commission:

> If the principle of self-determination means anything, the patient's refusal must be respected. There is therefore no need for any specific statutory provision.

Where a health professional had a conscientious objection to letting a person die in such circumstances, it would be advisable for him or her to raise the matter with a senior manager, who if possible could arrange the allocation of staff, so that his conscientious objections were respected. There is however no statutory right for the objector to insist upon that (as there is with a conscientious objection to participation in a termination of pregnancy or in fertilisation treatment), and in the event of a health professional failing to respect a valid advance decision refusing treatment, the health professional could face disciplinary action, fitness to practise proceedings before his or her registration body, civil proceedings and even criminal prosecution (see Chapter 11).

If necessary an application to the Court of Protection could secure the appointment of another person to take responsibility for the patient's health care under Section 17(1)(e).

Excluded decisions

The MCA excludes certain decisions being made on behalf of a person such as marriage or sexual relationships (S.27). Section 28 excludes the authorisation of medical treatment to a patient for mental disorder under the MCA from the Act, and Section 29 prevents reliance on the MCA for voting rights on behalf of a person. (These are considered in Chapter 5.)

Pregnant women

There is no specific statutory provision in the MCA covering the situation where P is pregnant. In the Law Commission's draft Mental Incapacity Bill[17] a clause was included that, in the absence of any indication to the contrary, made it a presumption that an advance refusal does not apply if it endangers the life of the fetus, of a pregnant woman. No such provision is included in the MCA, and therefore problems could arise. See Scenario F9.

Implications for health professionals and others

Criminal offences

Section 62 makes it clear that:

> For the avoidance of doubt, it is hereby declared that nothing in this Act is to be taken to affect the law relating to murder or manslaughter or the operation of section 2 of the Suicide Act 1961 (assisting suicide).

Vital to the legality of a health professional withholding or withdrawing treatment on the basis of a valid advance decision is the distinction in law between killing and letting die. Respecting the autonomy of a person expressed in an advance decision which explicitly refuses life saving treatment and on that basis withholding or withdrawing life-sustaining treatment, is not killing the patient, but letting the patient die. Nor is it an offence of aiding and abetting a suicide under the Suicide Act 1961. These distinctions are explored in Chapter 11.

Refusal to follow a valid, applicable advance decision

If a valid advance decision has been made and is applicable to a specific treatment, then a person who is aware of that advance decision but ignores it would be liable in civil and criminal law, just as they would if the person had the mental capacity to refuse that treatment at the time. Section 26(2) makes it clear that a person is not liable for carrying out or continuing to give the treatment unless he is satisfied that an advance decision exists which is valid and applicable to the treatment.

On the other hand, if treatment is withheld or withdrawn and the person concerned reasonably believed that a valid advance decision applied to the treatment, then that person does not incur liability.

Advance request to initiate or continue treatment

Burke decision

The facts of the Burke case are set out in Case F2.[18] Mr Burke challenged the guidance provided by the GMC (General Medical Council) on withholding or withdrawing treatment in respect of a mentally incapacitated adult, and claimed the right to insist that specific treatment were provided for him, even though it was contrary to the professional discretion of the medical staff. The Court of Appeal upheld the GMC's appeal against the High Court decision. The result is that a person has no legal right to insist on specific treatment being given at a later time, when he lacks the requisite mental capacity. Whilst a person can refuse specific treatments, a person cannot insist on specific treatments being given.

Assisted dying or suicide and mental incapacity

It is clear that a person when competent can draw up an advance directive which specifically refuses life-sustaining treatment, and can give specific instructions via a lasting power of attorney.

What is the situation however in relation to a request for assisted dying, i.e. when the patient wants a positive act to take place either to assist him to commit suicide (assisted suicide) or for that person to end his life (voluntary euthanasia)?

At present both of these actions are criminal offences. Lord Joffe introduced a third Bill into the House of Lords in 2005 which would make both assisted suicide and voluntary euthanasia lawful, provided several exacting conditions were satisfied. However in 2006 the House of Lords voted for the Bill to be postponed, thus effectively terminating it. Lord Joffe has declared a resolve to proceed with his campaign to introduce legislation to permit assisted suicide.

If an assisted dying or assisted suicide Bill is ever enacted, could it apply to those lacking mental capacity?

The Bill required the person to be mentally capable of requesting such a procedure, and this capacity must be confirmed by an attending physician, a consulting physician a solicitor and another witness.

Could the request for assisted suicide be made by way of an advance decision? The answer is 'no', because the patient must be mentally competent at the time the request is made, must have had advice from a palliative care specialist (either doctor or nurse) and complete a declaration. It is inconceivable that all this could be done in advance when the patient is mentally competent and then put into effect when the patient lacks mental competence. Assisted dying, as the last Bill envisaged, was therefore only for those who have proven mental capacity at the time the request is made and to be carried out. This discussion is of course hypothetical, since the Assisted Dying Bill has not been enacted.

Conclusions

Tragic cases such as those of Diane Pretty and Annie Linsall are likely to have raised the profile and the perceived value of advance decisions for those who are facing a chronic deteriorating illness. The use of advance decisions will probably increase. It is therefore important for health professionals, across all specialities, to be aware of the existence and implications of an advance decision. Early action may be necessary in the event of any doubts arising about the validity of the advance decision, or about its applicability to a given situation or to specific treatments, and in particular its validity and applicability in relation to life-sustaining treatments.

References

1   *Airedale NHS Trust* v. *Bland* [1993] AC 789.
2   *HE* v. *NHS Trust A and AE* [2003] EWHC 1017 (Fam).
3   Law Commission (1995) Report No. 231, *Mental Incapacity*. HMSO, London.
4   *Re W (a minor)(medical treatment)* [1992] 4 All ER 627.
5   In *Re B (Consent to treatment: Capacity)*, Times Law Report, 26 March 2002.
6   Code of Practice for the Mental Capacity Act 2005. Department of Constitutional Affairs February 2007 para 9.18. TSO, London.
7   *Ibid*. para 9.23.
8   *HE and (1) a Hospital NHS Trust and (2) AE (by her litigation friend the Official Solicitor)* [2003] EWHC 1017 (Fam).
9   Mental Capacity Act 2005 Explanatory Memorandum (2005). HMSO, London.
10 www.dca.gov.uk
11 National Council for Palliative Care (2005) *Guidance on the Mental Capacity Act 2005*. www.ncpc.org.uk
12 Code of Practice for the Mental Capacity Act 2005. Department of Constitutional Affairs February 2007 para 9.67. TSO, London.
13 *Ibid*. para 9.60.
14 Law Commission (1995) Report No. 231, *Mental Incapacity*. HMSO, London.
15 Code of Practice for the Mental Capacity Act 2005. Department of Constitutional Affairs February 2007 para 9.28. TSO, London.
16 *Re T (Adult: Refusal of Treatment)* [1993] Fam 95.
17 Law Commission (1995) Report No. 231, *Mental Incapacity*. HMSO, London.
18 *R. (on the application of Burke)* v. *General Medical Council and Disability Rights Commission and the Official Solicitor to the Supreme Court* [2005] EWCA Civ 1003; [2004] EWHC 1879; [2005] QB 424; [2005] 2 WLR 431; [2004] Lloyd's Rep Med 451.

Scenarios F
Advance Decisions

Introduction

Advance decisions, also known as living wills or advance refusals, had been recognised as valid at common law (i.e. judge made law or case law) but had not been placed on a statutory basis until the Mental Capacity Act 2005. These Scenarios should be read in conjunction with Chapter 9.

Scenario F1: The statutory provisions.

Rita Davis was suffering from multiple sclerosis and was anxious to ensure that as her disease progressed and she became incapable of making her own treatment decisions she would not receive artificial feeding and hydration and ventilation or be resuscitated. She therefore arranged to draw up a living will (i.e. advance decision) in which she gave an advance refusal of such treatments. The document was duly signed and witnessed. Only three months after signing the living will she was severely injured when she fell down some steps and was brought into hospital unconscious. She was carrying her living will in her handbag and doctors were concerned to know whether, if they operated and she required ventilation in intensive care, the advance decision would prevent their providing such treatment and care. What are the statutory provisions?

Rita Davis must have been 18 years and have had the requisite mental capacity at the time she signed the advance decision for it to be valid. If the document specifies that she had the necessary mental capacity and is signed and witnessed, there would be a presumption that it was valid, but this could be rebutted if evidence was produced to the contrary. However there are problems relating to the circumstances envisaged by Rita. She drew it up in the context of her multiple sclerosis and that condition deteriorating so much that she would not wish to receive life-sustaining treatments. This is not the situation which has occurred here. The doctors would therefore have very real doubts as to the applicability of Rita's advance decision to the situation following her fall. In this uncertainty they would be justified in taking any life saving measures, whilst an application to the Court of Protection for a declaration on the validity of her advance decision to the present situation was considered.

What situations would an advance decision cover?

See Scenario F2.

Scenario F2: A change of faith.

Jake, who belonged to a religious group which disagreed with any surgical procedures, drew up an advance decision which reflected these beliefs, and refused all surgical intervention in the event of his becoming mentally incapacitated and needing such treatments. Subsequently Jake was converted to another faith which did not hold those beliefs. It did not occur to him to change his advance decision. A few years later Jake lost the mental capacity to make treatment decisions. Doctors said that he required an appendectomy. A relative showed his advance decision to the staff and pointed out that for the last few years Jake had gone to a different church which was not opposed to surgery. Does the fact that Jake had not destroyed the advance decision mean that it is still valid and reflects views which he would still have held and expressed had he not lost his mental capacity? Alternatively is it an oversight that Jake has not changed or destroyed his advance decision?

In such a situation as shown in Scenario F2, health professionals would probably have to apply to the Court of Protection for a declaration as to the validity of the advance decision. The court could take into account his change of religion and the new beliefs and decide if Jake would have intended the advance decision to apply to the situation in which he now found himself.

Applicability of an advance decision

Scenario F3: Applicability of an advance decision.

Peter drew up a living will shortly after he was diagnosed with a chronic debilitating disease. It stated that in the event of his losing his mental capacity he would not wish to be given life-sustaining treatment, even though he could die as a consequence. Ten years later the disease had progressed to the point where Peter no longer had the mental capacity to make any decisions relating to his care and treatment. His relatives ensured that the health professionals were aware of his advance decision. However in the ensuing years, significant progress had been made in curing the specific disease he suffered by genetic means and the doctors were hopeful that if he could be kept alive, then the new treatments would make considerable improvements to his mental and physical well-being. They therefore wished the advance decision to be ignored or overruled.

In a situation like that in Scenario F3 an application would be made to the Court of Protection to determine the validity of the advance decision in the changing circumstances. Evidence would have to be taken as to whether Peter was aware of the scientific progress before he lost his mental capacity. In the meantime treatment could be given to him to sustain him, until the court had made its decision.

Life-sustaining decisions

Scenario F4: Advance decision completed in hospital.

Polly was seriously ill with cancer and feared a prolonged, painful death. Staff nurse Davidson asked her about whether she would wish to be resuscitated in the event of a cardiac arrest. Polly said that she would welcome such an event and would not wish to be resuscitated. Staff nurse Mavis Davidson wrote this up in Polly's records and asked her to sign it. She said that she felt too ill to write or sign anything. Mavis therefore wrote a note in Polly's records that she would not wish to be resuscitated in the event of an arrest, and said that she would sign it in Polly's name with her approval. Polly agreed to that and Mavis wrote that she was completing it on behalf of Polly and asked another nurse, Beryl, to witness what was happening. Polly gave a sign that she was happy with what was taking place. Beryl then wrote a note in the records that she had witnessed Polly acknowledging the decision and Mavis's signing on her behalf. Beryl signed the note. Subsequently Polly became very confused and dipped in and out of consciousness. The consultant queried what Mavis had done, and said that the decision against resuscitation should have been recorded on a hospital form, not just in Polly's records and doubted its validity. What is the law?

Whilst an advance decision relating to life-sustaining treatment must be in writing, the Act does not require the writing to be written by the person making the decision. The formalities are satisfied if a person writes it up on behalf of a mentally capacitated patient. The fact that Mavis wrote up Polly's wishes satisfies the legal requirements. In addition the fact that Polly did not sign it herself is acceptable provided that someone signed it on her behalf in her presence, and Mavis satisfies this requirement. The final formality that a witness should be present for the signing and that the witness signs this (or acknowledges it) in Polly's presence is satisfied by Beryl's presence and signature. The legal formalities required by Section 25(6) (a), (b), (c) and (d) are therefore all satisfied. The consultant would therefore be wrong in maintaining that the record of Polly's advance decision was invalid. In law it would be acceptable. It may of course be possible that Mavis did not follow the hospital procedures in what she did, but this is a separate issue and would not necessarily invalidate Polly's instructions in law. The issue of course may arise as to whether Polly had the requisite mental capacity at the time she gave her instructions, and Mavis would have to give evidence as to why she believed Polly to be capable at the time she recorded the advance decision. There would have been advantages in securing the opinion of an independent health professional on the issue of Polly's competence at the time. It is also advisable for the assessment of competence to be documented by the person who made it.

What would the situation be if the hospital used electronic records?

Writing would probably include electronic records. However there would have to be facilities for signatures to be incorporated as required by the conditions of Section 25(6)(b) and (d), where the advance decision referred to life-sustaining treatments.

Effect of an advance decision

Scenario F5 explores the situation where staff were not aware of the existence of an advance decision.

Scenario F5: Advance decision unknown.

In a Canadian case,[1] an unconscious patient was given a life-saving blood transfusion, in spite of the fact that she was carrying a card refusing such treatment. She was awarded C$20 000. The doctor had ignored her written request not to give her blood, and this constituted a trespass to her person. However, what would have been the situation if the nurse had not shown to the doctor the card on which the advance refusal was recorded and witnessed?

In such a revised situation, the doctor could not have been successfully sued for trespass to the person since he would not have known of the advance refusal, and therefore in fulfilling his duty of care to the patient he would not have realised that she had refused to have a blood transfusion. Action could of course be taken against the nurse if it was established that she had deliberately withheld information about the existence of an advance decision.

Disputes over advance decisions

Scenario F6: Relatives dispute.

Following a road traffic accident, Steve is brought unconscious into the A&E department. He is carrying a card which makes it clear that he would not wish to have any surgical intervention or blood. The card is not witnessed. His situation is life threatening and the doctor examining him knows that if he does not have blood or surgery within the next few hours, he will die. He consults the directorate manager on the validity of the card and is told that it is a valid advance decision. He therefore does not give Steve a transfusion or arrange for an operation. Relatives who arrive in the Accident and Emergency (A&E) department are horrified to be told that Steve is dying and no operation has been carried out. They are prepared to sue for breach of the duty of care by the doctor.

In such a situation as Scenario F6, the relatives could argue that the statutory provisions for refusing life-sustaining treatments have not been satisfied by Steve, and the advance decision is not therefore valid. The doctor could rely upon the statement of the directorate manager that the advance decision is valid. However it fails to comply with the statutory requirements of refusing life-sustaining treatments. It does not appear that Steve has mentioned that he is refusing these treatments, even though his life is at risk and the statement has not been witnessed. The doctor might be able to maintain that he had a reasonable belief in its validity and applicability, and therefore was not liable under the Act. If the directorate manager had queried the validity or the applicability of the advance decision of Steve and referred the issue of its validity to court, then the doctor could have continued life-sustaining treatment until the court had ruled on its validity.

Court ruling on validity of an advance decision

Scenario F7: Keeping alive.

A woman who was a Jehovah's Witness drew up an advance decision, which stated that if at a future time she no longer had mental capacity she would not wish to be given blood, even in a life saving situation. After the advance decision was created she changed her faith. She did not however withdraw or alter the advance decision. She was seriously injured in a road accident and needed a life saving blood transfusion. There was concern by her family and friends because she was no longer a Jehovah's Witness as to whether her advance decision was still valid. An application to the court to consider the validity of the advance decision was made.

In Scenario F7 it would be possible under Section 26(5) for life-sustaining treatment to be carried on whilst the decision of the court is awaited. This section enables action to be taken to provide life-sustaining treatment, or to do something which is reasonably believed to be necessary to prevent a serious deterioration in P's condition. However in the circumstances giving blood would completely defeat the wishes of the woman, if subsequently the court were to declare her advance decision was valid. In such circumstances it is hoped that the woman could be kept alive with non-blood products, and the court in an emergency session could make a very speedy declaration on the validity of the advance decision. In Case F1 the judge had to decide if an advance decision was still valid.

Case F1: HE and (1) a Hospital NHS Trust and (2) AE 2003.[2]

AE was brought up as a Muslim, but following the separation of her parents went to live with her mother and became a Jehovah's Witness. She signed a pre-printed form refusing a blood transfusion in February 2001. She suffered from a congenital heart defect. She was taken seriously ill in April 2003 and admitted to hospital. Her mother told the hospital that AE was a Jehovah's Witness and would not want to have a blood transfusion, and that the advance directive should be followed. AE's condition deteriorated and a blood transfusion became a life saving necessity. Her mother opposed a transfusion, but her father believed it should be given. He stated that his daughter had become engaged to a Muslim and agreed to give up her Jehovah's Witness faith as a condition of the marriage. She had subsequently ceased to attend Jehovah's Witness meetings. The father applied to court for a declaration that a blood transfusion could be given. AE was represented by the Official Solicitor.

The judge held that there was no reason in law why an advance directive could not be withdrawn without any formalities. He stated that it is fundamental that an advance directive is, of its very essence and nature, inherently revocable. He accepted the father's evidence that, as a matter of fact, AE had ceased to be a Jehovah's Witness. The burden of proof lay on those who sought to establish the continuing validity and applicability of the advance directive. Where life is at stake the evidence must be scrutinised with especial care. Clear and convincing proof is required. The continuing validity and applicability of the advance directive must be clearly established by convincing and inherently reliable evidence. If there is doubt, that doubt falls to be resolved in favour of the preservation of life. Once it was held that the advance directive was no longer valid, then the doctors had to treat AE in the way that in their clinical judgment best accorded with her interests, and her best interests required her to have the blood transfusion. The judge made a declaration accordingly.

   As a postscript the judge criticised the fact that the father was compelled to take action himself, and considered that, where there was a doubt as to the validity of an advance directive, then the doctors and health authorities should not hesitate to apply to the courts for assistance. This case was heard before the implementation of the Mental Capacity Act (MCA), but similar principles would apply. However from 1 October 2007 the case would be heard in the Court of Protection.

What can be refused?

> ### Scenario F8: Refusing pain management.
>
> Patrick is a Buddhist and believes in mind over matter. He had drawn up an advance decision which stated that if he were to be in a situation where he no longer had mental capacity to make his own decisions, he would not wish to be given any treatment including life-sustaining treatments, including ventilation or resuscitation. He is in the late stages of pancreatic cancer and had refused all pain relief. He gradually lost his mental capacity to make decisions and was clearly in severe pain. Health professionals caring for him were aware of his advance decision, but felt that it would not cover the administration of pain relief. A dispute arose between the clinical team and his relatives over whether pain relief could be administered.

Had the earlier draft of the Mental Incapacity Bill been enacted, there would have been no difficulties in deciding what action to take in Scenario F8, since Patrick could not, through an advance direction, advance decision or advance refusal refuse pain relief. However in the absence of such provision in the MCA, the court would have to determine whether Patrick's advance decision could include alleviation of pain. Account would have to be taken of the Buddhist views on pain management.

The Code of Practice makes it clear that an advance decision can only cover 'treatment' and not care (see Chapter 9). There is no statutory definition of 'care' and the definition of 'treatment' in Section 64 states that it 'includes a diagnostic or other procedure'. If pain relief is considered to be 'care' then the fact that Patrick has included it in his advance decision does not mean that it cannot be given, since an advance decision can only cover 'treatment'. However if pain relief is seen as a 'treatment' then its inclusion within an advance decision would be appropriate and, if all the other statutory requirements are satisfied, then pain relief could be withheld from Patrick.

Pregnant women and advance decisions

This is discussed in Scenario F9.

> ### Scenario F9: Refusal of blood.
>
> Pamela, a Jehovah's Witness, drew up an advance decision stating that if a situation arose where she lacked the mental capacity to make a decision she would

not want to be given a blood transfusion, even it is was a life-sustaining necessity. The document was signed and witnessed. Several years later she was involved in an explosion and was severely injured and incapable of making decisions. On arrival at the A&E department, the consultant stated that she was pregnant and if she did not have blood the fetus would die. Is the advance decision binding upon the health professionals?

The situation in Scenario F9 is another example where it may be necessary to seek a declaration from the court, since it is not clear from the advance decision whether or not it would cover the situation where Pamela is pregnant. However since it does cover a life saving situation, the court is likely to hold that it is valid and binding in those current circumstances. The fact that it does not explicitly refer to the possibility of a pregnancy would not necessarily invalidate its effect. It would be a different situation if there were specific statutory provision as the Law Commission had recommended in 1995. However, good practice in drawing up advance decisions would suggest that women of childbearing age should take into account the possibility of their being pregnant at the time an advance decision came into effect and decide, in drawing up the document, the effect of the pregnancy on their advance decision.

The Explanatory Memorandum[3] suggests that

The reference to 'life' includes the life of an unborn child. [Para 89]

However, as discussed in Chapter 9 this is open to a different interpretation by the courts.

Advance decisions and best interests

A valid and applicable advance decision where P is unable to make his own decisions removes the possibility of using the best interests criteria to determine what treatments P should have. It may be difficult for health and social services professionals and relatives to accept, but they have no option other than to ensure that the wishes of P are carried out, as Scenario F10 illustrates.

Scenario F10: Contrary to her best interests.

Rachel was 19 years old and her lungs were severely damaged by cystic fibrosis. She was assisted by the mother of another patient in drawing up an advance decision. In this she stated that in the event of her losing her mental capacity to make her own treatment decisions and in the event of her facing the terminal stage of her illness, she would not wish to be resuscitated, have any operative procedure or be given artificial nutrition and hydration, even though her life was at stake. She arranged for this statement to be witnessed. She agreed to have surgery under a mild anaesthetic for the insertion of a shunt to take future treatments of antibiotics. During the operation she regurgitated some substance into her lungs and had to be placed on a ventilator. The staff were aware of her advance decision. However her relatives were anxious that she should be kept alive. In addition it appeared that compatible lungs were available for transplant. Should Rachel be kept on a ventilator and be transferred for the transplant to take place?

The answer to this question depends entirely upon the clarity of the advance decision which Rachel signed and how apparent it is that it applies to the situation she is now in. She became mentally incapacitated because of a mishap during surgery, not because of her underlying condition. Does this mean that the advance decision is not applicable? From the staff and relatives point of view it would appear to be in Rachel's best interests for her to be kept alive. However this does not appear to accord with her wishes as set out in the advance decision. Section 25(4)c states that if there are reasonable grounds for believing that circumstances exist which P did not anticipate at the time of the advance decision and which would have affected his decision had he anticipated them, then the advance decision is not applicable to the treatment in question. This may be the situation in this Scenario. The Court of Protection would have to determine the question of its applicability, and in the meantime steps could be taken to keep Rachel alive.

Withdrawing or altering an advance decision

Scenario F11: A change of mind.

Bill had drawn up an advance decision which stated that in the event of his suffering from cancer he would not wish to be resuscitated or receive artificial nutrition and hydration (ANH). He was told that cancer of the throat had been diagnosed and was advised that he would need a gastric tube to be inserted for food. He told the nurse that in that case he would change his advance refusal so that the refusal of ANH would be deleted. Before he had a chance of changing the document, he became unconscious. The health professionals are in conflict over what treatments Bill should be given. The consultant considers himself to be bound by the advance refusal; the staff nurse holds that his instructions by word of mouth were sufficient to change the advance decision.

The MCA permits a person to withdraw or alter an advance decision at any time when he has capacity to do so. If Bill had the requisite mental capacity at the time that he told the staff nurse that he was prepared to accept the gastric tube to be inserted, then this would constitute an alteration to his advance decision and would be valid. A withdrawal (including a partial withdrawal) need not be in writing, nor need an alteration of an advance decision be in writing. However if the alteration of the advance decision meant that P was now wishing life-sustaining treatments to be refused by means of the advance decision, then the requirements of Section 25(5) would apply (see Scenario F4 and **Life sustaining decisions**, page 209).

Requesting treatments by advance decision

The statutory provisions only cover refusals. Should they have been extended to cover the request of a patient, when mentally incapacitated, to have specific treatments provided at a subsequent time when he or she was without capacity? The issue was discussed in the Burke Case F2.

Case F2: Burke case.[4]

A patient suffering from cerebellar ataxia, a progressive degenerative condition, and of full capacity, challenged the General Medical Council guidelines, *Withholding and Withdrawing Life-prolonging Treatments: Good Practice in Decision-making*. He argued that the guidelines were contrary to the Articles of the European Convention on Human Rights. He applied for judicial review and sought clarification as to the circumstances in which ANH would be withdrawn. He did not want ANH to be withdrawn until he died of natural causes.

The judge granted judicial review, holding that once a patient had been admitted to an NHS hospital there was a duty of care to provide and go on providing treatment, whether the patient was competent or incompetent or unconscious. This duty of care, which could not be transferred to anyone else, was to provide that treatment which was in the best interests of the patient. It was for the patient if competent to determine what was in his best interests. If the patient was incompetent and had left no binding and effective advance directive, then it was for the court to decide what was in his best interests. To withdraw ANH at any stage before the claimant finally lapsed into a coma would involve a clear breach of both Articles 8 and 3, because he would thereby be exposed to acute mental and physical suffering. The GMC (General Medical Council) guidelines were therefore in error in emphasising the right of the claimant to refuse treatment, but not his right to require treatment.

The GMC appealed against this ruling and the Court of Appeal's reserved judgment was given on 29 July 2005. The Court of Appeal held that doctors are not obliged to provide patients with treatment that they consider to be futile or harmful, even if the patient demands it. Autonomy and the right of self-determination do not entitle the patient to insist on receiving a particular medical treatment regardless of the nature of the treatment. However where a competent patient says that he or she wants to be kept alive by the provision of food and water, doctors must agree to that. Not to do so would result in the doctor not merely being in breach of duty but guilty of murder.

Checklist to determine whether one is bound by an advance decision

- Is there evidence that P had the requisite mental capacity when making the advance decision?
- Was P at least 18 years at the time he made the advance decision?
- Is P now lacking the mental capacity to make decisions for himself?
- Does the advance decision cover the situation which P is now in?
- Does the advance decision cover the treatments which have been recommended as being in P's best interests?
- Is there any evidence that the advance decision has been withdrawn or altered?
- Has P drawn up a lasting power of attorney?
- If so, was it drawn up before or after the advance decision?
- If it was drawn up after the advance decision, does it cover the same treatment and circumstances as the advance decision, and does it conflict with the advance decision?
- Is life-sustaining treatment being refused?
- If so, has P specified in writing in the advance decision that the refusal is to apply to such treatment, and are the statutory requirements for such a refusal satisfied?
- Is there a reasonable doubt about the validity or applicability of the advance decision?
- Is immediate treatment necessary to keep the patient alive whilst a declaration on the validity or the applicability of the advance decision is being sought from the Court of Protection?

References

1   *Malette* v. *Shulman* (1991) 2 Med LR 162.
2   *HE and (1) a Hospital NHS Trust and (2) AE by her litigation friend the Official Solicitor* [2003] EWHC 1017 (Fam).
3   Mental Capacity Act 2005 Explanatory Memorandum (2005). TSO, London.
4   *R. (on the application of Burke)* v. *General Medical Council and Disability Rights Commission and the Official Solicitor to the Supreme Court* [2005] EWCA Civ 1003; [2004] EWHC 1879; [2005] QB 424; [2005] 2 WLR 431; [2004] Lloyd's Rep Med 451.

10 Research

Introduction

The Joint Committee of Parliament[1] considered the issue of medical research and the adult who lacks mental capacity, and was concerned at the absence of any provision in the draft Mental Incapacity Bill relating to research, since it considered that if properly regulated research involving people who may lack capacity was not possible then treatments for incapacitating disorders would not be developed. The Joint Committee examined the importance of local research ethics committees for the protection of the rights of those participating in research, and the significance of the Helsinki Declaration by the World Medical Association in 1964 (and subsequently updated) to prevent the abuse of vulnerable people through medical experimentation. Those principles relating to research on those who lack the capacity to give a valid consent set out in the Helsinki Declaration (as revised in Edinburgh in 2000) are shown in Box 10.1. The full Declaration can be found in the appendix to (DH) guidance on local research ethics committees[2] and on the World Medical Association website.[3]

Box 10.1: Research principles set out in the Helsinki Declaration relating to those unable to give consent.

23. When obtaining informed consent for the research project the physician should be particularly cautious if the subject is in a dependent relationship with the physician or may consent under duress. In that case the informed consent should be obtained by a well-informed physician who is not engaged in the investigation and who is completely independent of this relationship.

---

24. For a research subject who is legally incompetent, physically or mentally incapable of giving consent or is a legally incompetent minor, the investigator must obtain informed consent from the legally authorised representative in accordance with applicable law. These groups should not be included in research unless the research is necessary to promote the health of the population represented and this research cannot instead be performed on legally competent persons.

25. When a subject deemed legally incompetent, such as a minor child, is able to give assent to decisions about participation in research, the investigator must obtain that assent in addition to the consent of the legally authorised representative.

26. Research on individuals from whom it is not possible to obtain consent, including proxy or advance consent, should be done only if the physical/mental condition that prevents obtaining informed consent is a necessary characteristic of the research population. The specific reasons for involving research subjects with a condition that renders them unable to give informed consent should be stated in the experimental protocol for consideration and approval of the review committee. The protocol should state that consent to remain in the research should be obtained as soon as possible from the individual or a legally authorised surrogate.

The Joint Committee's conclusion was that the inclusion of statutory provisions governing such research would enable the ethical requirements that must underpin research involving people with incapacity to be clearly enshrined in statute. It recommended that a clause should be included in the Bill to enable strictly-controlled medical research to explore the causes and consequences of mental incapacity and to develop effective treatment for such conditions. The clause should include rigorous protocols to protect incapacitated adults from being exploited or harmed.

The Joint Committee recommended that the Bill should set out the key principles governing research, such as those enshrined by the World Medical Association. These key principles should include the following:

- Research involving people who may be incapacitated must be reviewed by a properly established and independent ethics committee, and can only proceed if ethical permission is granted.
- Where a person has the capacity to consent, then his decision whether or not to partake in research must be respected.
- Considerable care should be taken to ensure that under these circumstances consent to participate was freely given and not a consequence of coercion.
- The inclusion of people in research, who lacked the capacity to consent, must only occur when such research has the potential for direct benefit to those with

that particular problem, and could not have been done through the involvement of those with capacity.

- Those undertaking research involving people lacking the capacity to consent must respect any indications that a person did not wish to participate (i.e. was dissenting).
- Any discomfort or risk involved in the research must be, at the most, minimal.

In addition the Joint Committee on Human Rights[4] questioned certain provisions in relation to research on persons lacking mental capacity. The Government response stated that:

> We want to achieve a balance between allowing important research to proceed whilst not exposing an extremely vulnerable group of individuals to unacceptable interference with the rights and freedom of action or privacy. People who lack capacity must not be denied the benefits that can be obtained through carefully regulated research. Without such research, the development of appropriate treatments and improvements in services may not be possible. [Para 53]
>
> The Government wishes to provide a strict but enabling system of safeguards to cover this entire breadth of research. [Para 54]

These recommendations were for the most part incorporated into the Bill, and were subsequently included in the statutory provisions.

The Joint Committee also recommended that the Codes of Practice should set out specific issues that ethics committees should be obliged to consider when any research includes people who may be incapacitated, including whether the involvement of mentally incapacitated persons is justified, whether issues of consent and consultation had been properly considered, and any other relevant matters. The Codes of Practice should also define the duties of research ethics committees in relation to incapacitated adults.

The eventual provisions in the Act are in accordance with long-standing international standards, for example those laid down by the World Medicine Association and the Council of Europe Convention on Human Rights and Biomedicine (Explanatory Memorandum Para 96).

Statutory provisions

Sections 30–34 contain the provisions relating to research and the mentally incapacitated adult.

Conditions for intrusive research

The Mental Capacity Act (MCA) prohibits intrusive research being carried out on, or in relation to, a person who lacks the capacity to consent unless certain conditions are met. These conditions are shown in Box 10.2.

> **Box 10.2: Conditions required for research on those lacking the requisite mental capacity to give consent.**
>
> - that the research is part of a research project
> - which is approved by an appropriate body as defined in Section 31
> - complies with the conditions laid down in Section 31 (see Box 10.3), and
> - complies with conditions relating to the consulting of carers and additional safeguards (i.e. Sections 32 and 33; see below).

Scenario G1 illustrates the implications of these provisions.

Intrusive research

Intrusive research is defined in Section 30(2) as:

> research which would be unlawful if carried out on a person capable of giving consent, but without that consent.

Clinical trials which come under the clinical trials regulations are excluded from the statutory provisions.[5] These are considered below.

The Code of Practice[6] notes that the Act does not have a specific definition for 'research' and it quotes the definitions used by the DH and National Assembly for Wales (NAW) publications, *Research Governance Framework for Health and Social Care*:

> research can be defined as the attempt to derive generalisable new knowledge by addressing clearly defined questions with systematic and rigorous methods.[7]

The Code of Practice points out that research may:

- provide information that can be applied generally to an illness, disorder or condition
- demonstrate how effective and safe a new treatment is
- add to evidence that one form of treatment works better than another
- add to evidence that one form of treatment is safer than another, or
- examine wider issues (for example, the factors that affect someone's capacity to make a decision).

The Code of Practice notes that:[8]

> It is expected that most of the researchers who ask for their research to be approved under the Act will be medical or social care researchers. However, the Act can cover more than just medical and social care research. Intrusive research which does not meet the requirements of the Act cannot be carried out lawfully in relation to people who lack capacity.

Non-intrusive research

Non-intrusive research could include research of anonymised records or the use of anonymous tissue or blood left over after it had been collected for use in other procedures. Whilst such research is excluded from the provisions of the Mental Capacity Act 2005, it could come under other legislative provisions such as the Data Protection Act 1998 and regulations under the Data Protection Act and the Human Tissue Act 2004 (see Chapter 14).

Requirements for approval

The appropriate body (i.e. the person, committee, or other body specified by the Secretary of State in regulations)[9] may not approve a research project relating to a person lacking the capacity to consent unless the conditions shown in Box 10.3 are present.

Box 10.3: Conditions for approval of a research project relating to a person lacking the capacity to consent (Section 31)

- (2) The research is connected with an impairing condition affecting P (the person lacking mental capacity) or its treatment.
- (3) An impairing condition is defined in Section 31(3) as a condition which is (or may be) attributable to, or which causes or contributes to, the impairment of, or disturbance in the functioning of, the mind or brain.
- (4) There must be reasonable grounds for believing that the research would not be as effective if carried out only on, or only in relation to, persons who have the capacity to consent to taking part in the project.
- (5)(a) The research must have the potential to benefit P without imposing on P a burden that is disproportionate to the potential benefit to P, or
- (5)(b) be intended to provide knowledge of the causes or treatment of, or of the care of persons affected by, the same or a similar condition.
- (6) If 5(b) applies and not 5(a), there must be reasonable grounds for believing – (a) that the risk to P from taking part in the project is likely to be negligible, and (b) that anything done to, or in relation to, P will not – (i) interfere with P's freedom of action or privacy in a significant way, or (ii) be unduly invasive or restrictive.
- (7) There must be reasonable arrangements in place for ensuring that the requirements of Sections 32 and 33 are in place. [See **Consulting carers** and **Additional safeguards** on pages 224 and 225].

Scenario G1 illustrates the workings of the conditions shown in Box 10.3.

Impairing condition

The Code of Practice discusses the meaning of impairing condition and the underlying cause:[10]

It is the person's actual condition that must be the same or similar in research, not the underlying cause. A *'similar condition'* may therefore have a different cause to that suffered by the participant. For example, research into ways of supporting people with learning disabilities to live more independently might involve a person with a learning disability caused by a head trauma. But its findings might help people with similar learning disabilities that have different causes.

The Code of Practice gives the example of a man with Down's syndrome who appears to be showing the symptoms of Alzheimer's disease, and his consultant is seeking to involve him in a research project to investigate the cause and treatment of dementia in people with Down's syndrome.
  The Code of Practice also notes that:[11]

Benefits may be direct or indirect (for example, the person might benefit at a later date if policies or care packages affecting them are changed because of the research). It might be that participation in the research itself will be of benefit to the person in particular circumstances. For example, if the research involves interviews and the person has the opportunity to express their views, this could be considered of real benefit to a particular individual.

Balancing risks against benefits

These provisions require ethical committees to be sure that the research on the mentally incapacitated person is justified in terms of its scientific value, and there is no valid alternative by carrying out the research on a person who does have the capacity to give consent. There must be a balancing exercise in contrasting the risks against the benefits to the mentally incapacitated person.
  The Code of Practice in discussing this balancing of the risks against the benefits of research involving adults who lack capacity gives the following examples of possible benefits:[12]

Potential benefits of research for a person who lacks capacity could include:

- developing more effective ways of treating a person or managing their condition
- improving the quality of healthcare, social care or other services that they have access to
- discovering the cause of their condition, if they would benefit from that knowledge, or
- reducing the risk of the person being harmed, excluded or disadvantaged.

The research could include both an analysis of the disease which has caused the mental incapacity and also the effects of the mental incapacity on his health and day-to-day life.[13]
  Paragraph 101 of the Explanatory Memorandum suggests the following interpretation of Subsections 5 and 6 of Section 31, which deal with the anticipated benefits and risks of the research:

There are two alternatives: either the research has the potential to benefit the person without imposing a burden disproportionate to that benefit (this type of research is sometimes called 'therapeutic research'); or the research is to provide knowledge of the causes of the person's condition, its treatment or the care of people who have the same or similar condition now or who may develop it in the future. In relation to this latter category, there must be reasonable grounds for believing that the risk to the person is negligible and the research must not interfere with the person's freedom of action or privacy in a significant way or be unduly invasive or restrictive. This latter category of research might include indirect research on medical notes or on tissue already taken for other purposes. It may also include interviews or questionnaires with carers about health or social-care services received by the person or limited observation of the person. And it could include taking samples from the person, e.g. blood samples, specifically for the research project.

The potential benefit to P is perhaps more loosely defined that some would wish. The Government justified departing from the Oviedo Convention (to which the United Kingdom is not a signatory) because it was too narrow in coverage. The Government did not accept the criteria from the Oviedo Convention that research must be of real and direct benefit to P, because for some research such as clinical and in a wider social care setting, it may be hard to show that it will definitely benefit a person directly, even though it may generate valuable knowledge about their condition.

Consulting carers (Section 32)

The researcher 'R' is required to take reasonable steps to identify a person who is not engaged in a professional capacity nor receiving remuneration, but is engaged in caring for P or is interested in P's welfare and is prepared to be consulted by the researcher under Section 32.

Subsection (7) makes it clear that the fact that a person is the donee of a lasting power of attorney given by P, or is P's deputy, does not prevent that person from being the person consulted under Section 32.

If such a person cannot be identified, then R must, in accordance with guidance issued by the Secretary of State or the Welsh Assembly, nominate a person who is prepared to be consulted by R but has no connection with the project.

At present there appears to be no provision for the health service body or local authority to be required to instruct the Independent Mental Capacity Advocacy service to provide a person to support and represent the person incapable of giving consent to participation in research, before research can be carried out using that person. The guidance to be produced might recommend an IMCA, but subordinate legislation would be necessary if it were to become a requirement that an IMCA should be appointed (in the absence of an appropriate person) where the person was being involved in research to which he or she could not give consent.

R must provide the carer or nominee with information about the project and ask him for advice as to whether P should take part in the project and what, in his opinion, P's wishes and feelings about taking part in the project would be likely to be if P had capacity in relation to the matter. If the person consulted advises R that in his opinion P's wishes and feelings would be likely to lead him to decline to take part in the project (or to wish to withdraw from it), if he had the capacity, then R must ensure that P does not take part, or if he is already taking part, ensure that he is withdrawn from it.

If treatment has commenced it is not necessary to discontinue the treatment if R has reasonable grounds for believing that there would be a significant risk to P's health if it were discontinued.

Scenario G2 illustrates this situation.

Urgent research (S.32(8)(9))

Special provisions apply where treatment is to be provided as a matter of urgency and R considers that it is also necessary to take action for the purposes of the research as a matter of urgency, but it is not reasonably practicable to consult under the above provisions of this section.

In these circumstances R must have the agreement of a registered medical practitioner who is not concerned in the organisation or conduct of the research project or where it is not reasonably practicable in the time available to obtain that agreement, he acts in accordance with a procedure approved by the appropriate body at the time when the research project was approved under Section 31. When R has reasonable grounds for believing that it is no longer necessary to take the action as a matter of urgency, he cannot continue to act in reliance on these urgent provisions (S.32(10)).

Scenario G4 discusses the implications of the provisions relating to urgent research.

Additional safeguards (Section 33)

There are additional safeguards to protect the interests of the person lacking the requisite mental capacity:

- nothing may be done to, or in relation to a person taking part in the research project who is incapable of giving consent,
- to which he appears to object (whether by showing signs of resistance or otherwise) except where what is being done is intended to protect him from harm or to reduce or prevent pain or discomfort, or
- which would be contrary to an advance decision of his which has effect or any other form of statement made by him and not subsequently withdrawn and R is aware of this.

Scenario G.3 illustrates the effect of resistance by a research participant who lacks the requisite mental capacity.

The MCA expressly states (S.33(3)) that the interests of the person must be assumed to outweigh those of science and society.

Scenario G5 illustrates the conflict between the interests of society and those of the participant.

If P indicates (in any way) that he wishes to be withdrawn from the project he must be withdrawn without delay. He must also be withdrawn without delay if R has reasonable grounds for believing that one or more of the requirements set out in Section 31(2)–(7) (see Box 10.3) are no longer met in relation to the research being carried out on P.

The research is not to be discontinued under Section 33(4) or (5) if R has reasonable grounds for believing that there would be a significant risk to P's health if it were discontinued.

Loss of capacity during research project

Section 34 applies if P had consented to take part in a research project begun before the commencement of Section 30 (1 April 2007) but, before the conclusion of the project, loses capacity to consent to continue to take part in it. In such a situation regulations may provide that despite his loss of capacity, research of a prescribed kind may be carried out on, or in relation to, P if:

a. the project satisfies the prescribed requirements
b. any information or material relating to P which is used in the research is of a prescribed description and was obtained before P's loss of capacity, and
c. the person conducting the project takes in relation to P such steps as may be prescribed for the purpose of protecting him.

The regulations may make provision about when, for the purposes of the regulations, a project is to be treated as having begun and include provisions similar to any made by Sections 31, 32 and 33.

Regulations[14] covering the situation where an adult who had given consent to participation in research lost the requisite mental capacity during the research project, were published and consulted upon in June 2006 and enacted in 2007. They provide that in such circumstances, despite P's loss of capacity, research for the purposes of the project may be carried out using information or material relating to him if certain specified conditions exist:

(a) the project satisfies the requirements set out in Schedule 1
(b) all the information or material relating to P which is used in the research was obtained before P's loss of capacity, and
(c) the person conducting the project ('R') takes in relation to P such steps as are set out in Schedule 2.

Schedule 1 is shown in Box 10.4.

Box 10.4: Schedule 1 to the Regulations on loss of capacity during the research project.

Requirements which the project must satisfy:

1. A protocol approved by an appropriate body and having effect in relation to the project makes provision for research to be carried out in relation to a person who has consented to take part in the project but loses capacity to consent to continue to take part in it.
2. The appropriate body must be satisfied that there are reasonable arrangements in place for ensuring that the requirements of Schedule 2 will be met [see Box 10.5 for Schedule 2].

Schedule 2 of the Regulations is shown in Box 10.5.

Box 10.5: Schedule 2 to the Regulations on loss of capacity during the research project.

Steps which the person conducting the project must take:

1. R must take reasonable steps to identify a person who – (a) otherwise than in a professional capacity or for remuneration, is engaged in caring for P or is interested in P's welfare, and (b) is prepared to be consulted by R under this Schedule.
2. If R is unable to identify such a person he must, in accordance with guidance issued by the Secretary of State, nominate a person who – (a) is prepared to be consulted by R under this Schedule, but (b) has no connection with the project.
3. R must provide the person identified under paragraph 1, or nominated under paragraph 2, with information about the project and ask him – (a) for advice as to whether research of the kind proposed should be carried out in relation to P, and (b) what, in his opinion, P's wishes and feelings about such research being carried out would be likely to be if P had capacity in relation to the matter.
4. If, any time, the person consulted advises R that in his opinion P's wishes and feelings would be likely to lead him to wish to withdraw from the project if he had capacity in relation to the matter, R must ensure that P is withdrawn from it.
5. The fact that a person is the donee of a lasting power of attorney given by P, or is P's deputy, does not prevent him from being the person consulted under paragraphs 1 to 4.
6. R must ensure that nothing is done in relation to P in the course of the research which would be contrary to – (a) an advance decision of his which has effect, or

---

(b) any other form of statement made by him and not subsequently with-drawn, of which R is aware.

7.   The interests of P must be assumed to outweigh those of science and society.

8.   If P indicates (in any way) that he wishes the research in relation to him to be discontinued, it must be discontinued without delay.

9.   The research must be discontinued without delay if at any time R has reason-able grounds for believing that one or more of the requirements set out in Schedule 1 is no longer met or that there are no longer reasonable arrange-ments in place for ensuring that the requirements of this Schedule are met in relation to P.

10. R must conduct the research in accordance with the provision made in the protocol referred to in paragraph 1 of Schedule 1 for research to be carried out in relation to a person who has consented to take part in the project but loses capacity to consent to take part in it.

Under Section 65(4) a statutory instrument containing regulations made by the Secretary of State under Section 34 may not be made unless a draft has been laid before and approved by resolution of each House of Parliament. This is known as the affirmative procedure in Parliament for enacting statutory instruments.

Ethics committees

The research must be approved by an appropriate body for the purposes of a research project. This has been defined in the Regulations[15] as a committee (or other body) –

(a) established to advise on, or on matters which include, the ethics of research investigations of the kind conducted, or intended to be conducted, as part of the project, including the ethics of intrusive research in relation to people who lack capacity to consent to it; and

(b) recognised for those purposes by or on behalf of the Secretary of State.

The regulations defining appropriate body came into force on 1 July 2007 for the purpose of enabling applications for approval to be made and on 1 October 2007 for all other purposes.

NHS research ethics committees

Local research ethics committees were established by the DH in 1991.[16] Multi-centre research ethics committees (MRECs) were established in 1997.[17] A central office for NHS research ethics committees (COREC) was established in 2000. The following year the DH published the Research Governance Framework for Health and Social Care. A policy document, *Governance Arrangements for NHS Research Ethics Committees*, was published in August 2001.[18] COREC was placed under the National Patient Safety Agency in 2005 and relaunched as the National Research Ethics Service in March 2007.

An ad hoc advisory group was set up to review the operation of National Health Service research ethics committees. Its report[19] was published in June 2005. Its conclusions ranged widely over the need to change the system of research ethics committees (RECs), the need to address perceived weaknesses in the REC system, and provide better support for Chairs, members and administrative staff. The aim of its recommendations was to raise the status and profile of RECs, and lay the firm foundation for a REC system that can be more responsive to changing requirements in the future in a UK-wide context. It recommended that significant changes to the National Health Service research ethics committee system should be made, which are shown in Box 10.6. Changes are being implemented under the new National Research Ethics Service (see NPSA website).

Box 10.6: Recommendations of the Advisory Group on the Operation of NHS Research Ethics Committees.

1. The remit of NHS RECs should not include surveys or other non research activity if they present no material ethical issues for human participants. COREC should develop guidelines to aid researchers and committees in deciding what is appropriate or inappropriate for submission to RECs.
2. RECs should not reach decisions based on scientific review. In the unusual situation of an REC having reservations about the quality of the science proposed, they should be able to refer to COREC for scientific guidance.
3. The recently introduced managed operating system has been well received. Its use of IT points the way to further efficiency and quality improvements. We believe that responsibility for site-specific assessment should be transferred to NHS hosts as soon as acceptable mechanisms for quality assurance are in place.
4. The application form and application process call for improvement. The form should take more explicit account of differences between types of research and should also give more space and attention to ethical issues.
5. We strongly encourage NHS research hosts to adopt common national systems. Substantial improvement to local research and development (R&D) procedures and their interaction with ethical review, including the ability to make multiple use of information supplied once, is required in order to reduce bureaucracy and timescales. This is the most pressing of all our recommendations.
6. We believe that a smaller number of RECs, perhaps one for each Strategic Health Authority, with a limited number of exceptions would be more appropriate. Their operations would be more intense than at present, with a greater use of electronic communications. The time commitment required of members and support staff for training should be more formally recognised, as should the time taken in committee hearings and preparation. This implies paying REC members appropriately, either directly or through compensating their employers.

7.　Research Ethics Committees must represent the public interest as well as patient perspectives on research. This means that membership needs to be drawn from a wider mix of society, and that all members need to be supported by appropriate training. We believe that our recommendation, that we move towards a system of fewer, paid RECs, will support this objective.

8.　The issue of excessive inconsistency amongst committees should be addressed by concentrating on the provision of appropriate training, and on capturing and sharing good practice where issues and arguments have already been explored. The newly introduced system of quality assurance by peer review amongst committees and their members should assist this process and should be further developed.

9.　We propose the creation of 'Scientific Officers' in COREC to support the work of committees. They might undertake much of the preliminary assessment required, and review reports. Chairs, for whom it is a major burden, currently undertake this work.

Clinical trials

Clinical trials which come under the Clinical Trials Regulations are excluded from the statutory provisions of the Mental Capacity Act 2005 Section 30(3). These are the regulations drawn up as a consequence of the European Directive.[20] Article 5 makes provisions for clinical trials on incapacitated adults not able to give informed legal consent. The regulations were enacted in 2004.[21] The exclusion covers any future regulations to be enacted for the purposes of this section.

The Clinical Trial Regulations Schedule 1 states that if any subject:

(a)　is an adult unable by virtue of physical or mental incapacity to give informed consent, and

(b)　did not, prior to the onset of incapacity, give or refuse to give informed consent to taking part in the clinical trial,

then the conditions and principles specified in Part 5 apply in relation to that subject.

Part 5 of Schedule 1 to the Clinical Trials Regulations is shown in Box 10.7.

Box 10.7: Part 5 of Schedule 1 to the Clinical Trial Regulations.

CONDITIONS AND PRINCIPLES WHICH APPLY IN RELATION TO AN INCAPACITATED ADULT

Conditions

1.　The subject's legal representative has had an interview with the investigator, or another member of the investigating team, in which he has been given the opportunity to understand the objectives, risks and inconveniences of the trial and the conditions under which it is to be conducted.

2. The legal representative has been provided with a contact point where he may obtain further information about the trial.

3. The legal representative has been informed of the right to withdraw the subject from the trial at any time.

4. The legal representative has given his informed consent to the subject taking part in the trial.

5. The legal representative may, without the subject being subject to any resulting detriment, withdraw the subject from the trial at any time by revoking his informed consent.

6. The subject has received information according to his capacity of understanding regarding the trial, its risks and its benefits.

7. The explicit wish of a subject who is capable of forming an opinion and assessing the information referred to in the previous paragraph to refuse participation in, or to be withdrawn from, the clinical trial at any time is considered by the investigator.

8. No incentives or financial inducements are given to the subject or their legal representative, except provision for compensation in the event of injury or loss.

9. There are grounds for expecting that administering the medicinal product to be tested in the trial will produce a benefit to the subject outweighing the risks or produce no risk at all.

10. The clinical trial is essential to validate data obtained –
    (a) in other clinical trials involving persons able to give informed consent, or
    (b) by other research methods.

11. The clinical trial relates directly to a life-threatening or debilitating clinical condition from which the subject suffers.

Principles

12. Informed consent given by a legal representative to an incapacitated adult in a clinical trial shall represent that adult's presumed will.

13. The clinical trial has been designed to minimise pain, discomfort, fear and any other foreseeable risk in relation to the disease and the cognitive abilities of the patient.

14. The risk threshold and the degree of distress have to be specially defined and constantly monitored.

15. The interests of the patient always prevail over those of science and society.

Implementation of research provisions

Originally Sections 30–34 of the MCA were to come into force on 1 April 2007,[22] but this was subject to two qualifications. The dates were delayed by an amending Statutory Instrument:[23]

a. 1 July 2007: Sections 30–34 for the purpose of enabling applications for approval in relation to research to be made to and determined by an appropriate body.

b. 1 October 2008: Sections 30–34 in respect of any research which is carried out as part of a research project which began before 1 April 2007 and was approved before 1 April 2007 by a committee established to advise on, or on matters which include, the ethics of research in relation to people who lack capacity to consent to it.

c. 1 October 2007: the other provisions of sections 30–34 (research).

Conclusions

It remains to be seen if the MCA has achieved the balance wanted by the Government, between allowing important research to proceed whilst not exposing an extremely vulnerable group of individuals to unacceptable interference with their rights and freedom of action or privacy. Monitoring of the work of research ethics committees may show the extent to which the MCA protects the interests of those lacking the mental capacity to give consent to research participation. However there needs also to be extensive involvement by those consulted under Section 32 to ensure that the participation or the discontinuation of those lacking the requisite mental capacity is closely monitored.

References

1 House of Lords and House of Commons Joint Cttee on the Draft Mental Incapacity Bill, Session 2002-3, HL paper 189-1; HC 1083-1 Chapter 15.

2 Department of Health (2001) *Governance Arrangements for NHS Research Ethics Committees*, London; replaces HSG(91)5 (the red book) and HSG(97)23 on multi-centre research ethics committees. See www.doh.gov.uk/research/rd1/researchgovernance/corec.htm

3 www.wma.net/e/policy/b3.htm

4 Joint Cttee on Human Rights letter 18 November 2004, as published in their 23rd Report. Available from DCA website.

5 The Medicines for Human Use (Clinical Trials) Regulations 2004 (SI 2004/1031).

6 Code of Practice for the Mental Capacity Act 2005. Department of Constitutional Affairs February 2007 para 11.2. TSO, London.

7 www.dh.gov.uk/PublicationsAndStatistics/Publications/PublicationsPolicyAndGuidance/PublicationsPolicyAndGuidanceArticle/fs/en?CONTENT_ID=4008777&chk=dMRd/5 and www.wales.gov.uk/content/governance/governance-e.htm

8 Code of Practice (reference 6 above) para 11.5.

9 Mental Capacity Act 2005 (Appropriate Body)(England) Regulations 2006 (SI 2006/2810); Mental Capacity Act 2005 (Appropriate Body)(England)(Amendment) Regulations 2006 (SI 2006/3474).

10 Code of Practice (reference 6 above) para 11.17.

11 Code of Practice (reference 6 above) para 11.15.

12 *Ibid.* para 11.14.

13   Explanatory Memorandum on the MCA para 100.
14   The Mental Capacity Act 2005 (Loss of Capacity during Research Project) (England) Regulations 2007 (SI 2007/679).
15   Mental Capacity Act 2005 (Appropriate Body)(England) Regulations 2006 (SI 2006/2810); Mental Capacity Act 2005 (Appropriate Body)(England)(Amendment) Regulations 2006 (SI 2006/3474).
16   HSG(91)5; see www.dh.gov.uk
17   HSG(97)23; see www.dh.gov.uk
18   Department of Health (2001) *Governance Arrangements for NHS Research Ethics Committees.*
19   Department of Health (2005) *Report of the Ad Hoc Advisory Group on the Operation of NHS Research Ethics Committees.*
20   Directive 2001/20/EC.
21   Medicines for Human Use (Clinical Trials) Regulations 2004 (SI 2004/1031).
22   Mental Capacity Act 2005 (Commencement No 1) Order 2006 (SI 2006/2814).
23   Mental Capacity Act 2005 (Commencement No 1)(Amendment) Order (SI 2006/3473).

Scenarios G
Research

Statutory protection of those unable to give a valid consent to research was introduced at a late stage into the Mental Capacity Act (MCA) draft legislation. These Scenarios should be read in conjunction with Chapter 10.

Scenario G1: Research on mood swings.

Donald who has Down's syndrome has been asked to take part in a research project designed to determine whether a form of behavioural therapy would be effective in controlling his mood swings. The researcher, Ben, is studying for a PhD under a research grant provided by a charity. Donald's mother is concerned because she considers that Donald does not have the capacity to give consent. What is the legal situation?

Mental capacity of the proposed research data subject

The first issue to be determined is the mental capacity of Donald. Preferably (though this is not a statutory requirement) an independent person (one who is not involved in the research project) who is trained to test mental capacity should be asked to assess Donald's mental competence.

Capacity to consent exists

If the assessment results in a conclusion that Donald has the mental capacity to give consent, then the common law relating to the giving of consent, including the right to withdraw consent at any time, would apply. The rules relating to the approval of the research by the local research ethics committee (REC) must also be followed. All relevant information about any risks or benefits of the research must also be provided to Donald.

Lack of capacity to consent

If on the other hand the assessment concludes that Donald lacks the capacity to give consent, then the provisions of the Mental Capacity Act 2005 apply. It is assumed that behavioural therapy does not come within the definition of clinical trial (if it does then the Clinical Trials Regulations will apply – see page 230).

Conditions necessary for the research to proceed

The research must have been approved by a regional or local ethics committee established by the appropriate body

The appropriate body is defined in the Regulations and means the REC.[1] It cannot approve the research involving those lacking capacity to consent unless the following conditions are satisfied.

Is the research intrusive?

If the research would be unlawful if it were carried out without the consent of a mentally capacitated person, then it is intrusive. Would carrying out behavioural research on a mentally capacitated person require that person's consent? The answer to that question would be 'yes'. The other statutory provisions must therefore be followed.

The research can only proceed with Donald as a research subject, if the following can be shown:

- The research must be connected with
  (a)   an impairing condition affecting Donald, or
  (b)   its treatment.

Is Down's syndrome an 'impairing condition'? 'Impairing condition' means a condition which is (or may be) attributable to, or which causes or contributes to (or may cause or contribute to), the impairment of, or disturbance in the functioning of, the mind or brain.

Down's syndrome would appear to come within that definition.

Could the research be carried out on others who were capable of giving consent?

Are there reasonable grounds for believing that research of comparable effectiveness cannot be carried out if the project has to be confined to, or relates only to, persons who have capacity to consent to taking part in it?

This is difficult to answer, since there may well be others who have Down's syndrome who are capable of giving consent to involvement in this behavioural research. However they may not suffer from the mood swings which is the area of research. How thorough a search must be made for alternative data subjects? In practice of course, it is the local ethics committee which has had to answer these questions, since unless it is satisfied that all the statutory conditions are met, it cannot approve the research proposal.

Will Donald benefit?

It must be shown that the research has the potential to benefit Donald without imposing on Donald a burden that is disproportionate to the potential benefit to Donald.

The answer to this in relation to Donald would depend upon the exact details of the behavioural research: would it involve time out (see glossary)? Would he be subjected to any negative or upsetting treatment? The ethics committee approved under the regulations would have to question the researcher on the detailed contents and implications of the research proposals.

Benefit to others affected by the same or a similar condition

If the balance of benefits to burdens is not favourable to Donald, then it must be shown that the research is intended to provide knowledge of the causes or treatment of, or of the care of persons affected by, the same or a similar condition. In this situation there must be reasonable grounds for believing that there are negligible risks to Donald from taking part and that anything done to, or in relation to, Donald will not interfere with Donald's freedom of action or privacy in a significant way, or be unduly invasive or restrictive.

However there is an additional safeguard set out in S.33(3) that:

> the interests of the person must be assumed to outweigh those of science and society.

It could not therefore be argued that the potential benefits to society from the research are such that Donald's own interests and rights can be ignored (see Scenario G5).

Consultation with others

Ben, the researcher must take reasonable steps to identify a person who, otherwise than in a professional capacity or for remuneration, is engaged in caring for P or is interested in P's welfare, and is prepared to be consulted by R about Donald being involved in this research. Donald's mother would be the obvious person to consult with, but if for some reason she was not willing to be consulted, then Ben would have to find someone else who was involved in caring for Donald or interested in Donald's welfare, and was prepared to be consulted (but who was not a professional nor paid carer).

If there were no such person, then Ben would have to look further afield. He would have to nominate a person who is prepared to be consulted by him, but has no connection with the project. Guidance is to be issued on how the process and procedures for this nomination should be undertaken.

The person consulted could be the donee of a lasting power of attorney given by Donald (unlikely in this situation since Donald has probably not had the requisite capacity to appoint one) or a deputy appointed by the Court of Protection for Donald.

What must Ben tell the person who is consulted or nominated?

Ben must inform Donald's mother if she has agreed to be consulted or any person who has been nominated for consultation about the project. There are no statutory provisions governing the kind of information which must be made known by the researcher, but it is likely to be covered by guidance from the Department of Health (DH) or contained within the revised code of practice.

What are the effects of the consultation?

Ben must ask those consulted for advice as to whether Donald should take part in the project, and what, in their opinion, Donald's wishes and feelings about taking part in the project would be likely to be if Donald had capacity in relation to the matter.

If the opinion given to Ben is that Donald would not wish to take part, then Ben would have to accept that refusal. He would have an obligation to make sure that Ben did not take part.

Withdrawal from project

If however Donald has already been involved in the research project and Ben is advised by any one who has been consulted that Donald would wish to withdraw from it if he were able to make his own decisions on participation, then Ben must ensure that the withdrawal takes place immediately. For example if Donald indicates by showing signs of resistance or in any other way that he objects to the research, then he must be withdrawn from the project without delay. There is a major exception to this immediate withdrawal:

The immediate withdrawal of Donald from the project is not required if Ben has reasonable grounds for believing that there would be a significant risk to Donald's health if his involvement in the project were discontinued.

The advice from the person consulted by Ben, whether a carer or an independent person specifically nominated, can be given at any time whilst the research is taking place. It is not just a once-and-for-all opinion given at the start of the involvement of Donald in the research project. There must therefore be practical arrangements for those giving their advice to the researcher on the involvement of the person without the requisite mental capacity, to be in contact whenever necessary throughout the whole of Donald's participation. Whilst the wishes and feelings of Donald could probably be more easily monitored by a carer, the nominated independent person would have to ensure that they are kept advised of Donald's situation and of his wishes and feelings.

An example of the discontinuation of research is given in Scenario G2.

Scenario G2: Carer advises in favour of the discontinuation of research.

Bob has Prader-Willi syndrome and Tom, a researcher, has received a grant to consider a dietary regime which is designed specifically for those persons who have this condition and is aimed at reducing their appetite. It is claimed that the research would assist in the treatment and care of such sufferers.

Bob lives with four residents who have similar disorders in a community home, and Tom approaches the home manager to assess whether Bob could take part in the research. Tom consulted the home manager John but, since John was a paid carer, Tom was advised to seek out Bob's sister, Joan, who was a regular visitor to him. Joan says that it is clear that Bob could not give consent himself and she was concerned to see the research ethics committee's approval for the project and have further information about the research.

Joan is given all the information she requests and notifies Tom that it is her opinion that had Bob had the mental capacity to make his own decision, Bob's wishes and feelings would be in favour of his taking part. She therefore advises Tom that Bob could take part in the project.

After one week, it is clear that Bob is becoming very distressed by being on the dietary regime and wants to come off it. There is no evidence at this stage that Bob's appetite has been reduced. Tom says that it is still early days and too soon to see any result, and urges Joan to let him continue with the diet for another three days. What does Joan do?

Joan has the responsibility of deciding if in her opinion Bob's wishes and feelings would be likely to lead him to wish to withdraw from the project if he had capacity in relation to the matter. She should advise Tom if she considers that this is the case. Tom would therefore have to assess whether coming off the diet straightaway would cause harm to Bob.

Tom has the responsibility of removing Bob from the research project immediately. However if Tom has reasonable grounds for believing that there would be a significant risk to Bob's health if it were discontinued, then Bob could continue to stay on the research project until that risk is removed. Joan should be consulted on the need to continue the treatment in order to prevent harm to Bob.

Additional safeguards

Evidence of resistance

Scenario G3: Evidence of resistance (S33(2) Safeguard in practice).

A research project conducted by Tony has been approved for the reduction of head banging in clients suffering from severe learning disabilities. The project involves the use of a special helmet which makes head banging more uncomfortable. Brian is taking part in this research and gives signs that he is not happy to be wearing the helmet. Tony, the researcher, claims that the research is designed to protect him from harm and should continue despite his resistance. What action should be taken?

Tony has the responsibility for deciding if the research is intended to protect Brian from harm or to prevent Brian suffering pain and discomfort. He would have to contact the person he consulted when it was first agreed that Brian could take part. The fact that science and society would benefit from the knowledge which this research project could generate would be irrelevant. If Brian shows that he wishes to withdraw from the project, and it is not established that the project is designed to protect him from harm or prevent pain and discomfort, then he should be withdrawn without delay. Only if Tony has reasonable grounds for believing that there would be a significant risk to P's health if it were discontinued could Brian's involvement continue.

Constant monitoring

The researcher must be constantly watchful to ensure that all the conditions, which had to be met before the research ethics committee could approve the research project, are still present. If for example it becomes apparent that research of comparable effectiveness could be carried out using persons who have the capacity to consent, then the research using a person incapable of giving consent should be discontinued. Only if the researcher had reasonable grounds for believing that there would be a significant risk to P's health if it were discontinued, could the project be carried on.

Urgent research

Scenario G4: Situation of urgent treatment which is also research.

Mohammad has been severely injured in a road traffic accident and has suffered head injuries and damage to the lungs. It is clear that he requires an immediate operation but Howard, the anaesthetist, is uncertain about which method of anaesthesia would be preferable, given his lung damage. Howard is currently researching a particular kind of equipment, and believes that this would be beneficial to Mohammad. He therefore wishes to include Mohammad in his research project. Can he take the benefit of Sections 32(8) and (9) relating to urgent treatment and research?

Clearly the operation which Mohammad requires is urgent, and therefore a decision on the appropriate means of carrying out the anaesthetic is urgent. It is necessary to take action for the purposes of the research as a matter of urgency. Is it reasonably practicable for Howard to consult Mohammad's informal carer or an independent nominated person? The use of the word 'reasonable' means that the time, the cost, and the likelihood of success can all be taken into account in determining whether the person should be consulted.

Clearly any delay in carrying out a vital operation may have serious consequences for Mohammad. If Howard decides that it is not reasonably practicable to consult the appropriate person, then he has to have the agreement of a registered medical practitioner who is not involved in the organisation or conduct of Howard's research project on methods of anaesthetic administration. If it is not reasonably practicable in the time available to obtain that agreement, then Howard can continue the research if he acts in accordance with a procedure approved by the research ethics committee (i.e. the appropriate body) at the time when the research project was approved. Once the emergency is over, Howard cannot continue to rely on these 'urgency' provisions.

Personal vis-à-vis benefits to science and society

The Mental Capacity Act 2005 expressly states (S.33(3)) that the interests of the person must be assumed to outweigh those of science and society.

Scenario G5: Exploited for society's benefit.

Jim Hansom, the owner of a residential care home for those with severe learning disabilities, was told by a water company, Cleaneau, that he would obtain a financial benefit if Cleaneau could supply the home with water from its new water processing plant. It believed that the residents would benefit from the different methods of water purification. There was a possibility that the new process could also reduce gastro-enteric diseases in the residents. Jim Hansom offered the carers of potential residents a discount to the usual fees because of the income provided by the water company. A parent challenged the owner on the legal basis of this project and the owner stated that he did not consider that it was a research project, but the home was being offered a benefit not yet available to the general population. It was simply a new service which he was receiving for the benefit of the residents.

Clearly in Scenario G5 the owner has not checked whether the project has been approved by the appropriate research ethics committee, because he does not believe it to be a research project. Yet a new product is being tested out and those without the capacity to consent are being used as the data subjects. Before the home commenced receiving the water it should have obtained approval from the appropriate research ethics committee. All the conditions in Sections 30–34 of the MCA should be satisfied. Since the research could be carried out with those with the capacity to give consent, and it is not directly related to the learning disabilities of the residents, it is unlikely that approval could be given. The fact that society would benefit from this project is irrelevant.

Checklists

1. Participation in research

- Does P have the requisite mental capacity to make his own decisions on participation in a research project?
- If so, the decision as to whether or not to participate can be left to P (if P gives consent but subsequently loses capacity during the research project – see checklist below).
- Has P drawn up an advance decision or made an advanced statement when competent, opposing participation in such a research project?
- If so, the research should not proceed.
- If P does not have the requisite mental capacity and has not made an advance decision or advance statement covering the research, then the following questions must be asked:
- Does the research come under the definition of a clinical trial?
- If so, then it is subject to the clinical trial regulations.
- If not, then the following questions must be asked:
- Has the research ethics committee approved the project and therefore been satisfied that the statutory conditions are met?
- Is the research connected with a condition which affects P (the person lacking mental capacity)?
- Is the research connected with an impairing condition affecting P or its treatment? (An impairing condition is defined in Section 31(3) as a condition which is (or may be) attributable to, or which causes or contributes to, the impairment of, or disturbance in the functioning of, the mind or brain.)
- Are there reasonable grounds for believing that the research would not be as effective if carried out only on, or only in relation to, persons who have the capacity to consent to taking part in the project?
- If 'no', then there would be no justification in using a person who lacks the capacity to give consent.
- If 'yes':
  - Does the research have the potential to benefit P without imposing on P a burden that is disproportionate to the potential benefit to P (this condition can be dispensed with if the risk to P is negligible and anything done to P will not interfere with his freedom of action or privacy in a significant way or be unduly invasive or restrictive), or
  - Are the benefits to P greater than the burdens in participating?

- Is the research intended to provide knowledge of the causes or treatment of, or of the care of persons affected by, the same or a similar condition?
- Are any risks to P from taking part likely to be negligible?
- Will anything to be done to or in relation to P interfere with his freedom of action or privacy in a significant way, or be unduly invasive or restrictive?
- Is there a carer who could be and is prepared to be consulted?
- If not, can a nominated independent person be consulted?
- Has the consultee been given the appropriate information?
- What is the opinion of the consultee on what P's wishes and feelings would have been had he had the requisite mental capacity?

2. Once the research has commenced

- Does P appear to object by showing signs of resistance or otherwise?
- If 'yes', is this because what is being done is intended to protect him from harm or to reduce or prevent pain or discomfort?
- Does P indicate that he wishes to be withdrawn from the project?
- If so, he must be withdrawn without delay unless R has reasonable grounds for believing that there would be a significant risk to P's health if it were discontinued.
- Is the researcher satisfied that the conditions for the research to be carried out on a person who lacks capacity are still present?
- If 'no', then P must be withdrawn from the project without delay (subject to the proviso about risks to his health).

3. Loss of capacity during research project

- If P loses capacity during the research project, it can only be continued if it satisfies the regulations.
- Has Schedule 1 of the Regulations[2] as shown in Box 10.4 been complied with (see Chapter 10, page 227)?
- Is Schedule 2 of the Regulations, as shown in Box 10.5 relating to the steps which the person conducting the project must take, complied with (see Chapter 10, page 227)?
- Is any information or material relating to P and used in the research of a prescribed description and was it obtained before P's loss of capacity?

4. Urgent research

- Is treatment being or about to be provided for P as a matter of urgency?
- Does R consider that, having regard to the nature of the research and of the particular circumstances of the case, it is also necessary to take action for the purposes of the research as a matter of urgency?
- Is it reasonably practicable to consult an informal carer or nominee?

- If 'yes', then the consultation must take place.
- If 'no', then R may take action if either he has:
  - the agreement of a registered medical practitioner not involved in the organisation or conduct of the research project, or
  - it is not reasonably practicable in the time available to obtain that agreement,
  - but he acts in accordance with a procedure set by the appropriate body, i.e. the ethics committee at the time the research project was approved.
- Does the action continue to be required as a matter of urgency?
- If no, then R can no longer act in reliance on these provisions.

References

1 Mental Capacity Act 2005 (Appropriate Body)(England) Regulations 2006 (SI 2006/2810); Mental Capacity Act 2005 (Appropriate Body)(England)(Amendment) Regulations 2006 (SI 2006/3474).
2 The Mental Capacity Act 2005 (Loss of Capacity during Research Project) (England) Regulations 2007 (SI 2007/679).

11 Protection of Vulnerable Adults and Accountability

Introduction

In its Mental Incapacity Bill,[1] following on from its consultation paper[2] the Law Commission drafted statutory provisions for vulnerable adults to provide a similar framework for protection as that provided for children under the Children Act 1989. However these provisions were not included within the Mental Capacity Bill. The Mental Capacity Act 2005 does however introduce a new criminal offence of ill-treating or wilfully neglecting a person who lacks capacity. This chapter explores this new offence and also considers those existing laws, both criminal and civil, which provide some protection for the mentally incapacitated adult. It also considers the accountability of those involved in the care of those lacking mental capacity.

Ill-treatment or neglect

Under Section 44(2) it is an offence to ill-treat or wilfully neglect a person who lacks capacity. The offence arises if a person D:

a. has the care of a person P who lacks, or whom D reasonably believes to lack, capacity
b. is the donee of a lasting power of attorney, or an enduring power of attorney (within the meaning of Schedule 4), created by P, or
c. is a deputy appointed by the court for P (S.44(1)).

A person who is guilty of an offence under Section 44 is liable on summary conviction to imprisonment for a term not exceeding 12 months or a fine not exceeding the statutory maximum or both; on conviction on indictment, to imprisonment for a term not exceeding five years or a fine or both.

The Joint Committee recommended that the scope of the new offence should be extended to include the misappropriation of the person's property and financial assets[3] (and not just physical ill-treatment), but they appreciated the difficulties of obtaining evidence when the victim lacks mental capacity.[4] It urged the Home Office and other departments to continue to co-operate to ensure that the state's positive obligation to provide for the protection of vulnerable people is complied with.[5]

Comment on this provision

As noted above the new offence is not so extensive as might be thought, since it does not explicitly cover financial abuse of a mentally incapacitated person. There are also some uncertainties which will eventually be resolved by case law, as disputes arise over the interpretation of the section.

Care of the mentally incapacitated person

There is no definition of 'a person who has the care of P' in the Mental Capacity Act (MCA). Whilst it is clear that the term would cover all professional and paid carers, and would also cover relatives who provide care and others who live with the person lacking mental capacity, would the term cover an individual who did the occasional shopping for a person living in a flat on the floor below? See Scenario H1.

'Carer' in the Carers (Recognition and Services) Act 1995 is defined as 'an individual who provides or intends to provide a substantial amount of care on a regular basis for the relevant person' (S.1(1)(b)), and this same definition is used in the Carers and Disabled Children Act 2000, where the individual is over 16 years and provides a substantial amount of care on a regular basis for another individual aged 18 or over (S.1(1)(a)). In the absence of a statutory definition within the MCA, case law will determine whether a substantial amount of care (and if so what is meant by substantial) is required for the offence to be committed.

What is covered by ill-treatment and wilful neglect?

The Code of Practice cites many forms of abuse, but not all of them would come under the provisions of this new offence.[6]

- **Financial abuse:** such as theft, fraud, undue pressure or the misuse or dishonest gain of property, possessions or benefits.
- **Physical abuse:** such as slapping, pushing and kicking. It also includes the misuse of medication (for example giving someone a high dose of medication in order to make them drowsy) and inappropriate punishments (for example not giving someone a meal because they had been 'bad').
- **Sexual abuse:** such as rape and sexual assault. It also includes sexual acts without consent (this includes if a person is not able to give consent or the abuser used pressure).

- **Psychological abuse:** such as emotional abuse, threats of harm, restraint or abandonment, refusing contact with other people, intimidation, and threats to restrict someone's liberty.
- **Neglect and acts of omission:** such as ignoring the person's medical or physical care needs, failing to get healthcare or social care and withholding of medication, food or heating.

The draft Code of Practice also listed **discriminatory abuse** such as racist or sexist abuse or abuse that is based on a person's disability, and other forms of harassment, slurs or similar treatment. This would have included making decisions based upon an unfavourable view of a person's sex, age, race, or religion. This type of abuse may arise as an aspect across all the forms mentioned above.

Not all of these forms of abuse would be covered by the new offence, but could come under existing criminal offences (see **Acts in connection with care or treatment**, page 247).

Multi-agency co-operation

The Code of Practice describes the multi-agency co-operation in protecting vulnerable adults.[7] Guidance on protecting vulnerable people from abuse has been issued by the DH for England, namely *No Secrets*,[8] and by the National Assembly for Wales, namely *In Safe Hands*.[9] Both documents define abuse as:

> Any violation of an individual's human and civil rights by any other person or persons.

Both documents describe a variety of forms of abuse, such as sexual, physical, verbal, financial or emotional abuse. It can be a single act, a series of repeated acts or failure to act, or neglect. Abuse can take place in any setting, for example in a person's own home, a care home or a hospital. *No Secrets* and *In Safe Hands* set out multi-agency procedures that must be followed when allegations of abuse are made or suspected.

A Dignity in Care campaign was launched in November 2006 by the Minister for Care Services.[10] The campaign aims to stimulate a national debate around dignity in care and create a care system where there is zero tolerance of abuse and disrespect for older people. An online practice guide has been developed with the Social Care Institute for Excellence (SCIE) and the Care Services Improvement Partnership (CSIP), and is available from the DH website.[11]

Fraud Act

The Fraud Act 2006 (which came into force in 2007) creates a new offence of 'fraud by abuse of position'. This new offence may apply to a range of people, including:

- attorneys under a lasting power of attorney (LPA) or an enduring power of attorney (EPA), or
- deputies appointed by the Court of Protection to make financial decisions on behalf of a person who lacks capacity.

Attorneys and deputies may be guilty of fraud if they dishonestly abuse their position, intend to benefit themselves or others, and cause loss or expose a person to the risk of loss. People who suspect fraud should report the case to the police.[12]

Acts in connection with care or treatment

Section 5 protects a person from civil and criminal action when they act under the provisions of the MCA in providing care and treatment for an adult lacking mental capacity. However Section 5(3) states that nothing in Section 5 excludes a person's civil liability for loss or damage, or his criminal liability resulting from his negligence in doing the act. The means that a person could still face civil or criminal proceedings because of their actions. This is explained below and see also Scenario H4.

Valuing people

The White Paper on learning disabilities, *Valuing People: A New Strategy for Learning Disability for the 21st Century*,[13] calculated that there are about 210 000 people with severe learning disabilities in England, and about 1.2 million with a mild or moderate disability. Health and social services expenditure on services for adults with learning disabilities stands at around £3 billion. The White Paper recognised four key principles, Rights, Independence, Choice and Inclusion, as lying at the heart of the Government's proposals. The White Paper is described by the Government as taking a life-long approach, beginning with an integrated approach to services for disabled children and their families, and then providing new opportunities for a full and purposeful adult life. The proposals should result in improvements in education, social services, health, employment, housing and support for people with learning disabilities and their families and carers.

The White Paper set out the aim of investing at least £1.3 million a year for the next three years, to develop advocacy services for people with learning disabilities in partnership with the voluntary sector, in order to enable people with learning disabilities to have as much choice and control as possible over their lives and the services and support they receive. The eligibility for direct payments was to be extended through legislation. In addition a national forum for people with learning disabilities was to be set up to enable them to benefit from the improvement and expansion of community equipment services now under way. New guidance on person-centred planning was to be issued with resources for implementation through the Learning Disability Development Fund.

To ensure implementation of the White Paper, the following initiatives were envisaged:

- Learning Disability Task Force
- Implementation Support Team
- Learning Disability research initiative: People with Learning Disabilities: Services, Inclusion and Partnership.

In February 2005 the DH announced that £41 million (double the amount for 2004) was to be made available to Primary Care trusts to provide services through the Learning Disabilities Development Fund.[14] Priorities for the spending included advocacy, person-centred planning and leadership from 2004, and new priorities for 2005 including day services modernisation, National Health Services campuses reprovision (redevelopment of the residential services developed by the NHS as a result of the contraction or closure of NHS hospitals) and support for people with learning disabilities from black and minority ethnic communities.

Eligibility criteria for continuing care

The DoH announced the implementation of a national framework for long term NHS healthcare to begin in October 2007. A single system for determining people's eligibility for long-term NHS healthcare will be introduced, and should reduce the disputes between NHS and social services and individuals over the payment of fees.[15]

Protection of vulnerable adults

Protection of Vulnerable Adults (POVA) scheme in England and Wales for care homes and domiciliary care agencies: a practical guide (2004)[16] was provided for by Part 7 of the Care Standards Act 2000. At the heart of the POVA scheme is the POVA list. The POVA scheme acts like a workforce ban. From 26 July 2004, individuals should be referred to, and included on, the POVA list if they have abused, neglected or otherwise harmed vulnerable adults in their care or placed vulnerable adults in their care at risk of harm. By making statutory checks against the list, providers of care know which individuals cannot be offered employment in care positions. Those on the list who seek employment in care positions will be committing a criminal offence. POVA checks are requested as part of the disclosures from the Criminal Records Bureau.[17]

The Safeguarding Vulnerable Groups Act 2006 makes criminal record checks compulsory for staff who:

- have contact with service users in registered care homes
- provide personal care services in someone's home, and
- are involved in providing adult placement schemes.

Potential employers must carry out a pre-employment criminal record check with the Criminal Records Bureau (CRB) for all potential new healthcare and social care staff. This includes nursing agency staff and home care agency staff.[18]

Criminal law and mental capacity

There are many areas of the criminal law where specific account is taken of a person's mental capacity to ensure that an injustice does not occur. These include:

- police procedures on arrest
- making a confession
- standing for trial
- being a witness
- being on a jury.

Police procedures on arrest

The Code of Practice which has been drawn up under the Police and Criminal Evidence Act 1984 Code C Annex 1 Appendix A – 105 provides protection for the mentally disordered, mentally vulnerable and mentally incapable of understanding the significance of questions. The assessment as to whether a defendant is mentally handicapped should be made on the basis of medical evidence and police, not having expertise in the matter, should not be allowed to state their opinion with respect thereof.[19] An appropriate adult is required to be brought in to ensure that the accused fully understands his rights, that the interview is conducted correctly and that he clearly understands what is being said to him.

Making a confession

Under Section 77 of the Police and Criminal Evidence Act 1984, where the case against the accused depends wholly or substantially on a confession by him, and the court is satisfied that he is mentally handicapped and the confession was not made in the presence of an independent person, then the court must warn the jury that there is special need for caution before convicting the accused in reliance on the confession.

An independent person is defined as not including a police officer or a person employed for police purposes,[20] and mentally handicapped is defined as meaning that a person is in a state of arrested or incomplete development of mind, which includes significant impairment of intelligence and social functioning.

There is no rule that a confession obtained from a mentally handicapped person in the absence of a solicitor and an appropriate adult should automatically lead to exclusion under Section 77 of the Police and Criminal Evidence Act 1984.

A defendant's mental condition is one of the factors to be taken into account in deciding if the confession is unreliable, and nothing in the authorities limits or defines the particular form of mental or psychological condition or disorder. The disorder must not only be of a type which might render a confession unreliable, but there must also be a significant deviation from the norm shown; and there must be a history pre-dating making of admissions which is not based solely on a history given by the subject and which points to or explains the abnormality or abnormalities.[21]

Being a witness

No witness is competent to give evidence if he is prevented by reason of mental illness or mental handicap from giving rational testimony. Where it is contended that the witness falls in such a category, it is for the judge to ascertain whether the witness is competent to give evidence. Where the judge is satisfied that he is, the judge should allow the witness to be examined and leave to the jury the decision on the worth of his testimony.[22]

Being on a jury

Under the Juries Act 1974 Schedule 1 Part 1 the following persons are disqualified for jury services:

1. a person who suffers or has suffered from mental illness, psychopathic dis-order, mental handicap or severe mental handicap and on account of that condition either:
    a. is resident in a hospital or similar institution or
    b. regularly attends for treatment by a medical practitioner.
2. A person for the time being under guardianship under Section 7 of the Mental Health Act 1983.
3. A person who under Part 7 of that Act has been determined by a judge to be incapable, by reason of mental disorder, of managing and administering his property and affairs.

(The definition of mental handicap is as given in the Mental Health Act 1983 – see Chapter 13.)

Sexual Offences Act 2003

The Sexual Offences Act 2003 creates offences under Sections 30–33, designed to give protection to persons with a mental disorder which impeded choice. The offences are as follows:

*   Section 30   Sexual activity with a person with a mental disorder impeding choice.
*   Section 31   Causing or inciting a person, with a mental disorder impeding choice, to engage in sexual activity.
*   Section 32   Engaging in sexual activity in the presence of a person with a mental disorder impeding choice.
*   Section 33   Causing a person, with a mental disorder impeding choice, to watch a sexual act.

In a recent case a defendant appealed against his conviction under Section 30, argu-ing that the magistrates had been wrongly advised as to the nature of the offence. The victim C suffered from cerebral palsy and had a mental age well below that of her actual age of 27 years. The High Court held that there was evidence on which the magistrates could properly conclude that the victim had been unable to effectively communicate her wishes to the accused by reason of her mental condition.[23]

In addition the 2003 Act also creates offences in relation to providing inducements etc to persons with a mental disorder to engage in sexual activity. The offences are as follows:

- Section 34   Inducement, threat or deception to procure sexual activity with a person with a mental disorder.
- Section 35   Causing a person with a mental disorder to engage in or agree to engage in sexual activity by inducement, threat or deception.
- Section 36   Engaging in sexual activity in the presence, procured by inducement, threat or deception, of a person with a mental disorder.
- Section 37   Causing a person with a mental disorder to watch a sexual act by inducement, threat or deception.

In addition offences are created in relation to care workers and sexual activity with a person with a mental disorder. They are:

- S.38   Care workers: sexual activity with a person with a mental disorder.
- S.39   Care workers: causing or inciting sexual activity.
- S.40   Care workers: sexual activity in the presence of a person with a mental disorder.
- S.41   Care workers: causing a person with a mental disorder to watch a sexual act.

Section 42 defines care workers as follows:

a person (A) is involved in the care of another person (B) in a way that falls within section 42 if any of subsections (2) to (4) applies.

(2)   This subsection applies if –
   (a)   B is accommodated and cared for in a care home, community home, voluntary home or children's home, and
   (b)   A has functions to perform in the home in the course of employment which have brought him or are likely to bring him into regular face to face contact with B.
(3)   This subsection applies if B is a patient for whom services are provided –
   (a)   by a National Health Service body or an independent medical agency, or
   (b)   in an independent clinic or an independent hospital,
   and A has functions to perform for the body or agency or in the clinic or hospital in the course of employment which have brought him or are likely to bring him into regular face to face contact with B.
(4)   This subsection applies if A –
   (a)   is, whether or not in the course of employment, a provider of care, assistance or services to B in connection with B's mental disorder, and
   (b)   as such, has had or is likely to have regular face to face contact with B.
(5)   In this section –
   'care home' means an establishment which is a care home for the purposes of the Care Standards Act 2000 (c. 14);
   'children's home' has the meaning given by section 1 of that Act;
   'community home' has the meaning given by section 53 of the Children Act 1989 (c. 41);
   'employment' means any employment, whether paid or unpaid and whether under a contract of service or apprenticeship, under a contract for services, or otherwise than under a contract;

'independent clinic', 'independent hospital' and 'independent medical agency' have the meaning given by section 2 of the Care Standards Act 2000;
'National Health Service body' means –
(a)   a Health Authority,
(b)   a National Health Service trust,
(c)   a Primary Care Trust, or
(d)   a Special Health Authority;
'voluntary home' has the meaning given by section 60(3) of the Children Act 1989.

Sections 43 and 44 of the Sexual Offences Act 2003 provide exceptions where marriage occurs or where the sexual relationships pre-dated the care relationship.

These provisions are designed to provide more protection for vulnerable persons.

Protection in a contractual situation

In law a mentally competent adult has the right to enter into lawful contracts and once an offer has been accepted, then is bound by the terms of the contract. There is a presumption in law that a person over 16 years is mentally competent. However if the adult lacks the mental capacity to make the contract then, in certain circumstances, the contract is only binding upon him if the contract was for necessaries. 'Necessaries' would cover goods and services suitable to his actual requirements. By Section 3 of the Sale of Goods Act 1979 it is provided that where necessaries are sold and delivered to a person who by reason of mental incapacity is incompetent to contract, he must pay a reasonable price for them. 'Necessaries' is defined as goods suitable to the position in life of such a person, and to his actual requirements at the time of the sale and delivery.[24] Section 7 of the MCA states in relation to the payment for necessary goods and services that:

(1)   If necessary goods or services are supplied to a person who lacks capacity to contract for the supply, he must pay a reasonable price for them.
(2)   'Necessary' means suitable to a person's condition in life and to his actual requirements at the time when the goods or services are supplied.

The problems which can arise are illustrated by a letter to Margaret Dibben in the *Observer*,[25] which is considered in Scenario H2.

Provisions in the Consumer Credit Act 2006 give powers to the court to alter or even set aside a credit agreement if it determines the relationship between the creditor and the debtor to be unfair.

See Scenario H6 and abuse in relation to social security payments and the role of the Department of Works and Pensions.

Concerns about the protection of vulnerable adults

Joint Committee Recommendations[26]

The Joint Committee of the Houses of Parliament expressed concerns about the extent of abuse, and the need for specific powers for investigating allegations of abuse.

In place of new legislation, the DoH and the Home Office issued guidance in 1999 on developing multi-agency procedures for the protection of vulnerable adults.[27] Not all local authorities have implemented the guidance. There was concern that the new Office of the Public Guardian will have a similar remit to the existing Public Guardianship Office (PGO), with no additional powers. The Joint Committee stated that the PGO is currently looking at ways in which the work carried out by its investigation team can be made more effective.

Other organisations and initiatives such as CHAI (Commission for Healthcare Audit and Inspection), CSCI (Commission for Social Care Inspection), PALS (Patient Advocacy and Liaison Services) and the Independent Complaints Advisory Service (ICAS) were considered.[28] It was thought that Scotland had far more robust arrangements.[29] The Joint Committee stated:

> We recommend that the statutory authorities should be given additional powers of investigation and intervention in cases of alleged physical, sexual or financial abuse of people lacking the capacity to protect themselves from the risk of abuse.[30]

Switching the burden of proof

To protect vulnerable adults it has been suggested that the burden of proof should be switched, i.e. the other party should have to prove that the person was able to understand the nature and effect of his or her actions. In the Sexual Offences Act 2003, circumstances are specified from which if it is proved that the defendant did the act, then the absence of consent to the relevant act is to be conclusively presumed. For example if the complainant feared violence from any person before the relevant act or was asleep or stupefied by a substance administered by anyone, then it is conclusively presumed that there was no consent.

Conclusions on the protection of vulnerable adults

It remains to be seen whether the new offence under Section 44(2), together with the statutory duties placed upon local authorities and employers, provide sufficient protection for vulnerable adults. There are of course existing laws protecting those who lack specific mental capacities, and these are discussed below.

Criminal offences and mental capacity of the accused

It is a requirement of most criminal offences that a person has the mental capacity to form the intent to commit the offence. Where a person lacks the requisite mental capacity (known in law as the mens rea) then the person cannot be guilty of that offence. As noted above, the law provides different forms of protection for the person who lacks mental capacity, and Scenario H3 illustrates a possible situation.

Criminal Law and the Mental Capacity Act 2005

Section 5 provides protection for a person who acts on behalf of an adult whom he reasonably believes lacks the requisite mental capacity. However as a result of Section 5(3) that person could still be subject to the laws of civil and criminal liability, as a result of their negligence.

Scope of the Mental Capacity Act 2005

Section 62 makes it clear that:

> For the avoidance of doubt, it is hereby declared that nothing in this Act is to be taken to affect the law relating to murder or manslaughter or the operation of section 2 of the Suicide Act 1961 (assisting suicide).

Murder and manslaughter

Murder

In order to secure a conviction of murder, the prosecution have to prove beyond reasonable doubt that the defendant must either have intended to cause death or intended to cause grievous bodily harm. Unless a situation comparable to that of the Dr Shipman case, who was convicted of murdering 15 patients, exists, it would be very unusual to be able to prove the intent necessary to convict of murder in a case involving professional care. Following a conviction for murder, a judge at the present time has no discretion over sentencing but must sentence the convicted person to life imprisonment, i.e. a life sentence is mandatory. (The current law requiring judges to impose a mandatory life sentence following a conviction or plea of guilty to murder is under review at the time of writing.)

Involuntary manslaughter

This may arise where death results from the gross negligence of a health professional, where there is no intention to kill or to cause grievous harm. In such cases there may be a prosecution for involuntary manslaughter or there may be no prosecution at all. It depends upon the circumstances. If for example there is such gross negligence leading to the death, then there may be a prosecution for manslaughter.

In a manslaughter prosecution, the jury would have to be convinced beyond reasonable doubt both as to the existence of the gross negligence and also that it caused the death of the victim. (The grandmother of a child mauled to death by a pit bull terrier was charged with her manslaughter as a result of gross negligence and faces a Crown Court trial in September 2007 (*The Times* 11th Aug 2007).)

An example of a leading case involving gross negligence amounting to manslaughter is given in Case Study H1 on page 272.

Voluntary manslaughter

This term is used to cover the situation where the defendant has caused the death of a person with intent, but owing to special circumstances a charge or conviction of murder is not appropriate. The term covers:

- death as a result of the provocation of the accused
- death as a result of diminished responsibility of the accused
- killing as a result of a suicide pact.

Suicide

As a result of the Suicide Act 1961, to attempt to commit suicide ceased to be a crime. However the aiding and abetting of the suicide of another remained a criminal offence under Section 2(1). This is shown in Box 11.1.

Box 11.1: Section 2(1) of the Suicide Act 1961.

A person who aids, abets, counsels or procures the suicide of another, or an attempt by another to commit suicide, shall be liable on conviction on indictment to imprisonment for a term not exceeding 14 years.

The Mental Capacity Act 2005 has not changed the law on assisted suicide and it is still a criminal offence to assist a person to die. There are specific provisions in the Act covering the power of a person holding a lasting power of attorney or a person acting according to an advance direction to agree to the withholding of life saving treatment, and these are discussed in Chapter 6 and Chapter 9. The MCA recognises the right of a person when they have the requisite mental capacity to make their own decisions about treatment and refuse life saving treatment if they so wish at a future time when they do not have the requisite mental capacity.

Letting die and killing.

The law makes a distinction between letting die and killing, and this distinction is not changed by the Mental Capacity Act 2005. The difference is shown in the Tony Bland case and in the contrasting cases of Re B[31] and Diane Pretty.[32] See Case Studies H2–6, pages 271–6 and see Box 2.2 in Chapter 2 for Re B on page 11.

Pain relief and killing

It does not follow that providing appropriate pain relief which may incidentally shorten life is a crime, as the trial of Dr Bodkin Adams[33] made clear. See Case Study H5.

Levels of medication

Clearly it must be established that the dosages which are given to a patient in the terminal stages of cancer and other illnesses are in accordance with the reasonable practice of a competent practitioner. It frequently happens that the tolerance built up to some pain medication requires higher and higher doses which, given to persons without that tolerance, would be lethal, grossly negligent and probably amount to a criminal offence. There is considerable benefit when practitioners are treating persons at such high levels for them to discuss recommended practice with colleagues. The importance of following competent medical practice is shown in the Annie Lindsell case (see Case Study H6).

Other criminal offences

Any paid or informal carer could also be liable to other criminal offences such as the offence of causing grievous bodily harm, or offences of theft.

Civil liability

Section 5 does not exclude liability for a civil wrong as Section 5(3) states that nothing in Section 5 excludes a person's civil liability for loss or damage, resulting from his negligence in doing the act. The usual rules of the law of negligence therefore apply to those taking responsibility for the care and treatment of persons lacking mental capacity.

Negligence and other civil wrongs

An action for negligence is the most frequent civil action brought in order to obtain compensation. It is one of a group of civil wrongs known as 'torts'. An action would be brought in the county court where less than £50 000 was being claimed. Claims above that amount would be brought in the High Court – the Queen's Bench Division. Other torts or civil wrongs are set out in Box 11.2.

Box 11.2: Civil wrongs i.e. torts.

– action for negligence
– action for breach of statutory duty
– action for trespass to the person, goods or land (this is considered in Chapter 2 on page 10)
– an action for nuisance
– an action for defamation (which includes libel and slander).

Liability in negligence

To obtain compensation in an action for negligence, the claimant must establish the elements shown in Box 11.3. See Scenario H5.

Box 11.3: Elements in an action for negligence.

1. The defendant owed a duty of care to the claimant.
2. The defendant was in breach of that duty of care, and
3. as a reasonably foreseeable result of that breach,
4. harm recognised by the courts as subject to compensation was caused.

The burden is on the claimant to establish on a balance of probabilities that each of the four elements shown in Box 11.3 are present.

Duty of care

Usually it is fairly clear if the law would recognise a duty of care as being owed to an individual in the context of healthcare. The health professional clearly has a duty of care towards all his clients. This may include others for whom he is not directly responsible but is asked to care for. It may also, depending upon the contract of employment, require him or her to return from off duty in a crisis. The duty will certainly involve the need to communicate with the client, relatives and colleagues. The duty to inform the mentally incapacitated person and the informal carer about significant risks is as much part of the duty of care as treatment and other procedures.

The definition of the duty of care was raised in a House of Lords case in 1932.[34] It was concerned with the question of whether a manufacturer owed a duty of care to the ultimate consumer, regardless of who had paid for the product.

The facts in this case were that the claimant alleged that she had drunk ginger beer which contained the decomposed remains of a snail, and held the manufacturers liable for the harm she suffered. The case went to the House of Lords over the issue of whether the manufacturers owed a duty of care to her. In a majority decision, the House of Lords decided in her favour. This may seem very remote from the duty of care owed by the carer of a person with mental capacity problems, but the statement of Lord Justice Atkins is very important in defining the duty of care. He said:

> You must take reasonable care to avoid acts or omissions which you can reasonably foresee would be likely to injure your neighbour. Who then, in law, is my neighbour? The answer seems to be persons who are so closely and directly affected by my act that I ought reasonably to have them in contemplation as being so affected when I am directing my mind to the acts or omissions which are called in question.

Usually there is no dispute that a duty of care is owed by a health professional to his clients. However, there can be situations where the existence of a legal duty of care is disputed. For example, it follows from the statement quoted above that the health professional would have a duty of care to ensure that reasonable care was taken of mentally incapacitated adults who came into a clinic where there were cupboards containing dangerous substances, that they should not be left unlocked and within reach. However, it also follows that no person has a duty to volunteer help, if a duty of care does not already exist. Once, however, this duty is assumed, then liability could arise. In Scenario H1 on page 270 a situation where Janice did shopping for a person sharing the same house is discussed. If Janice undertook to help her neighbour on a regular and substantial basis, it may be that the law would consider her to have assumed a duty of care.

Is there a duty to volunteer?

The law does not require an individual to volunteer help unless there is a pre-existing duty. Thus, if a health professional on holiday were to notice that an adult who appeared to have severe learning disabilities was in danger of drowning, there would be no duty in law to go to that person's assistance. The existence of a duty of care owed by the holidaying health professional to the adult with mental incapacity issues would not be established in law. However, the Nursing and Midwifery Council has made it clear in its *Code of professional conduct: standards for performance, conduct and ethics*[35] that there is professional duty upon the registered practitioner at all times. Para 8.5 states:

> In an emergency, in or outside the work setting, you have a professional duty to provide care. The care provided would be judged against what could reasonably be expected from someone with your knowledge, skills and abilities when placed in those particular circumstances.

This means that failure to volunteer help in certain situations could be seen as evidence of lack of fitness to practise. Of course, once a practitioner, or any other person, volunteers to take on a duty of care, then he is required in law to follow the reasonable standard of care and could be held accountable for any failures. It is unlikely that her employer would accept vicarious liability for such Good Samaritan acts, so a health professional would require professional indemnity insurance cover.

Of what does the duty consist?

The duty of care would include not only duties in relation to treatment and care, and in giving information, but also duties relating to the keeping of satisfactory records, duties in relation to management of the situation, of supervision and delegation to other staff, and all actions necessary to ensure that the client will be reasonably safe. A duty would also be held to exist in relation to colleagues, to ensure that they are reasonably safe.

The Court of Appeal has held that an ambulance service could owe a duty of care to an individual member of the public, once an emergency phone call providing personal details of that person had been accepted by the service.[36] The London Ambulance Service was held liable when the ambulance took 38 minutes to arrive to assist a pregnant woman who was asthmatic. The time of arrival had been falsely recorded. As a result of the delay, the woman suffered respiratory arrest with catastrophic results, including substantial memory impairment, personality change and a miscarriage.

In 2005 the Court of Appeal ruled that council education officers were professionals who owed a duty of care towards the child with special educational needs[37] if it was established that damage was reasonably foreseeable, the test of proximity was satisfied and the situation was one in which it was fair, just and reasonable that the law should impose a duty of care. On the facts of the case however the Court of Appeal held that there was no evidence of a breach of that duty of care.

Duty to parents

The House of Lords (in a majority verdict) has held that healthcare and other child care professionals did not owe a common law duty of care to parents against whom they had made unfounded allegations of child abuse and who, as a result, suffered psychiatric injury.[38] The same principles would apply where abuse of a mentally incapacitated adult was reasonably feared and reported.

The House of Lords has also held[39] that the police owed no duty of care to victims or witnesses. It confirmed an earlier decision[40] in a case brought by the mother of one of the Yorkshire Ripper's later victims, that whilst ethically police should treat victims and witnesses properly and with respect, this ethical duty was not converted into a legal duty of care. The prime function of the police was the preservation of the Queen's peace.

Standard of care

The claimant (formerly known as the plaintiff, i.e. the person suing for compensation) has to show that the defendant acted in breach of the duty of care. This is the 'fault element' which is required under the present laws to obtain compensation. In order to show that there has been a breach, it is first necessary to establish what standard should have been followed and how the defendant's actions differed, if at all, from what it was reasonable to expect.

The courts use a test known as the 'Bolam Test' to determine the standard expected from professionals. The name derives from a case heard in 1957[41] where a psychiatric patient was given electro-convulsive therapy without any relaxant drugs or restraint. He suffered several fractures and claimed compensation against Friern Hospital Management Committee. Mr Justice McNair, in deciding how to determine the standard which should have been followed, said:

> When you get a situation which involved the use of some special skill or competence, then the test as to whether there has been negligence or not is . . . the

standard of the ordinary skilled man exercising and professing to have that special skill. A man need not possess the highest expert skill; it is well-established
that it is sufficient if he exercises the ordinary skill of an ordinary competent
man exercising that particular art.

He added later:

He is not guilty of negligence if he has acted in accordance with a practice accepted
as proper by a responsible body of medical men skilled in that particular art.

The Bolam Test relates to the standards which were reasonably expected at the
time the alleged negligent act took place. It thus enables the standards applied by
the courts to change, and for professionals to be judged against the standards of
the time of the alleged negligence acts, not the standards which existed at the time
of the court hearing which may be many years later.

In the actual case of Bolam, the patient lost his claim. However, were the same
facts to occur in the 21st century, there would probably be an offer to settle without any attempt to defend the case, since standards are much higher now.

What if there are different opinions over the standard which should be followed?

Mr Justice McNair in the Bolam case referred to the fact that there are sometimes differences of opinion and quoted from an earlier case (*Hunter* v. *Hanley* 1955):[42]

In the realm of diagnosis and treatment there is ample scope for genuine difference of opinion, and one man clearly is not negligent merely because his
conclusion differs from that of other professional men, nor because he has
displayed less skill or knowledge than others would have shown. The true test
for establishing negligence in diagnosis or treatment on the part of a doctor is
whether he has been proved to be guilty of such failure as no doctor of ordinary
skill would be guilty of, if acting with ordinary care.

This principle was followed in the case of *Maynard* v. *West Midlands Regional
Health Authority*.[43]

The House of Lords stated the following:

It was not sufficient to establish negligence for the plaintiff [i.e. claimant] to
show that there was a body of competent professional opinion that considered
the decision as wrong, if there was also a body of equally competent professional opinion that supported the decision as having been reasonable in the
circumstances.

Standards of care and national guidance

Clearly health and social services professionals would be expected to follow the
guidance issued nationally by the DH and other bodies, relating to procedures and
practice on the care and treatment of vulnerable adults. The fact that particular

advice and guidance was not followed would not in itself constitute evidence of negligent practice, since there may be special circumstances which justified not following that particular guidance. The national guidance would however constitute a presumption that it should be followed.

The MCA Code of Practice

The MCA places the guidance on the MCA provided by the Code of Practice on a different legal basis from that of other national guidance. Section 42 places a duty on specific persons or officers (informal or unpaid carers are not included in the list) to follow the code. The effect of failure to obey the code is that if it appears to a court or tribunal conducting any criminal or civil proceedings that a provision of a code or a failure to comply with a code is relevant to a question arising in the proceedings, the provision or failure must be taken into account in deciding the question (S.42(5)). (See further in Chapter 17 on implementation.)

A possible situation is considered in Scenario H4.

The situation with regard to informal carers is considered in Chapter 15.

Causation

It is not enough for the claimant to show that the duty of care which was owed was broken; the claimant must also show that there was a causal link between that breach of duty and the harm which has occurred. This is known as 'causation'. There must be factual causation as well as the link being reasonably foreseeable.

Factual causation

In one decided case[44] three night watchmen drank tea which made them vomit. They went to the casualty department of the local hospital. The casualty officer, on being told of the complaints by a nurse, did not see the men, but told them to go home and call in their own doctors. Some hours later, one of them died from arsenical poisoning. The court held that:

- The casualty department officers owed a duty of care in the circumstances.
- The casualty doctor had been negligent in not seeing them, but
- even if he had, it was improbable that the only effective antidote could have been administered in time to save the deceased, and
- therefore the defendants were not liable. The patient would have died anyway.

The onus is on the claimant to establish that there is this causal link between the breach of the duty of care and the harm which occurred.

See Case Study H7.

An intervening cause, which breaks the chain of causation, may also prevent causation being established and therefore cause the claimant to fail in her claim.

Loss of a chance

The House of Lords (in a majority ruling) ruled in January 2005[45] that where a doctor negligently failed to refer for investigation a patient with possible symptoms of cancer, with the result that there was a nine-month delay in treatment for the condition, the patient whose chances of survival during that delayed period had fallen from 42 % to 25 % could not recover damages for that loss of chance. The delay had not deprived that patient of the prospect of a cure because, on a balance of probability, he could probably not have been cured anyway, and loss of a chance was not in itself a recoverable head of damage for clinical negligence.

Harm

To obtain compensation for negligence it must be established that harm has resulted from the negligent act. Harm includes personal injury and death, loss and damage of property. What types of harm do the courts recognise as being subject to compensation? Some of the forms of harm are shown in Box 11.4.

Box 11.4: Harm recognised as subject to compensation in the civil courts.

– personal injury, pain and suffering
– death
– loss of the ability to have children
– loss of the opportunity to have an abortion
– having a child after being sterilised
– post traumatic stress syndrome or nervous shock
– loss or damage of property.

Where psychiatric harm has occurred as well as physical injury then that is compensatable if a breach of the duty of care and causation can be established. However, where nervous shock (or post-traumatic stress disorder as it is now known) has occurred on its own, compensation will only be paid if a duty of care can be established. The principles of liability for nervous shock were outlined by the House of Lords in the case of *McLoughlin* v. *O'Brian*.[46] More recently, the House of Lords has set out the principles in a series of cases, some involving post-traumatic stress disorder suffered by those who witnessed or assisted at the Hillsborough football stadium disaster. In *Alcock* v. *Chief Constable of South Yorkshire Police*[47] the House of Lords held that a person who suffers reasonably foreseeable psychiatric illness as a result of another person's death cannot recover damages unless he can satisfy three requirements:

– that he had a close tie of love and affection with the person killed, injured or imperilled

- that he was close to the incident in time and space, and
- that he directly perceived the incident rather than, for example, hearing about it from a third person.

In *Page* v. *Smith*[48] the House of Lords made a distinction between primary and secondary victims: a claimant who was within the range of foreseeable injury was a primary victim, all other victims must satisfy the requirements set out above.

  This was applied by the House of Lords in the case of *White* v. *Chief Constable of South Yorkshire Police and Others*,[49] where it decided by a majority that police officers who had assisted in the aftermath of the Hillsborough disaster could not obtain compensation because they were not primary victims, since they were not in the zone of danger, nor did they satisfy the requirements set out above of being secondary victims.

  In contrast, a girl who witnessed her mentally-ill brother stab their mother to death was given £500 000 compensation by the NHS trust who admitted liability for her severe mental breakdown.[50] An independent inquiry had found that he had been allowed to leave the ward, even though medical staff realised that he posed a danger to himself and others.

  In one case[51] the claimant suffered psychiatric illness, after her daughter died following an operation for the removal of her wisdom teeth. Due to negligence on the part of the defendant, the daughter never regained consciousness and was pronounced dead 48 hours after the operation had taken place. The mother failed in her claim on the basis that there was no evidence showing that the events at the hospital had induced a post-traumatic stress disorder, and the overwhelming factor in her psychiatric illness was the fact of the death of her daughter, rather than the events at the hospital. The claim therefore failed on the ground of causation.

  Harm may also include financial losses such as loss of earnings.

Burden of proof

The claimant, i.e. the person bringing the action, normally has the burden of proving that there was negligence by the defendant which caused harm to him. The standard of proof in the civil courts where an action for compensation would take place is 'on a balance of probabilities'. This contrasts with the standard of proof in a criminal case, which is 'beyond reasonable doubt'.

  However, where certain circumstances arise it is possible for the claimant to argue that 'the thing speaks for itself' and the defendant has the task of showing that he was not negligent. This is known as a 'res ipsa loquitur' situation.

  Where self-defence is being used as a defence in a civil case to a claim for compensation for assault and battery, the defendant had to prove on a balance of probability that his mistaken belief that self-defence was necessary was both honestly and reasonably held.[52] This contrasts with the criminal test, where the defendant only has to show that his mistaken belief was honestly held; he does not have to prove that it was reasonably held.

Vicarious liability

It would be usual in the case of an employed health or social services profes-sional for his employer to be sued in the event of him or her being negligent. For obvious reasons, the employer is more likely to be able to pay the compensation due as a consequence of any harm caused by his negligence. This applies even though the employer has not been negligent in any way. In order to ensure that an innocent victim obtains compensation for injuries caused by an employee, public policy dictates that the doctrine of vicarious liability applies. Under the doctrine of vicarious liability, the employer is responsible for compensation payable for the harm. The effect of vicarious liability is shown in the discussion of Scenario H4.

For vicarious liability to be established the elements shown in Box 11.5 must be established.

Box 11.5: Elements in vicarious liability.

- There must be negligence i.e. a duty of care which has been breached and, as a reasonably foreseeable consequence, has caused harm, or some other failure by the employee.
- The negligent act or omission or failure must have been by an employee.
- The negligent employee must have been acting in the course of employment.

Employee

Normally there is no difficulty in defining who is an employee for the purposes of vicarious liability. The term may well include bank or agency persons, but much would depend upon the contractual relationship established between them and the NHS trust or hospital. Self employers or independent practitioners are not employees. They may have an honorary contract to work in hospital or social ser-vices premises. This is unlikely to make the hospital legally liable for their actions. If the hospital were prepared to pay out compensation in respect of the negligence of an independent practitioner, it would probably be subject to the right of indem-nity by the trust against the practitioner.

An employer is not liable for the actions of an independent contractor unless he has authorised them or is at fault in his choice of contractor. Thus, if decorators come on site and harm is caused by the negligence of one of their employees, the occupier of the site or the person who arranged for the decorators to be con-tracted, will not normally be responsible for their activities.

Where volunteers provide charitable services for those in need, the organisa-tion making use of them would probably have insurance cover to ensure that any harm caused by the volunteer is compensated.

Course of employment

Not only must the negligent person be an employee but this person must have been acting in the course of employment. This phrase is wider than 'within the job description' or 'within the rules' or 'following procedures'. Even where the employee is deliberately disobeying the orders of the employer, that action could still be construed as being in the course of employment if it is part of the work that an employee is authorised to do. The House of Lords (in the case of *Lister and Others* v. *Helsey Hall Ltd*) has held that school owners, who were the employers of a warden, could be held liable for acts of sexual abuse committed by the warden of a school boarding house against pupils.[53] The reasoning was that the acts of abuse were sufficiently connected with the work that he had been employed to do that they could be regarded as having been committed within the scope of his employment, i.e. in the course of his employment.

Personal accountability of the employee

Even where the employer is held to be vicariously liable, the employee who is responsible for harm such as the death of a client, could be found guilty of manslaughter for the gross negligence which led to the death; could lose his job following disciplinary action and, if a registered practitioner, could also be struck off the register following a Nursing and Midwifery Council, Health Professions Council or other registration body's hearing on fitness to practise. A schoolmaster was sentenced to a year's imprisonment following the death of a boy on a school trip in the Lake District. The judge held that he was unbelievably foolhardy and negligent in allowing the boy to jump into a turbulent mountain pool.[54] Similar principles would apply to the care of vulnerable adults.

Procedural provisions for claims brought in the name of a mentally incapacitated adult

The Civil Procedure Rules set out the situation when children or patients (persons who by reason of mental disorder within the meaning of the Mental Health Act 1983 are incapable of managing and administering their property and affairs)[55] are involved in civil proceedings. Rule 21.2 requires any such patient to have a litigation friend to conduct proceedings on his behalf. The court can either appoint the litigation friend or a person may act as the litigation friend (either as claimant or defendant) if he can fairly and competently conduct proceedings on behalf of the patient. Such a person is required to follow the procedure set out in Rule 21.5. This includes filing with the court the authorisation or certificate of suitability. No settlement, compromise or payment can be made without the approval of the court. Where money is recovered for the patient, it must be held according to the directions given by the court. Any expenses incurred by a litigation friend on behalf of the patient can be recovered from the amount paid into court if it has been reasonably incurred and it is reasonable in amount. A case concerned with the definition of legal capacity for the purposes of being able to participate in legal proceedings heard before the MCA came into force held that vulnerability to exploitation was an aspect of personality and behaviour to be taken into account when assessing whether an individual had capacity.[56] The judge held that, since the claimant was unlikely to be able to deal with the advice he was likely to have to give or receive in legal proceedings, he was declared a patient within the meaning of Part VII of the 1983 Mental Health Act, and therefore came within Part 21 of the Civil Procedure Rules.

Disciplinary action

All employees also face the possibility of disciplinary action if they fail to provide a reasonable standard of care for those vulnerable adults in their care. Under the contract of employment, the employee has an implied duty to act with reasonable care and to obey reasonable instructions. Being negligent in the care of vulnerable adults, whether or not harm was caused, could be seen as being a breach of this contractual term. As a consequence, the employer could hold disciplinary proceedings and, if the conduct was held to justify dismissal, terminate the contract of employment. The employee may then, if he has the requisite length of continuous service, apply to the employment tribunal, alleging that the employer has unfairly dismissed him or her.

Professional conduct proceedings

Any registered practitioner could be reported to his registration body in the event of an untoward event occurring, where there is evidence of negligence or professional misconduct. Recent changes to the fitness to practise proceedings of the Nursing and Midwifery Council, the General Medical Council and Health Professions Council means that these bodies are operating upon similar lines, with comparable committees and procedures for determining if a registered practitioner should remain on the register, be cautioned or face interim suspension. In addition the establishment of the Council for the Regulation of Healthcare Professions (now known as the Council for Healthcare Regulatory Excellence) is likely to lead to even greater similarities between the workings of the different health registration bodies.

Confidentiality

The fact that an individual lacks mental capacity does not mean that their rights of confidentiality are not protected. Those who are capable of giving consent to the disclosure of information are permitted in law to do so. If they lack that capacity, then the provisions of the Data Protection Act and the regulations made under that Act provide them with the same protection. There are specific and limited occasions where disclosure of personal information is permissible in law without the consent of the individual. These exceptions to the duty of confidentiality are set out in Chapter 15 on informal carers, but the same principles apply to health and social services professionals.

Section 60 of the Health and Social Care Act 2001 (now Section 251 of the NHS Act 2006) enabled regulations[57] to be made to enable people to use confidential patient information without breaking the law of confidentiality. Applications must be made to the Patient Information Advisory Group for approval on behalf of the Secretary of State.[58] The duty of confidentiality on informal carers is considered in Chapter 15.

Complaints

The use of complaints procedures to challenge decisions made under the Act or challenge omissions in implementing the Act is considered in Chapter 17.

Conclusions

This chapter has considered the protection of the vulnerable adult and the different forms of accountability which apply to the work of health and social services professionals. They apply as much to the care of vulnerable adults as they do to the care of those without disabilities. The operation of the new criminal offence of ill-treating or wilfully neglecting a person who lacks capacity should be monitored to ensure that it provides the necessary protection for the vulnerable adult.

References

1   Law Commission (1995) Report No 231, *Mental Incapacity*. HMSO, London.
2   Law Commission (1993) *Mentally Incapacitated and Other Vulnerable Adults: Public Law Protection*. Consultation Paper No 130. HMSO, London.
3   Joint Cttee para 272.
4   *Ibid*. para 273.
5   *Ibid*. para 274.
6   Code of Practice for the Mental Capacity Act 2005. Department of Constitutional Affairs February 2007 para 14.3. TSO, London.
7   *Ibid*. para 14.27.
8   Department of Health and Home Office (2000) *No secrets: Guidance on developing and implementing multi-agency policies and procedures to protect vulnerable adults from abuse*. http://www.dh.gov.uk/assetRoot/04/07/45/40/04074540.pdf
9   National Assembly for Wales (2000) *In safe hands: Implementing adult protection procedures in Wales*. http://www.wales.gov.uk/subisocialpolicy/content/pdf/safehands_e.pdf
10 Department of Health (2006) About the Dignity in care campaign. Ref. No Gateway no 7386.
11 www.dh.gov.uk/PolicyAndGuidance/
12 Code of Practice (see reference 6 above) para 14.7.

13   Department of Health (2001) *Valuing People: A New Strategy for Learning Disability for the 21st Century*. White Paper CM 5086.

14   Department of Health (2005) *Increased funding for learning disabilities services unveiled today*. DoH 2005/0061.

15   Department of Health (2007) National Framework for NHS continuing healthcare. Ref. No Gateway no 8427. DH, London.

16   Department of Health (2004) *Protection of Vulnerable Adults (POVA) scheme in England and Wales for care homes and domiciliary care agencies: a practical guide.*

17   www.doh.gov.uk/vulnerableadults

18   Code of Practice (see reference 6 above) para 14.30.

19   Richardson, P.J. (ed) (2005) *Archbold Criminal Pleadings Evidence and Practice*. 15–490. Sweet and Maxwell, London.

20   Police and Criminal Evidence Act 1984, S.77(3).

21   Richardson, P.J. (ed) (2005) *Archbold Criminal Pleadings Evidence and Practice*. 15–368. Sweet and Maxwell, London.

22   *Archbold Criminal Pleadings Evidence and Practice*. 8–39 (see reference 21 above).

23   *Hulme* v. *DPP* [2006] EWHC 1347; (2006) 170 SJ 598.

24   (2004) *Chitty on Contracts*. 29th edn. Sweet and Maxwell, London.

25   *The Observer* (27 November 2005) *Money Writes*. Letter (from DR, Norwich) to Margaret Dibben column.

26   Joint Cttee of Houses of Parliament Chapter 14 paras 255–274.

27   Department of Health and Home Office (2000) *No secrets: Guidance on developing and implementing multi-agency policies and procedures to protect vulnerable adults from abuse.* DH 1999; DoH, London. www.doh.gov.uk/scg/nosecrets.htm

28   Joint Cttee of Houses of Parliament Chapter 14 para 261.

29   *Ibid.* para 264.

30   *Ibid.* para 266.

31   *In Re B (Consent to treatment: Capacity)*, Times Law Report, 26 March 2002; [2002] 2 All ER 449.

32   *R. (On the application of Pretty)* v. *DPP* [2001] UKHL 61; [2001] 3 WLR 1598.

33   *R.* v. *Adams (Bodkin)* [1957] Crim LR 365.

34   *Donoghue* v. *Stevenson* [1932] AC 562.

35   Nursing and Midwifery Council (2004) *Code of professional conduct: standards for performance, conduct and ethics.*

36   *Kent* v. *Griffiths (No 3)* [2001] QB 36.

37   *Carty* v. *Croydon London Borough Council*. The Times Law Report, 3 February 2005, CA.

38   *D.* v *East Berkshire Community Health NHS Trust and Another; MAK and Another v. Dewsbury Healthcare NHS Trust and Another; RK and Another* v. *Oldham NHS Trust and Another*. Times Law Report, 22 April 2005, HL.

39   *Brooks* v. *Commissioner of Police of the Metropolis and Others*. Times Law Report, 26 April 2005, HL.

40   *Hill* v. *Chief Constable of West Yorkshire* [1989] AC 53, HL.

41   *Bolam* v. *Friern Hospital Management Committee* [1957] 1 WLR 582.

42   *Hunter* v. *Hanley* [1955] SLT 213.

43   *Maynard* v. *West Midlands Regional Health Authority* [1985] 1 All ER 871.

44   *Barnett* v. *Chelsea HMC* [1968] 1 All ER 1068.

45   *Gregg* v. *Scott*. Times Law Report, 28 January 2005, HL [2005] UK HL 2.

46   *McLoughlin* v. *O'Brian* [1982] 2 All ER 298.

47   *Alcock* v. *Chief Constable of South Yorkshire Police* [1992] 1 AC 310.

48   *Page* v. *Smith* [1996] AC 155.

49   *White* v. *Chief Constable of South Yorkshire Police and Others* [1999] 1 All ER 1, HL.

50   Frean, A. Sister who saw killing wins record trauma sum. *The Times*, 5 November 2001, p 5.

51   *Ward* v. *The Leeds Teaching Hospitals NHS Trust* [2004] EWHC 2106.

52   *Ashley and Another* v. *Chief Constable of Sussex Police*, Times Law Report, 30 August 2006, CA.

53   *L. and Others* v. *Helsey Hall Ltd* [2001] UKHL 22; [2001] 2 WLR 1311.

54   Jenkins, R. & Owen, G. Jailing of teacher may spell the end for school trips. *The Times*, 24 September 2003.

55   Civil Procedure Rules 21.1(2)(b); www.dca.gov.uk/civil/procrules_fin/contents/parts/part21

56   *Lindsay* v. *Wood*. Times Law Report, 8 December 2006, QBD.

57   Health Service (Control of Patient Information) Regulations 2002 (SI 2002/1438).

58   www.advisorybodies.doh.gov.uk/PIAG

Scenarios H
Protection of Vulnerable Adults

These Scenarios should be read in conjunction with Chapter 11, which considers the protection of vulnerable adults and the accountability of those involved in their care.

Criminal offence to ill-treat or wilfully neglect a person who lacks capacity

A situation illustrating the offence is shown in Scenario H1.

Scenario H1: Carer or neighbour?

Janice lived in a house which was divided into six separate dwellings with shared bath and toilet facilities. She would occasionally do shopping for an elderly widow, Beryl, living in the basement flat and sometimes stop to have a coffee with her. Infrequently she would take her a hot meal if she had been cooking. She noticed that Beryl seemed to be becoming more absent minded. Janice was studying for examinations and had not seen her for several weeks, and was told by the police that she had died. The police were concerned to establish how often Janice had contact with Beryl and if she could be described as Beryl's carer.

It is unlikely in this situation that Janice could be seen as Beryl's carer, though the question arises as to whether the definition of carer could be seen simply as a question of frequency of contact. So that, for example, if Janice saw Beryl every day could she then be seen as a carer, but if her contact was less regular or frequent, would she not be seen as a carer? Given the fact that there was no other relationship between Janice and Beryl it is unlikely that Janice would be seen as a carer for the purposes of Section 44(2). However the mere fact that a person voluntarily takes on a duty of caring for a mentally incapacitated person, would not prevent that person becoming by law a carer and therefore liable to prosecution under Section 44(2) for failure to fulfil that duty. Even if Janice is defined as a carer of Beryl, it would still have to be established that her failure to provide care was 'wilful neglect'. 'Wilful' implies a knowledge of the result of her failure to care and a decision to neglect her, oblivious of the consequences.

Contractual liability and mental incapacity

Even if an adult lacks the requisite mental capacity to make a contract, he may be bound by a contract supplying him with necessities. The situation is illustrated by a letter to Margaret Dibben in *The Observer*,[1] which is considered in Scenario H2.

Scenario H2: Contracts and mental capacity.

The Halifax allowed my 22-year-old son to take out a £3000 personal loan. He has Asperger's syndrome and is identified by the authorities as a vulnerable adult. He receives disability benefits and lives in supported accommodation. He has no concept of the value of money. His carers take his rent and household expenses from his income, giving him the balance.

Within a few days, he spent the entire loan on a number of consumer items. Despite Halifax's claim that it followed proper procedures, there appears to have been little, if any check on my son's expenses.

The following answer was provided by Margaret Dibben:

Under common law, people cannot be held to a contract if they are unable to understand the consequences, unless they are buying necessities.

But again by law, every one must presume that people they deal with are capable and must not discriminate against anyone with disabilities. It's a fine line.

Initially, Halifax repeated that it had no reason to reject your son's application though it became concerned when it realised that he was unable to repay the debt.

I pointed out his inability to enter into the contract in the first place and, as a gesture of goodwill, Halifax has now agreed to write off the outstanding loan.

The above situation is fraught with difficulties as Margaret Dibben points out: to require proof of mental capacity from persons with disabilities may be seen as discriminatory. Yet there needs to be evidence of mental incapacity in order that the presumption of capacity can be rebutted.

Murder and manslaughter

Case Study H1.

Case Study H1: Manslaughter.

Dr Adomako,[2] the person charged, was, during the latter part of an operation, the anaesthetist in charge of the patient, who was undergoing an eye operation. At approximately 11.05am a disconnection occurred at the endotracheal tube connection. The supply of oxygen to the patient ceased and led to a cardiac arrest at 11.14am. During that period the defendant failed to notice or remedy the disconnection. He first became aware that something was amiss when an alarm sounded on the Dinamap machine, which monitored the patient's blood pressure. From the evidence it appeared that some four-and-a-half minutes would have elapsed between the disconnection and the sounding of the alarm. When the alarm sounded the defendant responded in various ways by checking the equipment and by administering atropine to raise the patient's pulse. But at no stage before the cardiac arrest did he check the integrity of the endotracheal tube connection. The disconnection was not discovered until after resuscitation measures had been commenced.

  Dr Adomako accepted at his trial that he had been negligent. The issue was whether his conduct was criminal. He was convicted of involuntary manslaughter but appealed against his conviction. He lost his appeal in the Court of Appeal and then appealed to the House of Lords.[3]

The House of Lords clarified the legal situation.

The stages which the House of Lords suggested should be followed were:

– The ordinary principles of the law of negligence should be applied to ascertain whether or not the defendant had been in breach of a duty of care towards the victim who had died.
– If such a breach of duty was established, the next question was whether that breach of duty caused the death of the victim.
– If so, the jury had to go on to consider whether that breach of duty should be characterised as gross negligence and therefore as a crime. That would depend on the seriousness of the breach of duty committed by the defendant in all the circumstances in which the defendant was placed when it occurred.
– The jury would have to consider whether the extent to which the defendant's conduct departed from the proper standard of care incumbent upon him, involving as it must have done a risk of death to the patient, was such that it should be judged criminal.

The judge was required to give the jury a direction on the meaning of 'gross negligence' as had been given in the present case by the Court of Appeal. The jury might properly find gross negligence on proof of:

- indifference to an obvious risk of injury to health, or
- actual foresight of the risk coupled with either
  - a determination nevertheless to run it, or
  - an intention to avoid it but involving such a high degree of negligence in the attempted avoidance as the jury considered justified conviction, or
- inattention or failure to advert to a serious risk going beyond mere inadvertence in respect of an obvious and important matter which the defendant's duty demanded he should address.

The House of Lords held that the Court of Appeal had applied the correct test and his appeal was dismissed.

It follows that if a paid or informal carer of a person who lacked mental capacity acted or omitted to act with such gross negligence that the client/patient died, then proceedings for manslaughter could be brought. Following such a conviction, the judge has full discretion over the sentencing, which could range from an absolute discharge to substantial time of imprisonment.

Distinction between killing and letting die

Tony Bland case[4]

The House of Lords in the Tony Bland case made it clear that there was in law a clear distinction between letting nature take its course when, in the light of the prognosis, it was in the best interests not to continue active interventions and killing the patient.

In the words of Lord Goff:

The law draws a crucial distinction between cases in which a doctor decides not to provide, or to continue to provide, for his patient treatment or care which could or might prolong his life and those in which he decides, for example, by administering a lethal drug, actively to bring his patient's life to an end.

The facts of Tony Bland are shown in Case Study H2.

Case Study H2: Tony Bland.

The patient was a victim of the football stadium crush at Hillesborough and it was established that although he could breathe and digest food independently, he could not see, hear, taste, smell or communicate in any way and it appeared that there was no hope of recovery or improvement. The House of Lords had to decide if it was lawful to permit artificial feeding to be discontinued in the case of a patient in a persistent vegetative state. The House of Lords decided that it would be in the best interests of the patient to discontinue the nasal gastric feed and he was later reported as having died.

A court in Bristol gave consent in a similar case a few months after the House of Lords decision in Tony Bland's case.[5]

Cases of Re B and Diane Pretty

Case Study H3: Case of *Re B*.[6]

Miss B suffered a ruptured blood vessel in her neck which damaged her spinal cord. As a consequence she was paralysed from the neck down and was on a ventilator. She was of sound mind and knew that there was no cure for her condition. She asked for the ventilator to be switched off. Her doctors wished her to try out some special rehabilitation to improve the standard of her care, and felt that an intensive care ward was not a suitable location for such a decision to be made. They were reluctant to perform such an action as switching off the ventilator without the court's approval. Miss B applied to court for a declaration to be made that the ventilator could be switched off.

Two experts examined Miss B and said that she had the mental capacity to make decisions about switching off the ventilator. In the light of that assessment, the judge had no option other than to declare that she was entitled to refuse life saving treatment. The case is considered in more detail in Chapter 2 on page 11. See also Box 2.2.

Diane Pretty[7]

Case Study H4: Case of Diane Pretty.

In a well-publicised case, Diane Pretty, a sufferer of motor neurone disease, appealed to the House of Lords that her husband should be allowed to end her life, and not be prosecuted under the Suicide Act 1961. The House of Lords did not allow her appeal. It held that if there were to be any changes to the Suicide Act to legalise the killing of another person, then these changes should be made by Parliament. As the law stood, the Suicide Act made it a criminal offence to aid and abet the suicide of another person, and the husband could not be granted immunity from prosecution were he to assist his wife to die. The House of Lords held that there was no conflict between the human rights of Mrs Pretty as set out in the European Convention on Human Rights. Mrs Pretty then applied to the European Court of Human Rights in Strasbourg, but lost. The court held that there was no conflict between the Suicide Act 1961 and the European Convention of Human Rights.

The Council of Europe issued a press release entitled *Chamber judgment in the case of Pretty v. the United Kingdom*, published on 29 April 2002. It stated that:

The European Court of Human Rights has refused an application by Diane Pretty, a British national dying of motor neurone disease, for a ruling that would allow her husband to assist her to commit suicide without facing prosecution under the Suicide Act 1961 section 2(1). The applicant is paralysed from the neck downwards and has a poor life expectancy, whilst her intellect and decision making capacity remain unimpaired. She wanted to be given the right to decide when and how she died without undergoing further suffering and indignity. The court unanimously found the application inadmissible with no violations under the European Convention of Human Rights under Art 2 the right to life, Art 3 prohibition of human or degrading treatment or punishment; Art 8 the right to respect for private life; Art 9 freedom of conscience and Art 14 prohibition of discrimination.

It was subsequently reported that Diane Pretty had died.

It is clear that Diane Pretty would have had the right to refuse natural or artificial feeding and hydration. However she stated that she did not wish to suffer a slow death by starvation and would prefer to have a pain-free, dignified and speedy death. In law she could lawfully attempt to commit suicide, but in practice she lacked the physical powers to do so. She therefore needed to have assistance. However to assist anyone to commit suicide is a criminal offence. (See Box 11.1 in Chapter 11, page 255.)

Levels of pain medication

Case Study H5 illustrates the difference between giving a dose of medication in order to bring about the death of the patient and giving medication to control the patient's pain.

Case Study H5: Dr Bodkin Adams.

Dr Adams was charged with the murder of a resident of a nursing home in Eastbourne. It was alleged that he gave her large quantities of morphia and heroin which caused her death.

In the case of Dr Bodkin Adams the trial judge, Patrick Devlin, directed the jury in the following words:

> If the first purpose of medicine – the restoration of health – can no longer be achieved, there is still much for the doctor to do, and he is entitled to do all that is proper and necessary to relieve pain and suffering even if the measures he takes may incidentally shorten life. . . . It remains a fact, and remains a law, that no doctor has the right to cut off life deliberately . . . (the defence counsel) was saying that the treatment given by the doctor was designed to promote comfort; and if it was the right and proper treatment of the case, the fact that incidentally it shortened life does not give any grounds for convicting him of murder.[8]

Dr Adams was found not guilty of murder.

Annie Lindsell case

> **Case Study H6: Controlling pain.**
>
> On 28 October 1997 Annie Lindsell,[9] who was terminally ill with motor neurone disease, applied to court for a declaration that her GP would not risk prosecution for murder if he gave her potentially lethal painkillers when her condition deteriorated. After hearing that a responsible body of medical opinion supported her GP's plan she withdrew her application for the court's intervention. In the case a clear distinction was made between pain relief whose principal purpose was to control her pain, even though incidentally it might shorten her life, and medication given to end her life.

After the Annie Lindsell hearing, the British Medical Association (BMA) stated that it was pleased with the outcome:

> it has confirmed that doctors working within the law, can treat the symptoms of terminally ill patients, even if that treatment may have a secondary consequence of shortening the patient's life.

Annie Lindsell died a month later.

Criminal liability and learning disabilities

Scenario H3 illustrates a situation where a person with severe learning disabilities is involved in criminal proceedings.

> **Scenario H3: Criminal proceedings and a mentally incapacitated offender.**
>
> Harry, a community nurse, was asked to attend the police station where one of his clients, Peter, from a community home for those with challenging behaviour, was being questioned. It appeared that Peter had been arrested in the street for exposing himself. Harry was asked to act as an appropriate adult whilst Peter was questioned and to provide information on Peter's background.

Whilst it would usually be unwise for a registered nurse to be identified as an independent advocate of a patient, in these circumstances there would be no obvious reason why Harry should not be able to provide the protection which Peter required. Harry should have had some training in what was required as the 'appropriate adult'. There would be clear advantages in Harry ensuring that Peter had legal representation. Most primary care trusts and social service departments should have established a procedure with the local police and criminal courts so that, in the event of a person lacking mental capacity being arrested, identified officers could be made available to attend the police station and the courts.

Civil liability

Scenario H4 discusses civil liability in failing to follow the Code of Practice.

Scenario H4: Failure to follow Code of Practice.

Justin was a staff nurse working in a community home for those with learning disabilities. One of his residents, Ollie, was complaining of toothache. Justin decided that Ollie was not capable of giving consent to the dental examination and therefore arranged for Ollie to be given an anaesthetic for the examination and extraction. Ollie's parents discovered belatedly that Ollie had had the extraction and complained to Justin's manager. They maintained that Ollie's consent should have been obtained. And if it was established that he was not capable of giving consent to dental treatment, then they should have been brought in to give consent. An investigation was carried out. It was discovered that Justin had failed to follow the guidance in the Code of Practice relating to the determination of capacity. He had just assumed that Ollie lacked the requisite capacity and he had not carried out any evaluation of Ollie's mental capacity. He had not attempted to try to minimise anxiety or stress by making Ollie feel at ease. Nor had he chosen the best location where Ollie felt most comfortable and the time of day when Ollie was most alert. Nor did he consider bringing in an expert to advise on Ollie's mental capacity to make the specific decision.

In this Scenario, not only has Justin failed to follow the Code of Practice, he has also failed to follow the basic principle of the Mental Capacity Act 2005, namely that:

A person must be assumed to have capacity unless it is established that he lacks capacity (Mental Capacity Act S.1(2)).

It is the duty of a person to have regard to any relevant code if he is acting in relation to a person who lacks capacity and is doing so in a professional capacity (S.42(4)(e)).

The effect of failure to obey the code is that if it appears to a court or tribunal conducting any criminal or civil proceedings that a provision of a code or a failure to comply with a code is relevant to a question arising in the proceedings, the provision or failure must be taken into account in deciding the question (S.42(5)).

What action could Ollie's parents bring in his name?

Failure to assess Ollie's capacity is a civil wrong, not just by Justin, but also by the dentist, who should have carried out his own test to determine whether Ollie could give consent. It could be argued that both have failed to follow the reasonable standard of care required of a professional as set down in the Bolam case. In addition, Justin's failure to follow the guidance in the Code of Practice could be used as evidence of a trespass to Ollie's person. In theory the parents could bring a civil action for trespass to the person in the name of Ollie. In practice it is more likely that they would pursue their grievance through the complaints procedure, and perhaps seek some disciplinary action against Justin. Justin's employers could be held vicariously liable for Justin's civil wrongs.

Causation

In the case shown in Case Study H7 the claimants failed to establish causation, and the House of Lords ordered a new hearing on the issue of causation.

Case Study H7: *Wilsher v. Essex Area Health Authority.*[10]

A premature baby was being treated with oxygen therapy. A junior doctor mistakenly inserted the catheter to monitor the oxygen intake into a vein rather than an artery. A senior registrar, when asked to check what had been done, failed to notice the error. The baby was given excess oxygen. The parents claimed compensation for the retrolentalfibroplasia that the baby suffered, but failed to prove that it was the excess oxygen which had caused the harm. They therefore failed in their claim. It was agreed that there were several different factors which could have caused the child to become blind, and the negligence was only one of them. It could not been presumed that it was the defendant's negligence which had caused the harm. The House of Lords ordered the case to be reheard on the issue of causation. In the event, the parties settled.

An example of negligence

If a person follows the principles of the Mental Capacity Act (MCA), establishes that a client/patient lacks the requisite mental capacity and acts in the best interests of that client according to the criteria set down in Section 4, then that person is protected against an action for trespass to the person. However their actions may still lead to civil and criminal proceedings, as Scenario H5 illustrates.

Scenario H5: Negligence.

Dawn was a care assistant working in a community home. She was asked to arrange for Kevin, one of the residents, to be taken to the shops. She had been trained in this activity and knew that two care assistants were required. However because her colleagues were busy, she decided to take him on her own. As they were about to cross the road, Kevin let go of her hand, rushed across the road in front of a lorry and was severely injured. Kevin's relatives are prepared to sue on his behalf.

In the situation in Scenario H5, Dawn is at fault in failing to follow the risk assessment and management procedures of the home which have been set down to ensure Kevin's protection. She would be held personally accountable for this, but it would be her employers who would have to pay compensation to Kevin. The employers are vicariously liable for the negligence of Dawn, an employee who was acting in the course of employment. Under Section 5(3) of the MCA there can still be liability for negligence, even though a person was acting under the powers of the MCA in making decisions in P's best interests.

See also Scenario B13 on page 78.

Financial abuse

Scenario H6: Financial abuse.

Martha, aged 74, leads a hermit-like existence and never leaves her home. She has an arrangement with a neighbour for her benefit to be collected on her behalf. A community nurse visits Martha and suspects that she is not receiving all the money she should be getting and that the neighbour is keeping some for herself. What action can she take?

It is uncertain from the facts of this case as to whether the neighbour has taken on the role of an appointee, i.e. a person appointed by the Department for Work and Pensions to receive and deal with the benefits of Martha, who lacks the capacity to do this for herself. It may be just an informal arrangement between the neighbour and Martha. Whatever the arrangement, the receiver of the money has a duty to use it entirely in the best interests of Martha.

The Code of Practice[11] states that the Department for Work and Pensions (DWP) can appoint someone (an appointee) to claim and spend benefits on a person's behalf if that person:

- gets social security benefits or pensions
- lacks the capacity to act for themselves
- has not made a property and affairs legal power of attorney (LPA) or an enduring power of attorney (EPA) and
- the court has not appointed a property and affairs deputy.

The DWP has a responsibility to check that an appointee is trustworthy, and can investigate any allegations that an appointee is not acting appropriately or in the person's interests. The community nurse could take up her query with the relevant DWP agency (i.e. since Martha is over 60, the Pension Service. If Martha were under 60, concerns could be raised with the local Job Centre). The DWP can remove an appointee who abuses their position. If the neighbour is not an appointee, then the DPW can take steps to appoint an approved person.

References

1   *The Observer* (27 November 2005) *Money Writes*. Letter (from DR, Norwich) to Margaret Dibben column.
2   *R* v. *Adomako*. The Times Law Report, 4 July 1994; [1994] 3 All ER 79, HL.
3   *Ibid.*
4   *Airedale NHS Trust* v. *Bland* [1993] AC 789.
5   *Frenchay Healthcare NHS Trust* v. *S* [1994] 2 All ER 403.
6   In *Re B (Consent to treatment: Capacity)*. The Times Law Report, 26 March 2002; [2002] 2 All ER 449.
7   *R. (On the application of Pretty)* v. *DPP* [2001] UKHL 61; [2001] 3 WLR 1598.
8   Bedford, S. (1961) *The Best We Can Do*. Penguin, Harmondsworth.
9   Wilkins, E. Dying woman granted wish for dignified end. *The Times*, 29 October 1997.
10 *Wilsher* v. *Essex Area Health Authority* [1988] 1 All ER 871, HL.
11 Code of Practice for the Mental Capacity Act 2005. Department of Constitutional Affairs February 2007 para 14.35–6.

12 Children and Young Persons

Introduction

Those under 16 years are in general excluded from the provisions of the Mental Capacity Act (MCA), since under Section 2(5) no power is exercisable in relation to a person under 16 years. However there is an exception to this principle in relation to property matters. In addition there are several provisions where a person must be at least 18 years to utilise some of the tools given in the Act. There are a few sections of the MCA relating to children, and for convenience these are brought together in this chapter and the general rules relating to decision making by and on behalf of children considered.

Children Act 1989

The Children Act 1989 makes provision for the care of children and young persons under 18 years, and this Act will continue to be the main source of law for those individuals. In addition children and young persons come under the inherent jurisdiction of the High Court, and if they suffer from mental disorder may come under the Mental Health Act 1983 (see Chapter 13).

Family Law Reform Act 1969 and children of 16 and 17

Young persons of 16 and 17 years have a statutory right to give consent to surgical, medical and dental treatment under Section 8 of the Family Law Reform Act 1969.

Like adults (those over 18 years), there is a presumption that they have the capacity to give consent. The presumption of capacity can be rebutted, i.e. removed, if there is evidence that the person lacks capacity to make a specific decision and the standard of proof is on a balance of probabilities. Even where the young person is considered to have the necessary capacity, a refusal to consent to life saving treatment can be overruled by the court if it is considered to be in the best interests of the young person to have the treatment[1] (see Scenario I1). For this reason a person must be over 18 years to be eligible to draw up an advance decision which would cover the situation if they subsequently lack capacity (see **Advance decision,** page 286 and Chapter 9 on advance decisions). A case involving the refusal of a young person of 16 and 17 to consent to treatment considered to be in his or her best interests where the young person had the requisite mental capacity would be heard in the High Court, not the Court of Protection. However where capacity was lacking or disputed the Court of Protection could have jurisdiction. (An example can be seen in Case I1.) As will be seen below, there is maximum flexibility to enable a case to be transferred from the High Court to the Court of Protection and vice versa, wherever that would be in the interests of justice.

Changes to the law on overruling the refusal of a young person of 16 or 17 years

Lord Howe introduced an amendment to the Mental Health Bill, amending Section 131 of the Mental Health Act 1983 for a 16- and 17-year-old patient's refusal to consent or resistance to admission/treatment for mental disorder not to be overridden by the giving of consent by a person who has parental responsibility. An amendment was made by Section 43 of the Mental Health Act 2007. Lord Hunt (for the Government) said that:

> There is clearly support for 16- and 17-year-olds capable of expressing their own wishes to have their consent or refusal to consent to treatment and admittance to hospital for mental disorder protected in the Bill. Where they consent to admission and treatment in hospital for mental disorder, their consent should not be overridden by a person with parental responsibility for them. Where they do not consent to admission and treatment in hospital for mental disorder, their lack of consent should not be overridden by a person with parental responsibilities for them.[2]

Such a change may have a significant effect in the recognition of the human rights of the 16- and 17-year-old.

Young persons and children under 16 years

As a consequence of the House of Lords ruling in the Gillick[3] case, those under 16 years are able to give a valid consent to treatment and examination, if they have the requisite capacity to make the specific decision. However in these circumstances there is no presumption of capacity: capacity has to be established in respect of each decision which is to be made.

The House of Lords in a majority ruling held that if a child has the maturity to understand the nature, purpose, and likely effects of any proposed treatment, then he or she could give a valid consent without the involvement of the parents. This has given rise to the expression 'Gillick competent' which is also known as the test of competence according to Lord Fraser's guidelines (Lord Fraser was one of the judges in the House of Lords which decided the Gillick case). Lord Fraser stated that:

> Provided the patient, whether a boy or a girl, is capable of understanding what is proposed, and of expressing his or her own wishes, I see no good reason for holding that he or she lacks the capacity to express them validly and effectively and to authorise the medical man to make the examination or give the treatment which he advises.

Whilst the Gillick case itself was concerned with family planning and treatment, the principle applies to other forms of treatment, including abortion, and can apply to boys as well as girls. The principle that the ascertainable wishes and feelings of the child concerned (considered in the light of his age and understanding) should also be taken into account, is also stated in the Children Act 1989 Section 1(3)(a) as one of the factors to which the court must have regard in determining what if any orders should be made or varied.

Parental rights and consent on behalf of young persons and children

Section 8(3) of the Family Law Reform Act 1969 preserves the right of a parent to give consent to treatment and examination on behalf of a young person of 16 or 17 years. If a young person of 17 came unconscious into a hospital's Accident and Emergency department after a road accident the parent(s) could give consent to treatment on his or her behalf. Where however there is a dispute between the young person and the parent, as for example where a young person of 16 has become a Jehovah's Witness and has refused to give consent to a life saving blood transfusion, and the parent is not of the same faith and wants blood to be given, then it would be preferable, in order to protect the rights of the child and parents, for an application to be made to court for a declaration on what is in the best interest of the young person.

Where the young person or child is under 16 years the parent has the right and duty to act in the child's best interests, and could be prosecuted for failure to act appropriately if harm is caused to the child as a consequence. Where there is a major decision to be made, it is preferable for a declaration of the court to be obtained. See case study I1, page 290, on the sterilisation of a young person less than 18 years and case I2, page 293, on the court overruling the refusal of a 15-year-old to have a heart transplant.

Court of Protection

Property and financial decisions

With the exception of the execution of a will, the powers of the Court of Protection under Section 16 can be exercised even though P has not reached 16, if the court considers that it is likely that P will still lack capacity to make decisions in respect of that matter when he reaches 18. Thus in the case of a young person with severe learning disabilities, a decision about his property and affairs can be made even though he is under 16 years if it seems unlikely that he will have the necessary mental capacity at 18 years. (See Scenario I2.)

The power under the MCA Section 18(3) for the Court of Protection to exercise the powers given under Section 16 in respect of a child who has not reached 16 years, prevents the need for new proceedings to be commenced once the child reaches adulthood, and continues the jurisdiction of the previous Court of Protection in relation to children under 16.

The Code of Practice notes that[4] the Court of Protection can:

- make an order (for example, concerning the investment of an award of compensation for the child), and/or
- appoint a deputy to manage the child's property and affairs and to make ongoing financial decisions on the child's behalf.

In making a decision, the court must follow the Act's principles and decide in the child's best interests as set out in chapter 5 of the Code.

Offence of ill-treatment and neglect

Section 44 covers the offence of ill-treatment or wilful neglect of a person who lacks capacity to make relevant decisions. This section also applies to children under 16 and young people aged 16 or 17. But it only applies if the child's lack of capacity to make a decision for himself or herself is caused by an impairment of, or disturbance that affects how his or her mind or brain works. If the lack of capacity is solely the result of the child's youth or immaturity, then the ill-treatment or wilful neglect would be dealt with under the separate offences of child cruelty or neglect.[5]

Jurisdiction over the 16- and 17-year-old

Link between Court of Protection and family courts

A case relating to a 16- or 17-year-old who lacks capacity could be heard either in a court dealing with family proceedings or in the Court of Protection. Under Section 21, the new Court of Protection has the power in certain circumstances to transfer cases concerning children to a court that has jurisdiction under the Children Act 1989. Moreover, a case started in a court having jurisdiction under the Children Act 1989, in which the main relief claim relates to a time after adulthood, can be transferred to the Court of Protection. The intention behind this is to ensure that cases involving vulnerable 16- and 17-year-olds are approached in the most appropriate way possible.

The Explanatory Memorandum gives the example of a case of a dispute over the property of a person lacking mental capacity under the age of 18 years.

> For example, if the parents of a 17-year-old with profound learning difficulties are in dispute about residence or contact then it may be more appropriate for the Court of Protection to deal with the case, since an order more under the Children Act 1989 would expire on the child's 18th birthday at the latest.[6]

Where the 16- or 17-year-old lacks mental capacity as defined in Sections 2 and 3 of the MCA, then proceedings could either be brought in the High Court or the Court of Protection, depending on which court appears to be the more appropriate.

The Code of Practice puts forward the following example of the considerations which should be taken into account in determining whether to use the powers set out under the MCA.[7]

- In unusual circumstances it might be in a young person's best interests for the Court of Protection to make an order and/or appoint a property and affairs deputy. For example, this might occur when a young person receives financial compensation and the court appoints a parent or a solicitor as a property and affairs deputy.
- It may be appropriate for the Court of Protection to make a welfare decision concerning a young person who lacks capacity to decide for themselves (for example, about where the young person should live) if the court decides that the parents are not acting in the young person's best interests.
- It might be appropriate to refer a case to the Court of Protection where there is disagreement between a person interested in the care and welfare of a young person and the young person's medical team about the young person's best interests or capacity.

Dispute in relation to care and treatment

The Code of Practice discusses the most appropriate court for determining care and treatment decisions in relation to a 16- or 17-year-old and states:[8]

> A case involving a young person who lacks mental capacity to make a specific decision could be heard in the family courts (probably in the Family Division of the High Court) or in the Court of Protection.
>
> If a case might require an ongoing order (because the young person is likely to still lack capacity when they are 18), it may be more appropriate for the Court of Protection to hear the case. For one-off cases not involving property or finances, the Family Division may be more appropriate.

The Act, therefore, allows the Lord Chancellor to make an order allowing for transfer of proceedings from the Court of Protection to the family courts, and vice versa (Section 21). The choice of court will depend on what is appropriate in the particular circumstances of the case. Regulations have been issued on the transfer of proceedings from the Court of Protection to a court having jurisdiction under the Children Act and vice versa.[9] Scenario I3 illustrates the situation.

Provisions of the Mental Capacity Act which are not available for use in respect of a 16- and 17-year-old

Lasting power of attorney

A person creating the power of attorney must have reached the age of 18 years in order to execute the instrument (S.9(2)(c)).

A donee or attorney of the lasting power of attorney must have reached 18 years (S. 10(1)(a)).

The implications of these two sections are that a young person under 18 years cannot delegate powers of decision making on property and finance or personal welfare until he or she has reached 18 years. It would be possible for the appropriate document to be drafted in advance and then await the 18th birthday for it to be signed i.e. executed by the donor. Even though the unsigned document would not be effective in law as a lasting power of attorney, it would provide a statement of the young person's wishes and feelings, and if for some reason it was never appropriately executed and the young person came under the provisions of the MCA, it could provide evidence for determining what was in his or her best interests by using the criteria set out in Section 4(6), and considering what his or her views and beliefs would have been.

Similarly the young person could not take on the role of donee under a lasting power of attorney until he or she became 18 years. Once again it would be possible to prepare documents in advance, to be executed on the 18th birthday of the donee.

Advance decision

A person making an advance decision to refuse treatment must have reached 18 years (S.24(1)).

As explained above, this is because of the thinking underpinning common law rulings in which refusals by those under 18 years have been overruled, because the refusal of life saving treatment was not considered to be in the best interests of the young person. However any views they have previously expressed, either orally or in writing, about treatment preferences or dislikes should be fully taken into account in deciding what may be in their best interests at a time when they may lack capacity to express those views (see Scenario 14).

Making a will

In keeping with the Wills Act, which requires a person to be over 18 years to make a will (apart from specific exclusions), the MCA Section 18(2) confirms that the Court of Protection has no power to make a statutory will on behalf of young people aged less than 18 years.

Court of Protection

No permission is required for an application to the court for the exercise of any of its powers under the MCA by anyone with parental responsibility for a person who has not reached 18.

Parental responsibility has the same meaning as in the Children Act 1989, and includes the mother, the married father (it is irrelevant whether or not they are now divorced or separated), and the unmarried father if he has taken the necessary steps to be recognised as the father who has parental responsibilities for the child. If the child is adopted, parental rights move from the natural parents to the adopted parents by operation of law.

Urgent cases

A Practice Note was issued by the Official Solicitor[10] giving guidance on the procedures to be followed in respect of urgent and out of hours cases in which a decision was sought by a judge of the Family Division. The correct procedure was to make contact with the security officer in the Royal Court of Justice who would then refer the matter to the urgent business officer who, in turn, would contact the duty judge. The judge could agree to convene a hearing in court, elsewhere, or by telephone via a tape-recorded conference call. Guidance was also given for medical treatment and welfare cases involving adults who lacked capacity to make their own decisions and children. In adult cases, urgent applications had to be made to the Official Solicitor at the earliest possible opportunity. Out of hours cases would de dealt with initially by the urgent business officer, who would then contact the Official Solicitor. The application could be made by a National Health Service (NHS) trust, a local authority, a relative, carer or the patient. A direction could be sought for anonymity in suitable cases.

Conclusion

The Act has attempted to ensure that there is maximum continuity in court proceedings for those aged 16 and 17 by giving jurisdiction to both the family courts and the Court of Protection, and also in ensuring that decisions can be made about property and affairs for a person lacking mental capacity who is under 16 years and whose incapacity is likely to continue beyond 18 years. An application should be made to the court which is most appropriate to deal with the needs of that young person. Monitoring of the situation once the MCA is implemented should demonstrate the extent to which these aims have succeeded. The change to the legal situation of not overruling the refusal of a 16- and 17-year-old to admission to a psychiatric hospital will have significant implications for their human rights and may in time be extended to all areas of health and social care.

References

1   *Re W (a minor) (medical treatment)* [1992] 4 All ER 627.
2   www.publications.parliament.uk/pa/ld200607/idhansard/text/70115-0016.htm
3   *Gillick* v. *West Norfolk and Wisbech AHA and the DHSS* [1985] 3 All ER 402; [1986] 1 AC 112.
4   Code of Practice for the Mental Capacity Act 2005. Department of Constitutional Affairs February 2007 para 12.4. TSO, London.
5   *Ibid.* para 12.5.
6   (2005) Explanatory notes to Mental Capacity Act 2005 para 79. TSO, London.
7   Code of Practice (see reference 4 above) para 12.7.
8   *Ibid.* para 12.23.
9   Mental Capacity Act 2005 (Transfer of Proceedings) Order 2007 Statutory Instruments 2007 No. 1899.
10 Practice Note (Official Solicitor, CAFCASS and National Assembly for Wales: urgent and out of hours cases in the Family Division) [2006] 2 FLR 354.

Scenarios I
Children and Young Persons

Young persons and children under 18 years

The Mental Capacity Act (MCA) applies to those over 16 years. However there is a distinction in law between the consent of those over 16 years and those over 18 years. It is an established principle of the common law (i.e. judge made law or case law), that a young person under 18 years cannot refuse life saving treatment if that treatment is in his or her best interests.[1] Scenario I1 gives an example of a possible situation.

Scenario I1: Overruling a young person.

Ben had cerebral palsy and had communication difficulties. When he was 17 years he was offered the chance of transferring from the family home to a community based home for young people with physical disabilities. He was assessed under the Mental Capacity Act 2005, and it was determined that he was capable of deciding on his accommodation and with assistance from a therapist of communicating his decision. He was taken on a visit to the new accommodation and shown the room which he would be given and told that it was his choice of furniture and furnishings.

He decided however that he preferred to stay in the family home, where his room had been adapted to meet his disabilities, and he disliked change. His family were considering selling the home and buying a smaller property, and the social workers considered that it was in Ben's best interests for the long term to move to the community home, in preparation for a time when his parents could no longer provide accommodation for him. Ben disagreed with that decision.

This is a situation where in theory the parents are able to make the decision for Ben and overrule his wish to stay in the family home. However since Ben has been assessed as having the requisite mental capacity it would be preferable if that decision were to be made in court, so that he would have an opportunity to be represented. Since it has been decided that he does have the requisite mental capacity, it would be likely that the issues would be heard in the Family Division of the High Court. It could not be considered by the Court of Protection, since its jurisdiction is confined to the determination of capacity and decision making once incapacity has been determined to exist. If however there were a dispute over Ben's capacity to make or communicate the decision, then an application could be made to the Court of Protection for a declaration on the capacity of Ben, and if it were decided that he lacked the requisite capacity, then a determination of what was in his best interests could be made. Chapter 12 considers the transfer of cases between the High Court and the Court of Protection.

Sterilisation in the best interests of a young person

Case study 11: *Re B (a minor)(wardship: sterilisation).*[2]

Jeanette was 17 years old but was described as having a mental age of 5 or 6. Her mother and the local authority, which held a care order on her, advised by the social worker, the gynaecologist and a paediatrician, considered it vital that she should not become pregnant. She had been found in a compromising situation in her residential home. She could not be relied upon to take or accept oral contraceptives. Jeanette was likely to move to an adult training centre at the age of 19, and it would not be possible to provide her with the degree of supervision she had at present.

The House of Lords decided that the paramount consideration was the interests of the girl and, taking account of all the medical evidence, decided that it was in her interests to be sterilised. They made no distinction between non-therapeutic and therapeutic care of the child and recommended that in future all such cases should come before the courts.

As a result of the Mental Capacity Act 2005, a non-therapeutic (i.e. one for social reasons as opposed to one caused by a physical condition such as cancer) sterilisation would come under the definition of serious medical treatment. Since Jeanette is over 16 years and lacking the requisite mental capacity, any decision about whether she should be sterilised could come under the MCA provisions and be heard in the Court of Protection. Alternatively, if there were advantages in the case being heard before the family courts under the provisions of the Children Act 1989, then it could be referred there. The MCA and the Court of Protection rules enable maximum flexibility in hearing cases concerning young people (see also Scenario 12 below on property matters).

Court of Protection and financial decisions

Scenario 12: Management of property.

James was severely injured in a road traffic accident when he was 12 years old. He was on a pedestrian crossing and the motorist was held entirely to blame. James was awarded a compensation package of over £2 million. His parents were separated and disagreed how the funds should be spent on his behalf. James was then 15 years old and it was agreed that an application should be made to the Court of Protection since it seemed unlikely that he would have the necessary mental capacity at 18 years.

The Court of Protection in Scenario 12 would be able to decide whether a deputy should be appointed to manage James' property or whether a single declaration by the Court of Protection was appropriate.

Under the Court of Protection rules the applicant must serve a copy of the application form on a specified list of persons. This includes, where the person who is alleged to be mentally incapacitated is under 18, (i) his parent or guardian, or (ii) if he has no parent or guardian, the person with parental responsibility within the meaning of the Children Act 1989.

The most appropriate court

There is a principle that cases relating to young persons who lack mental capacity as defined in the MCA should be **heard in the most appropriate court.**

The Code of Practice[3] gives an example of this principle.

Scenario 13: Hearing cases in the appropriate court.

Shola is 17. She has serious learning disabilities and lacks the capacity to decide where she should live. Her parents are involved in a bitter divorce. They cannot agree on several issues concerning Shola's care – including where she should live. Her mother wants to continue to look after Shola at home. But her father wants Shola to move into a care home.

In this case, it may be more appropriate for the Court of Protection to deal with the case. This is because an order made in the Court of Protection could continue into Shola's adulthood. However an order made by the family courts under the Children Act 1989 would end on Shola's eighteenth birthday.

Advance decision and the young person under 18 years

Scenario 14: Too young to refuse?

Ahmed was 16 years old and had been converted to being a Jehovah's Witness. He was diagnosed with leukaemia and told his parents that he would not wish to receive blood. They did not share his religious views. Ahmed drew up an advance statement concerning his refusal, and he signed it and it was witnessed by a member of his church. Following treatment in hospital, the consultants told his parents that he needed blood and they were prepared to give their consent. Ahmed was too ill to be able to make any decisions about his future treatment. The health professionals were aware of his advance decision, but the patients' services manager advised them that since Ahmed was younger than 18 years it was not binding on them and they should act in Ahmed's best interests.

Several issues arise in Scenario 14, assuming that it is correct that Ahmed is not able to make a decision at the present time. The first is the validity of the written document and, if it is not effective as an advance decision, the weight which should be attached to it in the decision making process. The second issue is the rights of Ahmed's parents, and the third the procedural measures which are required.

Validity of the advance decision

The patient services manager is correct in stating that under the MCA a person must be over 18 years to create a valid advance decision. The document does not therefore properly constitute an advance decision. However it could be seen as incorporating the wishes and beliefs of Ahmed, and should therefore be taken into account in determining what are his best interests under Section 4(6).

This requires the decision maker, in determining what are the best interests of a person lacking the requisite mental capacity, to:

consider, so far as is reasonably ascertainable –
(a)   the person's past and present wishes and feelings (and, in particular, any relevant written statement made by him when he had capacity).

Rights of Ahmed's parents

Ahmed's parents have the right to make decisions on his behalf until he is 18 years old. Under Section 8(3) of the Family Law Reform Act 1968 any consent which would have been valid prior to the passing of the Act continues to be valid, and this would include parental consent on behalf of a child or young person less than 18 years old.

However Ahmed comes under the provisions of the MCA and although his advance decision is not valid, since he was under 18 years when he drew it up, decisions must still be made in his best interests according to the criteria set out in Section 4, and the principles set out in Section 1 followed. Ahmed's views and beliefs should therefore be taken into account.

Procedural measures

It would be unwise for Ahmed's parents to overrule his advance statement and his expressed wishes without seeking a declaration from the court. A court hearing could be speedily arranged and Ahmed should be represented by the Official Solicitor. It is likely that the case would go to either the Court of Protection or the family courts for a declaration as to what was in the best interests of Ahmed. The Practice Note covering urgent and out of hours cases is considered in Chapter 12.

Case I2 illustrates a similar situation which took place before the implementation of the MCA and, even though the girl was only 15 years old, similar issues arise.

Case I2: Child refusing a transplant.[4]

A girl of 15 years old refused to consent to a transplant that was needed to save her life. She stated that she did not wish to have anyone else's heart, and she did not wish to take medication for the rest of her life. The hospital, which had obtained her mother's consent to the transplant, sought leave from the court to carry out the transplant.

The court held that the hospital could give treatment according to the doctor's clinical judgment, including a heart transplant. The girl was an intelligent person whose wishes carried considerable weight, but she had been overwhelmed by her circumstances and the decision she was being asked to make. Her severe condition had developed only recently and she had had only a few days to consider her situation. While recognising the risk that for the rest of her life she would carry resentment about what had been done to her, the court weighed that risk against the certainty of death if the order were not made.

References

1 *Re W (a minor) (medical treatment)* [1992] 4 All ER 627.
2 *Re B (a minor)(wardship: sterilisation)* [1987] 2 All ER 206.
3 Code of Practice for the Mental Capacity Act 2005. Department of Constitutional Affairs February 2007 para 12.25. TSO, London.
4 *Re M (medical treatment: consent)* [1999] 2 FLR 1097.

13 Mental Capacity and Mental Disorder

Introduction

A person is held to lack capacity in relation to a matter if at the material time he is unable to make a decision for himself in relation to the matter because of an impairment of, or a disturbance in the functioning of, the mind or brain (S.2(1)). The inability to make decisions is further explained in Section 3 (see Chapter 4). This contrasts with the remit of the mental health legislation which deals with mental disorder.

Mental disorder

Mental disorder is defined in Section 1 of the Mental Health Act 1983 (as amended by Section 1 of the Mental Health Act 2007) as 'any disorder or disability of the mind'. The previous classifications of mental illness, mental impairment and psychopathic disorder are no longer used in mental health law.

Under a new Section 2A of the 1983 Act, learning disability (which is defined as 'a state of arrested or incomplete development of the mind which includes significant impairment of intelligence and social functioning') is not considered to be mental disorder unless the disability is associated with abnormally aggressive or seriously irresponsible conduct.

Dependence on alcohol or drugs is not considered to be a disorder or disability of the mind for the purposes of the definition of mental disorder. 'Promiscuity or other immoral conduct, or sexual deviancy' are deleted from the Mental Health Act 1983 by the 2007 Act as not being a disorder or disability of the mind.

What are the main differences between the Mental Capacity Act 2005 and the Mental Health Act 1983 as amended by the 2007 Act?

- **Mental capacity:** the Mental Capacity Act 2005 applies only to those who are unable to make specific decisions;
  the Mental Health Act 1983 does not require a lack of capacity.
- **Mental disorder:** the Mental Capacity Act (MCA) does not apply to those who are mentally disordered unless they lack mental capacity;
  the Mental Health Act 1983 only applies if the patient is suffering from mental disorder as defined in the Act.
- **Best interests:** the MCA requires that all decisions are taken in the best interests of the patient as defined in the Act;
  the Mental Health Act (MHA) does not statutorily require decisions to be made in the best interests of the patient, and detention may be required for the protection of others.
- **Range of treatment and care:** the MCA enables whatever care and treatment is considered to be in the best interests of the patient to be given;
  the MHA only authorises the administration of treatment for a mental disorder. However this has had a wide definition and includes feeding and basic care.
- **Protections available:** the MHA has a wide range of protections for those persons who lose their liberty by being detained under the Act. These include a Mental Health Act Commission, which has a duty to visit detained patients and respond to their complaints; Mental Health Review Tribunals (MHRTs) to review the justification for their detention or continued detention; managers with responsibilities for making applications to the MHRTs if the patients have not done so themselves within a specified time limit; the rights for patients to be given specified information when detained or when their section is changed.
  The MCA provides protection through the Court of Protection, but an application has to be made to trigger its jurisdiction.
- **Restraint:** the MCA enables only limited restraint to be used in narrowly specified circumstances (see Chapter 5 on best interests). It originally did not permit a loss of liberty within the definition of Article 5 of the European Convention on Human Rights. However this provision was repealed in the Mental Health Act 2007 in order to fill the Bournewood gap (see **Reform of the Mental Capacity Act 2005 to fill the Bournewood gap**). As a consequence of the introduction of the Bournewood safeguards, it will be possible for loss of liberty to result from the provisions of the Mental Capacity Act.
  The MHA provides the legal framework within which a patient can lose his or her liberty and be restrained lawfully without any contravention of Article 5.
- **Decision making when capacity is lost:** the MCA recognises several devices for ensuring that decisions are made in accordance with the wishes of a person made when he or she had the requisite mental capacity, to cover situations when this capacity is lost. These include advance decisions and lasting powers of attorney.

The MHA, as amended, does take into account advance decisions. Clinical decisions are the responsibility of the responsible clinician (the 2007 Act substitutes 'responsible clinician' for 'responsible medical officer' (RMO)) and in certain circumstances where the patient is unable or unwilling to give consent to treatment for mental disorder, a second medical opinion must be sought before the treatment can be given.

Mental Capacity Act and exclusion of mental disorder

There are specific statutory provisions in the Mental Capacity Act 2005 which exclude mental health matters from the Act. Section 28(1) provides a general exclusion of detained patients and states:

Nothing in [the MCA 2005] authorises anyone

(a)   to give a patient medical treatment for mental disorder, or
(b)   to consent to a patient's being given medical treatment for mental disorder,

if, at the time when it is proposed to treat the patient, his treatment is regulated by Part 4 of the Mental Health Act 1983.

(2) Medical treatment and mental disorder and patient have the same meaning as in that Act.

(See **Mental disorder** on page 294.)

The Mental Health Act 2007 sets up a new treatment order for mental health patients in the community, and an amendment to the Mental Capacity Act by Section 35(5) of the MHA 2007 makes it clear that such patients are excluded from the Mental Capacity Act. Subsection 1B to Section 28 of the MCA is as follows:

Section 5 does not apply to an act to which section 64B of the Mental Health Act applies (treatment of community patients not recalled to hospital).

When is treatment regulated by Part 4 of the Mental Health Act 1983?

This section becomes complex in its application, since not all patients detained under the Mental Health Act 1983 come within the provisions of Part 4 of that Act, which deals with the provision of treatment for mental disorder.

Exclusion of short term detained patients

Amendments have been made to Part 4 of the Mental Health Act 1983 by the 2007 Act so that the following detained patients are excluded from the provisions of Part 4:

(a)   Patients detained under Section 4 (emergency application: only one medical recommendation);
(b)   Section 5(2) (patient held under the doctor holding power for up to 72 hours) or 5(4) (nurses holding power for up to 6 hours) or 35 (remanded to hospital

for a court report) or section 135 (removal to a place of safety) or 136 (removed from a public place by a police constable) of a direction under section 37(4) (directions to place of safety pending a place in hospital under section 37.

(c)   Patients who have been conditionally discharged under section 42(2) or section 73 or 74 and not recalled to hospital.

The consequences are that these patients could come within the provisions of the MCA. Scenario J1 considers a possible situation.

Treatment for physical disorders

Furthermore Section 28 only excludes treatment for mental disorder, since that is the remit of Part 4 of the Mental Health Act 1983. It would be possible for treatments for physical disorder to be covered by the MCA 2005, even though the patient is a detained patient. The definition of treatment under the Mental Health Act 1983 has been widely interpreted and basic care, including nutrition, has been given under the authority of Part 4 of the Mental Health Act 1983. There are even judgments where a Caesarean section has been regarded as treatment for mental disorder under the Mental Health Act 1983, but these are now considered to be too widely defined. Scenario J2 describes such a situation. There is a new definition of treatment provided by the Mental Health Act 2007 as follows:

'Medical treatment' includes nursing, psychological intervention and specialist mental health habilitation, rehabilitation and care. (S.145(1) of the MHA 1983 as amended by Section 7 of the Mental Health Act 2007.)

A case where a patient detained under Section 3 of the Mental Health Act 1983 was given treatment for an ovarian cyst against her will, on the grounds that she was incapable of making a decision and that the treatment was in her best interests, is considered in Scenarios B, Case B2.

Section 37 (the provision of serious medical treatment by an NHS body and appointment of an independent mental capacity advocate (IMCA))

Section 37 does not apply if P's treatment is regulated by Part 4 of the Mental Health Act 1983 (S.37(2)). (See Chapter 9.)

Section 38 (the provision of accommodation by an NHS body and the appointment of an IMCA)

This statutory requirement for the NHS body to instruct an independent mental capacity advocate does not apply if P is accommodated as a result of an obligation imposed on the NHS body under the MHA (S38(2)) (see Chapter 9).

A new Subsection 2A to Section 38 has been added to the MCA by the Mental Health Act 2007 (paragraph 4(1) of Schedule 9) as follows:

This section [i.e. section 38] does not apply if:

(a)   an independent mental capacity advocate must be appointed under Section 39A or 39C (whether or not by the NHS body) to represent P, and
(b)   the hospital or care home in which P is to be accommodated under the arrangements referred to in this section is the relevant hospital or care home under the authorisation referred to in that section.

Section 39 (the provision of accommodation by a local authority and the appointment of an IMCA)

This statutory requirement for the local authority to instruct an independent mental capacity advocate does not apply if P is accommodated as a result of an obligation imposed on him under the MHA (S.39(3)).

Section 39 only applies if the accommodation is to be provided in accordance with:

a.   Section 21 or 29 of the National Assistance Act 1948, or
b.   Section 117 of the Mental Health Act

as the result of a decision taken by the local authority under Section 47 of the NHS and Community Care Act 1990 (S.39(2)).

It is clear from this section that S.117 accommodation is not regarded as accommodation provided under an obligation set by the Mental Health Act 1983. This is discussed in Chapter 9 and is in accordance with the interpretation of the Code of Practice.

The Code of Practice[1] states that the duty to consult an IMCA in relation to serious medical treatment or accommodation does not arise if the treatment is to be provided under the Mental Health Act 1983.

> Nor is there a duty to do so in respect of a move into accommodation, or a change of accommodation, if the person in question is to be required to live in it because of an obligation under the MHA. That obligation might be a condition of leave of absence or conditional discharge from hospital or a requirement imposed by a guardian or a supervisor.
>
> The duty to instruct an IMCA would apply as normal if accommodation is being planned as part of the after-care under section 117 of the MHA following the person's discharge from detention (and the person is not going to be required to live in it as a condition of after-care under supervision). This is because the person does not have to accept that accommodation.

The duty to appoint an IMCA only arises if the person has no close relatives, friends or any other person to protect their interests. An amendment added by the Mental Health Act 2007 makes it clear that a person appointed under Part 10 of Schedule A1 of the MCA (as amended by the Mental Health Act) to be P's representative is not, by virtue of that appointment, engaged in providing care or treatment for P in a professional capacity or for remuneration.

Amendments to the MCA are made in the Mental Health Act 2007, which added three new sections to Section 39, i.e. Ss. 39A, 39B and 39C (see **Sections 39A,**

39B and 39B and 39C of the MCA as added by the MHA below). In addition a new Subsection 3A states that Section 39 does not apply if:

(a) an independent mental capacity advocate must be appointed under section 39A or 39C (whether or not by the local authority) to represent P, and

(b) the place in which P is to be accommodated under the arrangements referred to in this section is the relevant hospital or care home under the authorisation referred to in that section.

The following questions would have to be asked:

- Is this person (formerly detained under the MHA) under a duty to live in the accommodation provided under Section 117?
- If the answer to that is 'no', then the provisions relating to IMCAs apply.
- If the answer is 'yes', then the person comes under the MHA and the IMCA provisions do not apply.

See Scenarios J8 and J9.

Sections 39A, 39B and 39C of the Mental Capacity Act as added by the Mental Health Act 2007

These sections are shown in Box 13.1.

Box 13.1: New Sections 39A, 39B and 39C of the MCA as added by the Mental Health Act 2007 (Schedule 9 paragraph 6).

Section 39A

(1) This section applies if:
  (a) a person P becomes subject to Schedule A1, and
  (b) the managing authority of the relevant hospital or care home are satisfied that there is no person, other than one engaged in providing care or treatment for P in a professional capacity or for remuneration, whom it would be appropriate to consult in determining what would be in P's best interests.

(2) The managing authority must notify the supervisory body that this section applies.

(3) The supervisory body must instruct an independent mental capacity advocate to represent P.

(4) Schedule A1 makes provision about the role of an independent mental capacity advocate appointed under this section.

(5) This section is subject to paragraph of 152 of Schedule A1.

(6) For the purposes of subsection (1), a person appointed under Part 10 of Schedule A1 to be P's representative is not, by virtue of that appointment engaged in providing care or treatment for P in a professional capacity or for remuneration.

Section 39B

(1)   This section applies for the purposes of section 39A.
(2)   P becomes subject to Schedule A1 in either of the following cases.
(3)   The first case is where an urgent authorisation is given in relation to P under paragraph 69(2) of Schedule A1 (urgent authorisation given before request made for standard authorisation).
(4)   The second case is where the following conditions are met:
(5)   The first condition is that a request is made under Schedule A1 for a standard authorisation to be given in relation to P (the requested authorisation).
(6)   The second condition is that no urgent authorisation was given under paragraph 69(2) before that request was made.
(7)   The third condition is that the requested authorisation will not be in force on or before, or immediately after, the expiry of an existing standard authorisation.
(8)   The expiry of a standard authorisation is the date when the authorisation is expected to cease to be in force.

The third case is where, under paragraph 69 of Schedule A1, the supervisory body selects a person to carry out an assessment of whether or not the relevant person is a detained resident.

Section 39C Person unrepresented whilst subject to Schedule A1

(1)   This section applies if:
   a)   an authorisation under Schedule A1 is in force in relation to P
   b)   the appointment of a representative of P ends
   c)   the managing authority are satisfied that there is no appropriate person to consult about
(2)   The managing authority must notify the supervisory body that this section applies.
(3)   The supervisory body must instruct an independent mental capacity advocate to represent P.
(4)   Paragraph 159 of Schedule A1 makes provision about the role of an independent mental capacity advocate appointed under this section.
(5)   The appointment of an independent mental capacity advocate under this section ends when a new appointment of a person as P's representative is made in accordance with Part 10 of Schedule A1.
(6)   For the purposes of subsection (1), a person appointed under Part 10 of Schedule A1 to be P's representative is not, by virtue of that appointment, engaged in providing care or treatment for P in a professional capacity or for remuneration.

Guidance for deputies appointed by the court

A code provided for the guidance of deputies appointed by the court (S.42(1(d)) may contain separate guidance for deputies appointed by virtue of Para 1(2) of

Schedule 5 (Functions of deputy conferred on receiver appointed under the Mental Health Act – S.42(6)).

Which is the appropriate legislation to be used – MCA or MHA?

The above discussion on the differences between the MCA and the MHA may cause confusion over which is the appropriate Act to use. Chapter 13 of the Code of Practice provides some pointers as to which Act would be relevant.

Restraint

If there is a need to use restraint which would deprive a person of liberty then the MHA or other legislation might be considered appropriate. The MCA would not be appropriate unless the limited loss of liberty envisaged under the Bournewood amendments (see **Reform of the Mental Capacity Act 2005 to fill the Bournewood gap,** page 307) would apply. The Code of Practice[2] states that:

It might be necessary to consider using the MHA rather than the MCA if:

- it is not possible to give the person the care or treatment they need without carrying out an action that might deprive them of their liberty
- the person needs treatment that cannot be given under the MCA (for example, because the person has made a valid and applicable advance decision to refuse all or part of that treatment). (Authors note: this may now have to be amended since the new provisions of the Mental Health Act 2007 enable a person to draw up an advance decision which refuses ECT or other treatments set out in Regulations – see Scenario J3 on page 320)
- the person may need to be restrained in a way that is not allowed under the MCA
- it is not possible to assess or treat the person safely or effectively without treatment being compulsory (perhaps because the person is expected to regain capacity to consent, but might then refuse to give consent)
- the person lacks capacity to decide on some elements of the treatment but has capacity to refuse a vital part of it – and they have done so, or
- there is some other reason why the person might not get the treatment they need, and they or somebody else might suffer harm as a result.

Following the implementation of the Bournewood safeguards, there will be scope for using the MCA in some of the above situations, rather than the MHA.

Guardianship or community treatment order

Similar problems arise over whether the provisions of the MCA relating to the appointment of deputies should be used or the guardianship provisions of the MHA. This is discussed in the Code of Practice (paras 13.16–13.21).

A guardian can only be appointed under the Mental Health Act 1983 if it can be shown that the person is suffering from a mental disorder. The previous requirement that a person must be suffering from a specified form of mental disorder has been amended by the MHA 2007.

The after-care under supervision arrangements introduced in 1996 have been repealed by the Mental Health Act 2007 and a compulsory treatment in the community order introduced.

Court of Protection

Court of Protection visitors (S.61)

The Lord Chancellor can appoint a Court of Protection visitor to a panel of Special Visitors or a panel of General Visitors. (These Court of Protection visitors replace the current 'Lord Chancellors Visitors'.) (See Section 102 of the Mental Health Act 1983.)

This is further considered in Chapter 7.

Lasting powers of attorney and deputies of the Court of Protection

These powers can still be exercised even though the patient is detained under the MHA, and provided that the patient has the requisite mental capacity, he or she could create a lasting power of attorney (LPA), even though detained under the MHA. The Code of Practice[3] states that:

Being subject to the MHA does not stop patients creating new Lasting Powers of Attorney (if they have the capacity to do so). Nor does it stop the Court of Protection from appointing a deputy for them.

However the powers of both the LPA and a court appointed deputy are limited by the MHA and they would not be able to give consent to treatment on behalf of the patient, if the treatment is being given under the MHA. Nor, unless they happened to be the nearest relative, would they be able to exercise the powers which the MHA gives to the nearest relative in relation to the discharge of the patient.

In certain cases, people subject to the MHA may be required to meet specific conditions relating to:

- leave of absence from hospital
- after-care under supervision (now repealed by Mental Health Act 2007) or
- conditional discharge.

Conditions vary from case to case, but could include a requirement to:

- live in a particular place
- maintain contact with health services, or
- avoid a particular area.

If an attorney or deputy takes a decision that goes against one of these conditions, the patient will be taken to have gone against the condition. The

MHA sets out the actions that could be taken in such circumstances. In the case of leave of absence or conditional discharge, this might involve the patient being recalled to hospital.[4]

Attorneys and deputies may also be able to apply to the Mental Health Review Tribunal on behalf of the detained patient.

Since the hospital authorities might not be aware of the appointment of an LPA or deputy it would be good practice for the LPA or deputy to notify the hospital of their appointment and discuss with the health professionals both the implications and the limitations of their appointments.

Where the patient is not detained under the MHA, then the MHA provisions do not apply and the LPA and the deputy may have powers to give consent to the treatment for mental disorder.

See Scenario J4.

The Bournewood gap

(For the Bournewood case see also Chapter 3 on page 31.)

In November 2006 the Government introduced a draft Mental Health Bill which amended the Mental Health Act 1983 and also contained provisions to amend the Mental Capacity Act 2005 in order to provide protection for those persons caught in the Bournewood situation. The Bournewood case is set out in Box 13.2.

Box 13.2: Bournewood case.

L was born in 1949 and lived in Surrey. He was autistic, unable to speak and his level of understanding was limited. He was frequently agitated and had a history of self-harming behaviour. He lacked the capacity to consent to or object to medical treatment. For over 30 years he was cared for in a National Health Service trust hospital, Bournewood Hospital. He was an in-patient at the hospital's intensive behavioural unit from around 1987 to 1994, when he was discharged on a trial basis to paid carers, with whom he successfully stayed until July 1997. In 1995 he started attending a day-care centre on a weekly basis. On 22 July 1997, while at the day centre, he became particularly agitated, hitting himself on the head with his fists and banging his head against the wall. Staff could not contact his carers, so called a local doctor, who gave him a sedative. L remained agitated and, on the recommendation of a social worker, was taken to hospital. A consultant psychiatrist diagnosed him as requiring in-patient treatment. With the help of two nurses he was transferred to the hospital's intensive care unit as an informal patient. The consultant considered detaining him compulsorily under the MHA but concluded that it was not necessary, as he was compliant and had not resisted admission or tried to run away. His carers asked for his discharge, but his psychiatrist considered that it was not in his best interests to be discharged and that he should remain in hospital. The carers on his behalf challenged the legality of this decision, by seeking judicial review of the hospital's decision to admit him. They lost in the High Court, which held

> that L had not been detained but had been informally admitted in accordance with the common law doctrine of necessity. L appealed to the Court of Appeal which held that Section 131 of the MHA required a person to have the mental capacity to agree to admission; a person lacking the requisite capacity should be examined for compulsory admission under the Act. L had been detained in July 1997 and had therefore been unlawfully detained. The health care authorities appealed to the House of Lords. They succeeded in their appeal to the House of Lords, which held that an adult lacking mental capacity could be cared for and detained in a psychiatric hospital, using common law powers. L therefore had not been detained but had been lawfully admitted as an informal patient on the basis of the common law doctrine of necessity.

The claimants subsequently took the case to the European Court of Human Rights.[5]

The court held that the absence of procedural safeguards to protect an applicant against arbitrary deprivation of liberty on the ground of necessity after he had been compulsorily detained breached his right to liberty guaranteed by Article 5.1 of the European Convention on Human Rights. It also held unanimously that Article 5.4 had been breached, in that the applicant's right to have the legality of his detention reviewed by a court had not been ensured. (Article 5.4 of Schedule 1 of the Human Rights Act 1998 is shown in Chapter 3 and in Box 13.3.) The court considered that the violation of Articles 5.1 and 5.4 constituted sufficient just satisfaction for any non-pecuniary damage sustained. It awarded 29,500 euros for costs and expenses, less 2677 euros received in legal aid from the Council of Europe. As a consequence of this decision Parliament had to consider filling what has become known as the Bournewood Gap (or even chasm). The United Kingdom was obliged to provide protection for those adults who were incapable of giving a valid consent to admission but were being detained without being placed under the Mental Health Act. The Department of Health (DH) issued a Consultation Paper asking respondents to choose from various options put forward (see **DH options to fill the Bournewood gap**).

Box 13.3: Article 5.4 of the European Convention on Human Rights.

Everyone who is deprived of his liberty by arrest or detention shall be entitled to take proceedings by which the lawfulness of his detention shall be decided speedily by a court and his release ordered if the detention is not lawful.

The House of Lords debates on the Mental Capacity Bill and the Bournewood case[6]

The dilemma facing the Government over filling the Bournewood gap was clearly stated by Lord Carter in moving Amendment No. 23 to the Mental Capacity Bill. He analysed the problems presented by the Bournewood decision and summed up the options available to the Government to fill the Bournewood gap.[7] The option to amend the Mental Capacity Bill was not taken at that time, since fuller discussion was required.

Department of Health options to fill the Bournewood gap

The DH published a Consultation Paper in March 2005 seeking views raised by and consequent options for public policy arising from the judgment of the European Court of Human Rights, published on 5 October 2004 in the case of *HL* v *the United Kingdom*.[8]

As a result of the judgment it was clear that additional procedural safeguards were required for those incapacitated patients who are not subject to mental health legislation, but whose treatment nonetheless involves a deprivation of liberty. The four options put forward by the DH for consultation were:

Option 1:   Do nothing.
Option 2:   Protective care.
Option 3:   Extend the use of the Mental Health Act 1983.
Option 4:   Extend the use of existing 1983 Act powers to place people under guardianship.

Option 1 is in fact not an option, since the existing law and the use of common law powers of necessity have been criticised by the European Court of Human Rights, and therefore some changes must take place.

Option 2 would be a new system of 'Protective Care' to provide a legal basis for depriving of their liberty people of unsound mind who lack capacity, in order to provide care or treatment in their best interests. A new system, specifically for people who lack capacity, would be introduced to govern admission/detention procedures, reviews of detention and appeals. The patients would be treated in accordance with the principles and procedures set out in the MCA.

Options 3 and 4 are not mutually exclusive, and would make use of the existing powers to detain people of unsound mind under the Mental Health Act 1983 to cover those who lack capacity (perhaps cover the whole of the 'Bournewood group' through this route). Alternatively or in addition, the guardianship powers under Section 7 of the Mental Health Act 1983 could be extended to cover the Bournewood group.

In 29 June 2006 the DH published its report on the consultation and the Government's proposals.[9]

Proposals following Bournewood consultation

The key proposals of the DH were as follows:

- All involved will have to act in the best interests of the person in care and in the least restrictive manner.
- The criteria under which someone can be detained will be strengthened.
- An individual's rights will have to be respected and it will be easier to challenge the decision once someone has been detained.

- Every person will have someone independent to represent their interests.
- The proposals will cover both care homes and those being treated in hospitals.

It was the intention of the Government to amend the MCA to ensure that the European Court ruling was included in mental health legislation.

The outcome of the consultation suggested that minimum requirements in any legislation relating to the protective custody of the mentally incapacitated person were identified as:

- a clear and unambiguous definition of 'deprivation of liberty' (see **Deprivation of liberty** below)
- a clear definition of those liable to be made subject to these powers
- processes and timescales for tests of capacity
- admission procedures
- assessment, care planning and reviews
- the respective responsibilities of the various agencies involved
- the role of advocacy
- the rights of carers, relatives and friends, including a statutory requirement for 'appropriate persons to be consulted'
- the appeals process.

Deprivation of liberty

The Government decided not to give a statutory definition to the deprivation of liberty since 'what constitutes deprivation of liberty will depend on the specific circumstances of each individual case'. It would however include in the revised Code of Practice detailed guidance setting out the factors that would need to be taken into account when considering whether a person is, or needs to be, deprived of liberty.

Appeals process

Many respondents to the consultation considered that an appeal against detention should be to the Mental Health Review Tribunals. However the Government has stated that it considered the appropriate appeal process to be through the Court of Protection since that court, as the Court established by the Mental Capacity Act, is best placed to take on this role as part of its overall responsibility for the personal welfare of those who lack capacity. A relative, friend or carer will have the right to bring proceedings before the Court of Protection, and if there is not such a suitable person, an independent person (possibly an independent mental capacity advocate) will be appointed by the relevant local authority or Primary Care trust.

The suggestion that there should be a first tier review in the appeal process received a mixed response in the consultation. The Government concluded that because of the necessity to comply with Article 5.4 in any appeal process it would abandon the proposal, on the grounds that it might be seen as interfering with the right of appeal to a court and delay the speedy decision by such a court on the lawfulness of instances of deprivation of liberty.

Role of carers, friends, and relatives

Provision would be made to ensure that these are consulted in any decision relating to the deprivation of liberty. They will receive a copy of the authorisation to deprive of liberty and notification of the name of the person identified to act as representative of the person deprived of liberty.

Monitoring of implementation

The Government considered that the existing powers of the MHA Commission, the Healthcare Commission, the Commission for Social Care Inspection and the National Assembly for Wales are adequate for monitoring purposes, and no further functions or powers were necessary.

Link with the Mental Health Act 1983

The Government did not support the use of detention under the Mental Health Act 1983 as the mechanism for closing the Bournewood gap. It preferred the amendment of the Mental Capacity Act for such purposes. It stated that it is intended that the Bournewood powers should not extend to those within the scope of mental health legislation who indicate that they do not wish to be admitted to hospital for treatment for mental disorder or, if they raise no objection to admission, do not wish to receive such treatment.

Extension of guardianship

The Government did not believe that guardianship, even in an amended form, would best meet the needs of those coming within the Bournewood provisions.

Reform of the Mental Capacity Act 2005 to fill the Bournewood gap

The Mental Health Act 2007 provides a new Schedule A1 to the MCA, which sets out the provisions for the deprivation of liberty for persons in hospitals and residents in care homes. It also repeals Section 6(5) which stated that D does more than merely restrain P if he deprives him of his liberty within the meaning of Article 5(1) of the European Convention of Human Rights. Other consequential amendments have been noted throughout this book, and include the provision for an IMCA to be appointed under new Sections 39A and 39C, and new Sections

4A and 4B on deprivation of liberty which are shown in Boxes 3.3 and 3.4 in Chapter 3, pages 24 and 25.

Who will be covered by the Bournewood provisions?

- those over 18 years
- who suffer from a disorder or disability of mind
- who lack the capacity to give consent to the arrangements made for their care, and
- for whom such care (in circumstances that amount to a deprivation of liberty within the meaning of Article 5 of the European Convention on Human Rights) is considered after an independent assessment to be a necessary and proportionate response in their best interests to protect them from harm.

(The Government view was that in the main those protected by the Bournewood provisions would be mainly those with significant learning disabilities or elderly people suffering from dementia, but will include a minority of others who have suffered physical injury.)

The Bournewood safeguards

The Mental Health Act 2007 contains amendments to the MCA to introduce the safeguards necessary to justify loss of liberty of residents in hospitals and care homes. These are known as the 'Bournewood safeguards'. They are set out in the new Schedule A1 to the MCA as introduced by the Mental Health Act, and can be found in a Briefing Paper available from the DH.[10] The new Schedule A1 to the MCA details these safeguards (which are considered below). In addition a new Schedule 1A lists the persons who come under the MHA and are therefore ineligible to be deprived of liberty by the MCA. For example if P is subject to a hospital treatment regime and detained in a hospital under that regime, then he is ineligible to lose his liberty under the MCA.

Details of the Bournewood safeguards introduced by amendments to the MCA by the Mental Health Act 2007 Schedule 7

A. Authorisation of deprivation of liberty by a supervisory body

Where a hospital or care home identifies that a person who lacks capacity is, or risks, being deprived of their liberty, they must apply to the supervisory body for authorisation of deprivation of liberty. The supervisory authority will be the relevant local authority for those in care homes or the Primary Care trust for those in hospital. (In Wales, it will be the National Assembly for Wales.)

The Code of Practice will include a checklist of issues to consider to assist managers to assess whether a person is at risk of deprivation of liberty. DH guidance will build on that issued by the DH and Welsh Assembly Government (WAG) in December 2004 following the European Court of Human Rights (ECHR) decision.

Regulations will set out the information to be provided with a request for authorisation.

Normally authorisation will be sought in advance. However in urgent circumstances it will be possible for the hospital or care home to issue an urgent authorisation, giving their reasons in writing, and a standard authorisation must be obtained within seven days of the start of the deprivation of liberty.

B. Assessment required pre authorisation

The supervisory body must obtain the following assessments before granting an authorisation of deprivation of liberty:

1. Age assessment – they are aged 18 or over.
2. Mental health assessment – they are suffering a mental disorder.
3. Mental capacity assessment – they lack the capacity to decide whether to be admitted to or remain in the hospital or care home.
4. Eligibility assessment – a person is eligible unless they are:
    a. detained under the MHA
    b. subject to a requirement under the MHA which conflicts with the authorisation sought, e.g. a guardianship order requiring them to live somewhere else.
    c. subject to powers of recall under the MHA, or
    d. unless the application is to enable mental health treatment in hospital and they object to being in hospital or to the treatment in question.
5. Best interests assessment – the proposed course of action would constitute a deprivation of liberty and it is:
    a. in the best interests of the person to be subject to the authorisation and
    b. a proportionate response to the likelihood of suffering harm and the seriousness of that harm.
6. No refusals requirement – the authorisation sought does not conflict with a valid decision by a donee of a lasting power of attorney or a deputy appointed for the person by the Court of Protection and is not for the purpose of giving treatment which would conflict with a valid and applicable advance decision made by the person.

C. Effect of the six assessments

If any of the assessments conclude that the person does not meet the criteria for an authorisation to be issued, the supervisory body must turn down the request for authorisation. It must also notify the hospital or care home, the person concerned, any IMCA and all interested persons consulted by the best interests assessor of the decision and the reasons.

A person could be detained whilst a decision is sought from the Court of Protection about the lawfulness of authorising detention to enable life sustaining treatment or treatment believed necessary to prevent a serious deterioration in the person's condition to be given.

D. Duration of authorisation for deprivation of liberty

To be assessed on a case-by-case basis. The maximum period for authorisation would be 12 months, but it is expected that authorisations would be for shorter periods in many cases, and must be the shortest time necessary to protect them from harm.

E. Best interests assessment

If the best interests assessor concludes that deprivation of liberty is necessary in a person's best interests to protect them from harm, he will be required to recommend who would be the best person to be appointed to represent the person's interests.

F. Action to be taken by supervisory body after receiving assessments which show the criteria are met

- It must grant the authorisation of deprivation of liberty.
- It cannot be longer than the time period recommended by the best interests assessor nor longer than 12 months.
- The authorisation must be in writing and include the purpose of the deprivation of liberty, the time period, any conditions attached and the reasons that each of the qualifying criteria are met.
- A copy must be given to the hospital or care home, the person concerned, any IMCA appointed and all interested persons consulted by the best interests assessor.
- The person's representative must keep in touch with the person, support them in all matters concerning the authorisation, and request a review or make an application to the Court of Protection on their behalf where necessary.
- If there is no one available among friends or family then the supervisory body will appoint a person, who may be paid, to act as the representative for the duration of the authorisation.

G. Hospital and care home managers have the following duties

- To take all practical steps to ensure that the person concerned and their representative understand what the authorisation means for them and how they may appeal or request a review.
- To ensure that any conditions attached to the authorisation are met, and
- to monitor the individual's circumstances as any change may require them to request that the authorisation is reviewed.

Hospitals and care homes may apply for further authorisation when the authorisation expires.

H. Review of authorisation

An authorisation may be reviewed for the following reasons:

- The hospital or care home requests a review because the individual's circumstances have changed.
- The person or their representative requests a review.

The supervisory body must review an authorisation following such a request and obtain a new assessment where any of the criteria for authorisation are affected by the changed circumstances. Outcomes from the review include:

- termination of authorisation
- varying of the conditions attached to the authorisation
- changing the reason recorded that the person meets the criteria for authorisation.

Deprivation of liberty in other circumstances

The Court of Protection may make an order on a personal welfare matter which may lead to a deprivation of liberty (see Chapter 7 and the new powers of the Court of Protection under Section 21A).

The Mental Capacity Act 2005 as amended will make deprivation of liberty unlawful in cases where there is neither a Bournewood authorisation nor a relevant decision by the Court of Protection.

The person's representative

Draft regulations were published in January 2007,[11] which covered the appointment of a representative and who is eligible to be appointed. The eligibility criteria are shown in Box 13.4.

Box 13.4: Eligibility criteria for a representative.

a. 18 years of age
b. Able to keep in contact with relevant person
c. Not prevented by ill-health from carrying out the role of the representative
d. Willing to be the relevant person's representative
e. Not financially interested in the relevant person's managing authority
f. Not a close relative (see Box 13.5) of a person who is financially interested in the managing authority
g. Not employed by, or providing services to, the relevant person's managing authority where the relevant person's managing authority is a care home
h. Not employed to work in the relevant person's managing authority in a role that is, or could be, related to the relevant person's case, where the relevant person's managing authority is a hospital and
i. Not employed to work in the relevant person's supervisory body in a role that is, or could be, related to the relevant person's case.

The definition of 'close relative' is shown in Box 13.5.

Box 13.5: Close relative for the purpose of the draft regulations on representatives.

a. spouse, civil partner or partner
b. a parent or child
c. a brother or sister
d. a grandparent or grandchild
e. a child of a person falling within paragraphs a or c.
f. a stepfather or stepmother
g. a half-brother or half-sister.

The regulations also cover the process of selection (Part 2). The best interests assessor must determine whether the person has the capacity to select their own representative. If not then the regulations lay down in Part 3 the procedure to be followed, the formalities to be complied with and the termination of the representative's appointment. Part 4 of the regulations cover the monitoring of the representative's contact by the managing authority and payment. The representative can be paid where the best interests assessor has notified the supervisory body that they have not selected a nominated person to be a representative. In this situation the supervisory body may select a person to be a representative, who:

a. would be performing the role in a professional capacity
b. has satisfactory skills and experience to perform the role
c. is not a family member, friend or carer of the relevant person
d. is not employed to work in the relevant person's managing authority, where the relevant person's managing authority is a hospital, and
e. is not employed to work for the supervisory body.

Assessment

Part 5 of the draft regulations[12] also make provisions relating to the assessments. All assessments required for a standard authorisation must be completed within 21 days from the date the supervisory body receives a request for such an authorisation from a managing authority. Where the best interests assessor and the eligibility assessor are not the same person, then the former must provide the latter with any information he has. Where the managing authority and the supervisory body are the same, an employee of that body cannot be appointed as the best interests assessor.

Assessors

Draft regulations were published in January 2007 on the eligibility and selection of assessors.[13] These set out the eligibility criteria for mental health assessors, mental capacity assessors and best interests assessors. In addition general eligibility criteria require all assessors (other than the age assessor) to be insured in respect of any liabilities that might arise in connection with carrying out the assessment, and the supervisory body must be satisfied that they have the skills and experience and have undertaken training appropriate to the assessment they are to carry out. Mental health assessors must be approved doctors under Section 12 of the Mental Health Act 1983 or a registered medical practitioner who the supervisory body is satisfied has special experience in the diagnosis and treatment of mental disorder. Eligibility criteria for mental capacity assessors are shown in Box 13.6 and for best interests assessors in Box 13.7.

Box 13.6: Eligibility criteria for mental capacity assessors.

a. Approved under S.12 of the Mental Health Act 1983.
b. A registered medical practitioner who the supervisory body is satisfied has special experience in the diagnosis and treatment of mental disorder.
c. An approved mental health professional.
d. A social worker registered with the General Social Care Council or Care Council for Wales.
e. A first level nurse registered with the Nursing and Midwifery Council (NMC) with a recordable qualification in mental health nursing.
f. A first level nurse registered with the NMC with a recordable qualification in learning disabilities nursing.
g. A registered occupational therapist.
h. A chartered psychologist registered with the British Psychological Society and who holds a practising certificate issued by that Society.

Box 13.7: Eligibility criteria for best interests assessors.

a. An approved mental health professional.
b. A social worker registered with the General Social Care Council or the Care Council of Wales.
c. A first level nurse registered with the NMC with a recordable qualification in mental health nursing.
d. A first level nurse registered with the NMC with a recordable qualification in learning disabilities nursing.
e. A registered occupational therapist.
f. A chartered psychologist registered with the British Psychological Society and who holds a practising certificate issued by that Society.

Selection of assessors

A supervisory body may only select a person to carry out an assessment in any individual case where the person is not financially interested in the care of the relevant person, not a close relative of the relevant person and not a close relative of a person who is financially interested in the care of the relevant person. 'Close relative' has the same meaning as shown in Box 13.5. There are also regulations to ensure the independence of the best interests assessor, so that he or she cannot be involved in the care, or making decisions about the care, of the relevant person, and is not employed by the care home or hospital where the relevant person is to be detained.

Monitoring of assessors

The DH has published a statement of intent stating that regulations were to be published on the monitoring arrangements. The monitoring function will initially be given to the three existing inspectorates: the Healthcare Commission, the Commission for Social Care Inspection and the MHA Commission, but eventually these three bodies are to be merged (probably at the end of 2008, depending upon the passage of the legislation through Parliament). In the meantime the DH states that the expectation is that the existing inspectorates will work in a co-ordinated manner to avoid duplication of activity.

The monitoring role will include the following:

- monitor and report on the operation of the Bournewood safeguards
- visit hospitals and care homes
- visit and interview people in hospitals and care homes
- require the production of, and inspect reports.

The monitoring process will consider:

- Whether the provisions have been applied correctly and in line with guidance in the Code of Practice in cases where authorisation has been requested.
- Whether the guidance in the Code of Practice on identifying those at risk of deprivation of liberty and on avoiding deprivation of liberty is being complied with.
- Whether conditions attached to authorisation and requirements to request review if circumstances change are complied with.
- Whether appropriate steps are being taken in cases where authorisation has been refused.

Monitoring will not cover treatment and care (other than as it relates to the deprivation of liberty) nor will it cover the revisiting of individual assessments. Monitoring will not constitute an alternative review or appeal process.

A power is to be introduced to enable the monitoring body to require supervisory bodies and managing authorities of hospitals or care homes to disclose information to the monitoring body (including data on ethnicity).

The aim of the DH is for a monitoring regime to come on stream by April 2008.

Information to be provided with an application for authorisation

A statement of intent from the DH published in 2007 stated that regulations were to be published, setting out the information to be provided with an application for authorisation to enable the supervisory body to select suitable assessors, so that the assessments can be completed accurately and quickly. A standard form is to be developed to enable greater consistency across the country. This should assist care homes and hospitals which may be applying to different Primary Care trusts (PCTs) and different local authorities (LAs) in different cases.

The information to be included is shown in Box 13.8.

Box 13.8: Information to be provided in application for authorisation.

- The person, their age, their mental disorder and other relevant health information, ethnicity, issues relevant to carrying out the assessments (e.g. if the person was deaf).
- Purpose and nature of the proposed deprivation of liberty, including relevant care plans and needs assessment.
- Contact details for the care home or hospital and lead professionals involved and for the person if they currently reside somewhere else.
- Contact details for family friends and carers to contact for the best interests assessment.
- Whether an urgent authorisation has been issued.

Ordinary residence

A statement of intent published by the DH in 2007 stated that regulations will be published to authorise or require a LA in which the person is ordinarily resident to:

- act as the Supervisory Body to deal with the application, even though it may wish to dispute being the Supervisory Body
- become the Supervisory Body in place of another local authority, and
- to recover from another local authority expenditure incurred in exercising functions as a Supervisory Body.

The purpose of the regulations is to prevent any dispute about which LA is the Supervisory Body delaying decisions about whether the deprivation of liberty is authorised.

A case is discussed on page 328, Case J1, where a daughter refused to let her mother, who lacked the requisite mental capacity, be taken to a care home.[14] The judge made an order, using the inherent jurisdiction of the family courts, that it was lawful for the mother to reside in the care home and it was lawful, being in the mother's interests, for the local authority by its employees or agents to use reasonable and proportionate measures to prevent the mother from leaving the unit. It is unlikely that the introduction of the Bournewood safeguards would prevent the need for such an application in similar circumstances in the future.

Conclusions

The interface between mental health and mental capacity is extremely complex, and there is likely to be considerable confusion initially over the scope of the different Acts of Parliament. In addition it may be found that the measures taken to fill the Bournewood gap prove to be inadequate, too slow or bureaucratic to provide adequate protection to those lacking mental capacity and who risk losing their liberty. It is likely that there will be further amendments to both the MHA and MCA and the regulations made under it in due course.

Reform of the Mental Health Act 1983

The Mental Health Act 2007 makes significant changes to the Mental Health Act 1983. These are less radical proposals than had originally been proposed when a new MHA was envisaged, but even so have encountered opposition in the House of Lords in relation to the proposal that patients could be detained in a psychiatric hospital even though the 'treatability test' was not satisfied. The changes to the Mental Heath Act 1983 include:

- Amending the definition of mental disorder by replacing it with a new simplified definition, i.e. 'any disorder or disability of the mind' and by abolishing the four separate categories of mental disorder. This is discussed above (see **Mental disorder** on page 294). This will mean that some categories not covered by the Mental Health Act 1983 will be included under the definition of mental disorder, e.g. mental disorders arising out of injury or damage to the brain in adulthood. Learning disability will only be treated as a mental disorder for the purposes of the MHA if it is associated with abnormally aggressive or seriously irresponsible conduct on the part of the patient concerned. The definition of mental disorder no longer cites promiscuity, other immoral conduct and sexual deviancy as conditions excluded from its definition.
- The former treatability test used as the basis of detention for psychopathic disorder and mental impairment is replaced by a test of the availability of appropriate treatment, which must be satisfied before a patient can be detained.
- A new community treatment order is introduced for patients following a period of detention in hospital. It replaces the after-care under supervision provisions which were introduced by the Mental Health (Patients in the Community) Act 1995.
- The group of practitioners who can take on functions previously performed by the approved social worker (ASW) and responsible medical officers is broadened:
  - The new role replacing the ASW will be known as the approved mental health professional (AMHP), and he or she will have the same functions as the ASW as well as additional functions in relation to supervised community treatments. The AMHP may include suitably trained nurses, occupational therapists and chartered psychologists and, unlike the ASW, will not have to be employed by the local authorities.
  - The new role replacing the responsible medical officer will be known as the responsible clinician, and will be open to other suitably trained professionals such as chartered psychologists, nurses, social workers and occupational therapists, as well as registered medical practitioners. The responsible clinician will have overall responsibility for a patient.

- Enabling a patient to apply to the county court for the nearest relative to be displaced, and amending the definition of nearest relative to include a civil partner.
- Increasing the frequency with which the Mental Health Review Tribunal considers the cases of civil patients treated under the MHA.
- Ending finite restriction orders, so that the restrictions will remain in force for as long as the offender's mental disorder poses a risk of harm to others.

The amendments made by the Mental Health Act 2007 to the Mental Health Act 1983 will come into force in October 2008. A new Code of Practice for the Mental Health Act will be prepared which must include the fundamental principles set out in Section 8 of the Mental Health Act 2007.

On 10 September 2007 the Department of Health and the Ministry of Justice published two consultation papers: the Mental Capacity Act 2005 Deprivation of Liberty Safeguards and a draft addendum to the Mental Capacity Act Code of Practice. Consultation ends on 2 December 2007. The documents can be accessed on the Ministry of Justice website: www.justice.gov.uk/publications.

References

1 Code of Practice for the Mental Capacity Act 2005. Department of Constitutional Affairs February 2007 para 13.46. TSO, London.
2 *Ibid.* para 13.12.
3 *Ibid.* para 13.39.
4 *Ibid.* paras 13.40 and 41.
5 *HL v. United Kingdom (Application No 45508/99)*. Times Law Report, 19 October 2004. (2005) 40 EHRR 32; [2005] Lloyd's Rep Med 169.
6 House of Lords, 25 Jan 2005, columns 1246–1256.
7 House of Lords, 25 Jan 2005, columns 1250–2.
8 Department of Health (2005) *'Bournewood' Consultation. The approach to be taken in response to the judgment of the European Court of Human Rights in the 'Bournewood' case.*
9 Department of Health (2006) *Protecting the Vulnerable: the 'Bournewood' Consultation.*
10 Department of Health (2006) Bournewood Briefing Sheet. Gateway Reference 6794.
11 Draft Mental Capacity (Deprivation of Liberty: Appointment of Relevant Person's Representative and Assessment) Regulations 2007.
12 *Ibid.*
13 Mental Capacity (Deprivation of Liberty: Eligibility and Selection of Assessors) Regulations 2007.
14 *Re PS (an Adult) and the City of Sunderland and PS (by her litigation friend the Official Solicitor and CA* [2007] EWHC 623 (Fam).

Scenarios J
Mental Capacity and
Mental Disorder

Exclusion from Mental Capacity Act (MCA) of patients subject to Part 4 of the Mental Health Act (MHA)

> ### Scenario J1: Which jurisdiction – MCA or MHA?
>
> Huw was arrested by a police constable in the town centre after a crowd had gathered around him as he shouted verbal abuse. He was taken to the police station where the duty officer decided that he had been arrested under Section 136 of the MHA. He was placed in a cell and the police doctor summoned. The doctor decided that Huw needed immediate medication since he appeared to be in a diabetic coma resulting from alcohol consumption. Huw appeared unable to make any decisions for himself. What is the legal situation?

If it is clear that Huw is unable to make his own decisions, then the question arises as to whether action could be taken in his best interests under the Mental Capacity Act 2005, or whether he comes under the Mental Health Act 1983. The Mental Capacity Act 2005 excludes from its provisions those patients who are detained under the Mental Health Act 1983 and who come under the provisions of Part 4 of the Act. Accepting (though on the facts this is by no means certain) that Huw has been detained by the police using their powers under Section 136 of the Mental Health Act 1983, this does not mean that he comes under Part 4 of that Act. Part 4 enables treatment to be given for mental disorder to those who are detained under specified sections of the Mental Health Act 1983. Section 136 is excluded from those provisions (see page 296). It therefore follows that Huw cannot be treated under Part 4 of the MHA, so he is not excluded from the provisions of the Mental Capacity Act 2005.

It follows therefore that if Huw lacked the requisite mental capacity to make his own decisions, then the police doctor must act in Huw's best interests. He must follow the principles laid down in Section 1 of the Act and the criteria for determining best interests which are set down in Section 4 of the MCA. It would not appear that the situation comes within the definition of serious medical treatment, for which an independent mental capacity advocate would have to be appointed if there were no other appropriate person who could be consulted about Huw's best interests.

Treatment for a physical condition

A further example of the dilemma over which jurisdiction (MCA or MHA) applies can be seen in Scenario J2. See also Scenario J6.

Scenario J2: MCA 2005 or MHA 1983?

Chris is pregnant and as a result of a serious bout of bipolar disorder has been detained under Section 3 of the Mental Health Act 1983 for treatment for mental disorder. At times she appears to have the mental capacity to make her decisions, but there are other times when she is either so severely depressed that she is unable to communicate or so elated that she is unable to speak rationally. Her obstetrician has examined her and is of the view that it would be in her best interests to have a Caesarean section, since she had one for her child who is now 2 years old. The obstetrician is not clear as to whether she has the capacity to give consent to a Caesarean. What is the law if she is assessed as being incapable of giving consent?

In this situation of Scenario J2, Section 28 of the MCA would not apply, since, although Chris is detained under Section 3 of the MHA 1983, the proposed treatment is not for mental disorder, but for a Caesarean section. (There have been cases in the past when a detained pregnant woman has been given a Caesarean under the powers of Part 4 of the MHA, on the grounds that this was treatment for mental disorder.[1] However it is not thought that these decisions would survive the rulings made by the Court of Appeal in the cases of *Re MB*[2] and of *St George's NHS Trust*).[3]

If the view is taken that an operation to perform a Caesarean section is not treatment for mental disorder regulated by the Mental Health Act 1983, then although Chris is detained in a psychiatric hospital under Section 3 of the Act and comes under the provisions of Part 4 for treatment for her mental disorder, the decision on whether she should be given a compulsory Caesarean does not come under the Mental Health Act 1983 but under the Mental Capacity Act 2005, i.e. Section 28(1) of the MCA does not apply. See the discussion of Case B2 in Scenarios B on best interests (page 79).

If the MCA applies to Chris's situation then the following questions must be answered:

- Does Chris have the requisite mental capacity to make her own decision on the Caesarean section? The fact that she is under Section 3 of the MHA does not automatically mean that she lacks the capacity to give consent or refuse according to the definition of capacity in Sections 2 and 3 of the MCA. It would be preferable for this assessment to be carried out by a person qualified in determining mental capacity who is not a member of the multi-disciplinary team caring for Chris, so he or she can act independently of the team.
- If the assessment concludes that Chris lacks the mental capacity to make a decision about a Caesarean section, then the question of what is in Chris's best interests has to be answered. MCA provisions on best interests set out in Section 4 and the Section 1 principles would apply.
- Is a Caesarean section 'serious medical treatment'? Since a Caesarean section would appear to come within the definition of serious medical treatment as defined in Section 37(6) and in the regulations,[4] the National Health Service body, i.e. the NHS trust who is providing her care and treatment, is required to instruct an independent mental capacity advocate to represent Chris, in the absence of an appropriate person.
- Should an independent mental capacity advocate be appointed? Unless there is an appropriate person (who is neither paid nor working in a professional capacity) who can be consulted on what Chris's best interests are, the NHS trust must ensure that an independent mental capacity advocate (IMCA) is appointed.
- What is the consequence of the IMCA appointment? Once the independent mental capacity advocate had been instructed and met with Chris and considered all her views, and discussed the situation and Chris's best interests with family, friends, and paid carers and others, she or he would report back to the NHS trust, which has an obligation under Section 37(5) to take into account any information given or submissions made by the independent mental capacity advocate.
- Does urgent action need to be taken? If the obstetrician caring for Chris considers that there is urgent necessity for the caesarean Section to be carried out, and there is not time for the appointment of an IMCA, the NHS trust has the power under Section 37(4) to provide the treatment, even though it has not been able to appoint an IMCA. There may be time for an application to be made to the Court of Protection for an emergency declaration to be made as to what is in Chris's best interests.

The provision of independent mental capacity advocates is considered in Chapter 8.

Refusal of treatment by an advance decision

Scenario J3: Advance decision refusing ECT.

Jamie's mother was a chronic schizophrenic and, disturbed by the treatment she received when detained under the Mental Health Act, Jamie drew up an advance decision. In this he stated that if he were ever to be detained under the MHA he would not wish to be given electro-convulsive therapy. He later showed signs of severe depression and had to be detained under Section 3 of the MHA. Doctors recommended that he should receive electro-convulsive therapy (ECT). He refused to give consent to this and a second opinion doctor was appointed under the provisions of Part 4 of the MHA. The Second Opinion Appointed Doctor (SOAD) recommended that Jamie should receive compulsory ECT. The nurses were concerned because of Jamie's advance decision.

Jamie is detained under the Mental Health Act 1983, and his treatment for mental disorder is regulated by Part 4 of that Act. Although he has drawn up an advance direction, Section 28(1) excludes treatment being given under the Act when the person's treatment is regulated by Part 4 of the Mental Health Act 1983. Under Part 4, Section 58 of the MHA applies to the administration of ECT. Section 58 enabled (prior to the amendments of the 2007 Act (see below S.58A)) ECT to be given without the consent of the patient if a second opinion is obtained from an independent medical practitioner that the ECT should be given. Jamie's advance direction is therefore overruled.

This would appear to be contrary to Jamie's rights. If he, when mentally capacitated, states that he would never wish to receive certain forms of treatment for his mental disorder, surely there should be some recognition from his health professionals over his specified wishes.

This would appear to be contrary to Jamie's rights and amendments were made to the Mental Health Act 1983 by the Mental Health Act 2007.

Section 58A of the Mental Health Act

As a consequence of Section 27 of the Mental Health Act 2007, a new Section 58A is added to the 1983 Act as follows:

58A Electro-convulsive therapy, etc

(1) This section applies to the following forms of medical treatment for mental disorder –
  (a) electro-convulsive therapy; and
  (b) such other forms of treatment as may be specified for the purposes of this section by regulations made by the appropriate national authority.
(2) Subject to section 62 . . . , a patient shall not be given any form of treatment to which this section applies unless he falls within subsection (3) or (4) below.
(3) A patient falls within this subsection if –
  (a) he has consented to the treatment in question; and
  (b) either the approved clinician in charge of it or a registered medical practitioner appointed as mentioned in section 58(3) . . . has certified in writing that the patient is capable of understanding the nature, purpose and likely effects of the treatment and has consented to it.
(4) A patient falls within this subsection if a registered medical practitioner appointed as aforesaid (not being the approved clinician in charge of the treatment in question) has certified in writing –

    (a)   that the patient is not capable of understanding the nature, purpose and likely effects of the treatment; but

    (b)   that it is appropriate for the treatment to be given; and

    (c)   that giving him the treatment would not conflict with –

        (i)   an advance decision which the registered medical practitioner concerned is satisfied is valid and applicable;

        (ii)   a decision made by a donee or deputy or by the Court of Protection; or

        (iii)   an order of a court.

(5)   Before giving a certificate under subsection (4) above the registered medical practitioner concerned shall consult two other persons who have been professionally concerned with the patient's medical treatment (neither of whom shall be the responsible clinician or the approved clinician in charge of the treatment in question), and of those persons one shall be a nurse and the other shall be neither a nurse nor a registered medical practitioner.

(6)   Before making any regulations for the purposes of this section, the appropriate national authority shall consult such bodies as appear to it to be concerned.

(7)   In this section –

    (a)   a reference to an advance decision is to an advance decision (within the meaning of the Mental Capacity Act 2005) made by the patient;

    (b)   'valid and applicable', in relation to such a decision, means valid and applicable to the treatment in question in accordance with section 25 of that Act;

    (c)   a reference to a donee is to a donee of a lasting power of attorney (within the meaning of section 9 of that Act) created by the patient, where the donee is acting within the scope of his authority and in accordance with that Act; and

    (d)   a reference to a deputy is to a deputy appointed for the patient by the Court of Protection under section 16 of that Act, where the deputy is acting within the scope of his authority and in accordance with that Act.

(8)   In this section, 'the appropriate national authority' means –

    (a)   in a case where the treatment in question would, if given, be given in England, the Secretary of State;

    (b)   in a case where the treatment in question would, if given, be given in Wales, the Welsh Ministers.

This effect of the new S 58A is that if Jamie, when mentally capacitated, had stated in an advance decision that he would never wish to receive ECT or another treatment specified under Section 58A, then he cannot be given it.

The role of an LPA where the donor is detained under the MHA

Scenario J4: Role of LPA when patient detained under the MHA.

Beryl suffered from bipolar disorder and was frequently admitted to psychiatric hospital. She asked her mother if she would act as her attorney to make decisions on her care and treatment. Her mother accepted and the appropriate papers were completed and signed. Beryl was then admitted to the ward under Section 3 and her mother told the charge nurse that she had been appointed under an legal power of attorney (LPA). The charge nurse said that since Beryl was under section, the LPA was irrelevant and all decisions should be made by the multi-disciplinary team. Beryl's mother wished to challenge that statement.

The charge nurse is correct to a limited extent: if the treatment of a patient is regulated under Part 4 of the Mental Health Act 1983, then the provisions of the MCA do not apply to that treatment. However Part 4 only applies to treatment for mental disorder. There may be other treatments for a physical condition on which Beryl's mother could be consulted. The charge nurse should welcome Beryl's mother to the multi-disciplinary team meetings when Beryl's care and treatment is being discussed and her future accommodation and care being planned. Although the mother would have no legal right to make those decisions which come under Part 4, as the nominated representative of the patient her contribution to the planning of Beryl's care and treatment should be welcomed and, if Beryl lacks the requisite mental capacity to make her own decisions, Beryl's mother should be invited to give her views on the best interests of Beryl according to the criteria in Section 4.

Role of deputy when patient detained under the MHA

Scenario J5: Role of deputy when patient detained under the MHA.

Ivor was severely injured in a road accident and received over £3 million in compensation. The Court of Protection appointed his cousin Jane as a deputy to make decisions relating to his care and treatment, with powers to authorise expenditure from his account. One of the effects of the road traffic accident was serious brain damage which led him to be aggressive and dangerous without any warning. After attacking a stranger who was walking past his house, he was placed under Section 37 of the Mental Health Act 1983 with a restriction order and sent to a regional secure unit. Jane was uncertain of her role as deputy following Ivor's detention.

On her appointment Jane would have been given specific instructions as to the action she would be able to take on Ivor's behalf. If it was not a reasonably foreseeable event that Ivor should be placed under section, then it is clear that Jane's instructions need to be updated. She should consult with the Office of the Public Guardian as to whether there should be a further hearing by the Court of Protection to determine whether her appointment should continue and what new instructions she should be working under. Even though Ivor's treatment for mental disorder now comes under the Mental Health Act 1983, there are still other decisions which need to be made on his behalf, particularly in relation to his finances.

Scenario J6: Detained patient and physical illness.

Bob was a chronic schizophrenic who was periodically detained in hospital under Section 3 of the Mental Health Act 1983, often as a result of his failing to attend the health centre for his regular injections. During one admission he complained of severe stomach pain and was diagnosed as having an inflamed appendix. Immediate surgery was arranged, but Bob refused surgery on the grounds that he did not trust the doctors to do him no harm. Can he be compelled to have the surgery?

Bob comes under Part 4 of the Mental Health Act 1983, and therefore his treatment for mental disorder is regulated under that Act and is excluded from the Mental Capacity Act 2005. This does not apply to treatment for a physical disorder. Since doctors are proposing surgery for a physical condition the MCA would apply. The following questions therefore arise:

- Does Bob have the capacity to give or refuse consent to the appendectomy?
- If the answer is 'yes', then his decision will prevail.
- If the answer is 'no', then action must be taken in his best interests.

Since the appendectomy would probably come within the definition of serious medical treatment, an IMCA should be appointed if there is no appropriate person who could be consulted about Bob's best interests.

Scenario J7: Prophylactic care and a detained patient.

James and John were twins aged 35 years. James suffered from biopolar disorder which occasionally required in-patient admission. John had recently had a genetic test which showed that he had a probability of contracting stomach cancer in the future. He decided that on medical advice that he would have a prophylactic removal of his stomach. He recommended that James should have the same treatment to prevent the cancer occurring. James was detained under Section 3 of the MHA and it appeared that he was incapable of giving consent to the surgery.

In Scenario J7 the proposed surgery for James would not be considered as treatment for mental disorder, so it would not come under Part 4 of the MHA and would not therefore be excluded from the provisions of the MCA. James's competence to make the decision about surgery would have to be assessed. If the conclusion was that James had the requisite capacity then the decision could be left to him. If the conclusion was that he lacked the requisite capacity, it would have to be decided if he would be likely to have the necessary capacity in the future. If that was a possibility, then the decision could be left until then, since there seems to be no immediate danger of stomach cancer occurring. If however it is doubtful that James will recover the appropriate capacity, then a decision would have to be made in his best interests. The proposed surgery would probably come within the definition of serious medical treatment and if John is not seen as an appropriate person to consult, an independent mental capacity advocate would have to be appointed by the NHS trust before the treatment proceeded, unless there were an appropriate person amongst his family or friends who could be consulted on his behalf and act for him.

Section 117 accommodation

Scenario J8: Patient detained under the MHA and due to be discharged with Section117 after-care.

Sahra had been detained under Section 3 of the Mental Health Act 1983 and was due to be discharged. It was decided that there was no need for her to be placed under a community treatment order. The multi-disciplinary team met to consider provision for her after-care and decided that it was preferable if she stayed in a hostel, especially provided for those with mental health needs. This accommodation was offered to her. The approved social worker suggested that an independent mental capacity advocate should be appointed for her, since she had no immediate family or friends. The psychiatrist said that that was not a requirement of the legislation.

In this situation the local authority approved social worker is part of the multi-disciplinary team deciding upon Sahra's after-care. The accommodation is being discussed as part of the duty of the NHS trust and the local authority and voluntary groups under Section 117 of the MHA 1983. Section 39 applies where the local authority is providing accommodation under Section 117 of the MHA, as a result of its community care assessment under Section 47 of the NHS and Community Care Act 1990. Under Section 39 the local authority has a responsibility to ensure that an independent mental capacity advocate is appointed to support and represent Sahra if she has no appropriate person who could be consulted as to what was in her best interests. Section 39 will only apply if Sahra lacks the requisite mental capacity to make her own decisions on accommodation. Since Sahra is not under an obligation under the MHA to stay at the hospital, the provisions of Section 39 are not excluded.

The consultant is therefore wrong in assuming that the obligation to consider the appointment of an IMCA under Section 39 does not apply. It would have been a different situation had she been transferred to accommodation under Section 17 of the Mental Health Act 1983, where she had an obligation to remain (see Scenario J9).

This Scenario contrasts with the situation in Scenario J9.

Scenario J9: Patient detained under the MHA.

Jessica was detained under Section 3 of the Mental Health Act 1983 and it was agreed in the multi-disciplinary team that she should be given leave to stay at a home where there were fewer restrictions, as part of her rehabilitation progress. It was decided not to transfer her to the unit but that she should be given leave under Section 17, which would enable her to be returned to the psychiatric hospital and leave to be cancelled if the leave did not work well. Her approved social worker questioned whether an independent mental capacity advocate should be appointed for her, since she appeared to lack close family and friends.

In contrast with Scenario J8 Jessica is being placed in accommodation by the NHS trust as part of its functions and duty under the MHA. Where an NHS organisation is providing accommodation, Section 38(2) excludes the requirement to appoint an IMCA if the accommodation is being provided as the result of an obligation imposed under the MHA. There is therefore no requirement to appoint an IMCA under the MCA for Jessica. The fact that the statutory duty under Section 38 of the MCA does not apply to the situation does not, of course, mean that an advocate cannot be provided under any of the local advocacy schemes. However the fact that this advocate does not have the statutory powers and rights as an IMCA under the MCA could affect their effectiveness. (This is discussed in Chapter 8, page 176.)

Bournewood situation

Scenario J10: Patient held at common law in a Bournewood situation.

Maud had been living in a care home for several years. She suffered from Alzheimer's disease, and this had been accompanied by growing violence in recent months. Her mental capacity had greatly diminished and the home believed that she needed to be detained to prevent her leaving the home and possibly being a danger to other people. The relatives were opposed to her being detained under the MHA, and her psychiatrist believed that her detention need be for only a short time. The care home was registered to take mentally disturbed patients and was prepared to keep her there as long as it could exercise greater control over her movements. It therefore wished to apply for the power to restrict her movements.

Once the Bournewood provisions contained within the Mental Health Act 2007 are implemented, the care home must follow the procedure set out in Chapter 13.

1. Application for authorisation

The care home, i.e. the managing authority, must identify Maud as being a person who lacks capacity and who risks being deprived of her liberty.

It must apply to the supervisory body, i.e. the local authority in which Maud was ordinarily resident, for authorisation of deprivation of liberty.

2. Assessments required

1. Age assessment – Maud is over 18 years.
2. Mental health assessment – Maud is suffering a mental disorder.
3. Mental capacity assessment – Maud lacks the capacity to decide whether to be admitted to or remain in the hospital or care home.
4. Eligibility assessment – Maud is:
   a. Not detained under the MHA.
   b. Not subject to a conflicting requirement under the MHA.
   c. Not subject to powers of recall under the MHA, nor
   d. a treatment order in hospital to which Maud objects.
5. Best interests assessment – the authorisation would be in Maud's best interests and is a proportionate response to the likelihood of suffering harm and the seriousness of that harm.
6. There is no conflict between the authorisation sought and a valid decision by a donee of a lasting power of attorney or a deputy, and it does not conflict with a valid and applicable advance decision made by Maud.

3. Appointment of representative for Maud

If the best interests assessor concludes that Maud has the capacity to appoint her own representative, then she can do this. Otherwise the best interests assessor can appoint a representative. If the assessor notifies the supervisory body that a representative has not been appointed for her, then it can appoint a representative who can be paid to act as Maud's representative.

4. Authorisation granted

If all the assessments are satisfactory then authorisation by the supervisory body can be granted for the deprivation of Maud's liberty for up to 12 months.

5. Review and monitoring

The supervisory authority should keep under review Maud's deprivation of liberty, and the whole process of the assessments and authorisation will be monitored to ensure that all the required procedures were followed.

Inherent jurisdiction of the court

In spite of the MCA and the amendments resulting from the introduction of the Bournewood safeguards, it is likely that the court will still be required to use its inherent jurisdiction to protect adults who lack the requisite mental capacity. In a case heard before the implementation of the Bournewood safeguards, the court decided that its inherent jurisdiction to protect the welfare of adults who lacked mental capacity enabled the court to make an order to stop a daughter (who wanted her mother to return to her care) preventing the mother from being moved from a hospital to a care home. The move to the care home was considered to be in the best interests of the mother. The facts are shown in J1.

Case J1: Inherent powers of the court.[5]

PS was admitted to hospital on 22 January 2007. She was ready for discharge by 7 February 2007, but her daughter (CA) informed the hospital that she was intending to discharge her mother into her own care rather than into the care of the T unit, a residential care and elderly mentally infirm unit where P had lived since 28 July 2006. The T unit had been identified as suitable for meeting PS's permanent needs at a meeting, convened by the LA and attended by CA in November 2006. Concerns were increased by CA's request to the hospital that they should not inform the LA of what she was planning. The LA made an ex parte out-of-hours telephone application to a judge and he made an interim order for PS to be moved to the T unit over the weekend until a hearing on the following Tuesday. Mr Justice Munby of the Family Division made interim declarations that PS lacked the capacity 1. to litigate, 2. to decide where she should reside, 3. to decide whom she had contact with, 4. to decide on issues concerning her care and 5. to manage her financial affairs. [*5 separate declarations on capacity were required because capacity is always issue specific* authors note.] The judge made an interim order that it was lawful as being in her best interests that PS reside at the T unit. The local authority was concerned that CA might attempt to remove PS from the T unit and the judge granted an injunction, backed by a penal notice, restraining CA from doing anything to obstruct or prevent PS from remaining at the T unit. The local authority also sought an order permitting it to use appropriate means to stop CA removing PS. The judge was satisfied that the inherent jurisdiction of the court enabled it to protect vulnerable adults, and cited the House of Lords in *Re F.*[6] However he noted that any exercise of its inherent jurisdiction must be compatible with the various requirements of Article 5 of the European Convention on Human Rights. He suggested that the following minimum requirements must be satisfied in order to comply with Article 5:

1. The detention must be authorised by the court on application made by the local authority and before the detention commences.
2. Subject to the exigencies of urgency or emergency the evidence must establish unsoundness of a kind or degree warranting compulsory confinement.

In other words, there must be evidence establishing at least a prima facie case that the individual lacks capacity and that confinement of the nature proposed is appropriate.

3. Any order authorising detention must contain provision for an adequate review at reasonable intervals, in particular with a view to ascertaining whether there still persists unsoundness of mind of a kind or degree warranting compulsory confinement.

The judge made an order that it was lawful being in PS's best interests for the local authority by its employees or agents to use reasonable and proportionate measures to prevent PS from leaving the T unit.

There was also concern that CA, who was empowered to sign cheques on her mother's behalf, was not applying PS's modest savings appropriately in meeting PS's requirements. The judge therefore made an order that it was in PS's best interests that her financial affairs were managed by the Director of Adult Services (DS). DS was appointed to be receiver of the property, money and income of PS, and authorised to take all such steps as may be necessary to preserve the same with power to pay and apply the income to or for the benefit of PS. The fact that the Court of Protection had jurisdiction to make such an order did not prevent the court from making one. The judge considered that it would be an unnecessary burden and, in his judgment, wholly disproportionate to the very modest amounts involved to condemn the parties to the trouble and expense of separate proceedings in the Court of Protection.

A case such as J1 would now (since 1 October 2007) be heard in the Court of Protection, but similar orders are likely to be made. This case should be contrasted with *Re DE (an adult patient), JE and Surrey County Council*, which is considered in Chapter 3.[7] In that case the court declared that the actions of Surrey County Council in requiring a resident to remain in a care home were contrary to his Article 5 rights.

The High Court also used its inherent jurisdiction in a situation where a wife, in her 80s was objecting to the decision that her husband, who was 90, should live in a home for the elderly mentally infirm (EMI). Mrs S considered that he should live with her at home, with the assistance of a support package provided by the local authority and Primary Care trust.[8] The judge held that it was in Mr S's best interests to live in the EMI home and the without notice court application by the local authority was justifiable. However he listed the lessons to be learnt from such a situation and recognised the exceptional nature of without notice applications.

References

1 *Tameside and Glossop Acute Services Trust* v. *CH* [1996] 1 FLR 762; *Norfolk and Norwich (NHS) Trust* v. *W* [1996] 2 FLR 613; *Rochdale NHS Trust* v. *C* [1997] 1 FCR 274.
2 *MB(re) (Adult Medical Treatment)* [1997] 2 FLR 426.
3 *St George's NHS Trust* v. *S* [1998] 3 All ER 673.

4   The Mental Capacity Act 2005 (Independent Mental Capacity Advocates)(General) Regulations 2006 (SI 2006/1832) reg 4.

5   *Re PS (an Adult) and the City of Sunderland and PS (by her litigation friend the Official Solicitor and CA* [2007] EWHC 623 (Fam).

6   *Re F (Mental Patient: Sterilisation)* [1990] 2 AC 1.

7   *Re DE (an adult patient), JE and Surrey County Council* [2006] EWHC 3459.

8   *B Borough Council and Mrs S and Mr S (by the Official Solicitor)* [2006] EWHC 2584 (Fam).

14 Organ and Tissue Removal, Storage and Use

Introduction

Specific protections are provided for those adults incapable of giving consent to the removal and subsequent use of their tissue or organs by the Mental Capacity Act 2005 and the Human Tissue Act 2004 and regulations[1] made under that legislation.

Removal of tissue from deceased persons

The Human Tissue Act 2004 applies to this situation.

Where a person has died and has not given instructions relating to the removal of tissue or organs from his or her body after his death, then the provisions of the Human Tissue Act (HTA) apply. Guidance is provided by the Codes of Practice issued by the Human Tissue Authority (see **Code of Practice issued by the Human Tissue Authority** on page 334). The legality of the removal, use and storage of the tissue depends upon the reasons why it is required. No consent of relatives is required when a post mortem is ordered by a coroner and tissue is removed as a consequence of the post mortem. However there are now strict rules relating to the storage and retention of the tissue, once the post mortem is completed.

Deceased persons

Consent is required for:

- the continued storage or use of material no longer required to be kept for the coroner's purposes

- the removal, storage and use for the following scheduled purposes:
  - anatomical examination
  - determining the cause of death
  - establishing, after a person's death, the efficacy of any drug or other treatment administered to them
  - obtaining scientific or medical information, about a living or deceased person, which may be relevant to any other person now or in the future ('a future person')
  - public display
  - research in connection with disorders, or the functioning, of the human body
  - transplantation
  - clinical audit
  - education or training relating to human health
  - performance assessment
  - public health monitoring

  and

  - quality assurance.

Where the deceased person did not give consent pre death to any of these purposes, or was incapable of giving consent, then consent can be given firstly by a person nominated by the deceased for that purpose. If there is no such person, then consent can be given by a relative. The HTA sets out a hierarchy of relatives:

- spouse or partner* (including civil or same sex partner)
- parent or child (in this context a 'child' can be any age)
- brother or sister
- grandparent or grandchild
- niece or nephew
- stepfather or stepmother
- half-brother or half-sister
- friend of long standing.

It is to be noted that S.54(9) states for these purposes a person is another person's partner if the two of them (whether of different sexes or the same sex) live as partners in an enduring family relationship.

Consent is not required for:

- carrying out an investigation into the cause of death under the authority of a coroner
- keeping material after a post mortem under the authority of a coroner
- keeping material in connection with a criminal investigation or following a criminal conviction.

Removal of tissue from living persons

If tissue needs to be removed for diagnostic or treatment purposes it can only be done with the consent of that person or, where the person lacks the capacity to give the necessary consent, within the provisions of the Mental Capacity Act 2005. This means that the health professional, having a reasonable belief in the absence of the requisite capacity, must have a reasonable belief that the removal of the tissue is in the best interests of P according to the criteria laid down in Section 4 (see Chapter 5). Scenario K1 provides an example. If the removal is required in the course of intrusive research, then either the individual must have the requisite capacity to give consent or, if he or she lacks the capacity, will be protected by Sections 30–34 of the Mental Capacity Act 2005 which govern participation in intrusive research or by the clinical trials regulations (see Chapter 10 and Scenarios G).

Storage and use of tissue removed from living persons

Scheduled purposes (see Box 14.1)

The Human Tissue Act 2004 covers the situation where storage and use of tissue removed from living persons arises, and distinguishes between scheduled purposes where consent is required (or there are specific provisions where a person is incapable of giving consent) and other purposes where consent is not required. The definition of scheduled purposes is contained in Schedule 1 of the Human Tissue Act 2004 and is shown in Box 14.1.

Box 14.1: Schedule 1 to the Human Tissue Act 2004.

Specified purposes requiring consent: general

1. Anatomical examination.
2. Determining the cause of death.
3. Establishing after a person's death the efficacy of any drug or other treatment administered to him.
4. Obtaining scientific or medical information about a living or deceased person which may be relevant to any other person (including a future person).
5. Public display.
6. Research in connection with disorders, or the functioning, of the human body.
7. Transplantation.

Where a person lacks the specific capacity to give consent to the storage and use of tissue for the purposes set out in Box 14.1, then the provisions of Section 6 of the Human Tissue Act 2004 apply. Section 6 is shown in a simplified format in Box 14.2. Scenario K2 illustrates a situation involving the storage and use of tissue for a scheduled purpose.

> **Box 14.2: Section 6 Human Tissue Act 2004 (simplified).**
>
> Where –
>
> a.   an activity for the storage and use of material from a body of a person who
>
>   (i)   is an adult, and
>
>   (ii)   lacks capacity to consent to the activity, and
>
> b.   neither a decision of his to consent to the activity, nor a decision of his not to consent to it, is in force,
>
> there shall for the purposes of this Part be deemed to be consent of his to the activity if it is done in circumstances of a kind specified by regulations made by the Secretary of State.

Regulations for persons who lack capacity to give consent and transplant regulations came into force on 1 September 2006.[2] Regulation 3 provides for the storage and use of materials from adults who lack the capacity to give consent. It permits tissue to be stored and used without the consent of an adult lacking mental capacity if it is for:

1.   Obtaining scientific or medical information about a living or deceased person which may be relevant to any other person (including a future person) if it is reasonably believed to be in P's best interests.
2.   Transplantation if in P's best interests.
3.   A clinical trial which is authorised and conducted in accordance with the clinical trials regulations.
4.   is intrusive research and complies with S. 30(1)(a) and (b) of the Mental Capacity Act (MCA) (i.e. it is authorised by an appropriate body and complies with Sections 32 and 33 of the MCA).
5.   A situation where P lost capacity after the research had commenced and S.34 of the MCA applies.
6.   A situation where the research began before the research provisions of the MCA came into force and is ethically approved according to Regulation 8 (see Box 14.3).

Code of Practice issued by the Human Tissue Authority

The Code of Practice on consent in relation to the HTA[3] issued by the Human Transplant Authority gives guidance in relation to the use of human tissue taken from adults who are incapable of consent. It emphasises the importance of presuming that the adult is capable of giving consent and encouraging the person to understand the decision to be made:

> 38. The ability of adults with learning difficulties, or with limited capacity, to understand should not be underestimated. Where appropriate, someone who knows the individual well, such as a family member or carer, should be consulted as he/she may be able to advise or assist with communication.

It also points out that the storage and the use of tissue outside the provisions of the Human Tissue Act 2004 and the regulations may be a criminal offence.

Ethical approval for the purposes of Regulations 3–6

Regulation 8 states that research is ethically approved if approval is given by a research ethics authority in the circumstances shown in Box 14.3.

Box 14.3: Ethically approved research. The circumstances required by Regulation 8.

- the research is in connection with disorders, or the functioning of the human body
- there are reasonable grounds for believing that research of comparable effectiveness cannot be carried out if the research has to be confined to, or related only to, persons who have capacity to consent to taking part in it
- there are reasonable grounds for believing that research of comparable effectiveness cannot be carried out in circumstances such that the person carrying out the research is not in possession, and not likely to come into possession, of information from which the person from whose body the defined material has come can be identified.

An example of the workings of Regulation 8 is shown in Scenario K3.

Consent is not required for storage and use of tissue from living persons for specified purposes

Under Section 1(10) of the HTA the following activities are lawful and consent is not required for the storage for use and the use from living persons for the following purposes:

- clinical audit
- education or training relating to human health (including training for research into disorders, or the functioning, of the human body)
- performance assessment
- public health monitoring
- quality assurance.

Exceptions to the Licensing Regulations

Regulations came into force in September 2006[4] which define research as ethically approved where it is approved by a research ethics authority. They also except from licensing requirements the storage of relevant material by a person who intends to use it for a scheduled purpose in the following circumstances:

A.   Where it is to be used for any purpose specified in paragraphs 2–5 or 8–12 of Part 1 of Schedule 1 to the Act (i.e. determining the cause of death, establishing after a person's death the efficacy of any drug or treatment administered to him, obtaining information which may be relevant to another person, public display, clinical audit, education or the purpose of qualifying research.

B.   Storage of relevant material is excepted where

the person storing it is intending to use it for the purpose of transplantation and

it is an organ or part of an organ and the storage it for a period of less than 48 hours.

C.   Storage of relevant material from the body of a deceased person is excepted where:

it is for the purpose of research or

the relevant material has come from premises in respect of which a licence is in force, is stored by a person intending to use it for the sole purpose of analysis for a scheduled purpose other than research and

it will be returned to premises in respect of which a licence is in force when the analysis is competed.

Analysis of DNA (deoxyribonucleic acid) (regulation 5)

Where a person lacks capacity to consent to analysis of his DNA, the purposes for which his DNA may be analysed are shown in Box 14.4.

Box 14.4: Analysis of DNA (Regulation 5).

Analysis of the DNA of a person incapable of consenting is permitted for the following purposes:

a.   any purpose which the person carrying out the analysis reasonably believes to be in P's best interests;

b.   the purposes of a clinical trial which is authorised and conducted in accordance with the clinical trial regulations;

c.   the purposes of intrusive research which is carried out on or after the relevant commencement date in accordance with the requirements of Section 30(1)(a) and (b) of the Mental Capacity Act 2005 (approval by appropriate body) and compliance with Sections 32 and 33 of that Act;

d.   the purposes of intrusive research –

a.   which is carried out on or after the relevant commencement date

b.   in relation to which Section 34 of the Mental Capacity Act 2005 (loss of capacity during research project) applies, and

c.   which is carried out in accordance with regulations made under section 34(2) of that Act; or

e.   research which is carried out before the relevant commencement date and which, before that date, is ethically approved within the meaning of regulation 8 (see Box 14.3).

A situation involving the analysis of DNA is shown in Scenario K4.

Exceptions to the consent provisions and the analysis of DNA

An offence is not committed under this section if the results of the analysis are to be used for 'excepted' purposes. 'Excepted' purposes include:

- medical diagnosis of that person
- coroner's purposes
- criminal investigation or prosecution
- national security
- court order
- clinical audit, education and training, etc., and
- research, provided the sample is anonymised and the research is research ethics committee (REC) approved.

Transplants and the mentally incapacitated adult

Section 33 of the Human Tissue Act 2004 makes it a criminal offence to remove any transplantable material from the body of a living person intending that the material be used for the purpose of transplantation. However in certain circumstances approval can be given by the Human Tissue Authority to the transplantation of organs (or part of organs), bone marrow and peripheral blood stem cells. Regulations drawn up under the HTA specify the conditions which must be satisfied. Regulation 11 specifies the circumstances in which the restriction on transplants involving a live donor is lifted. The regulation is shown in Box 14.5.

Box 14.5: Regulation 11. Cases in which restrictions on transplants involving a live donor are lifted.

1. Sections 33(1) and (2) of the HTA (offences relating to transplants involving a live donor) shall not apply in any case involving transplantable material from the body of a living person if the requirements of paragraph 2–6 are met.
2. A registered medical practitioner who has clinical responsibility for the donor must have caused the matter to be referred to the Authority.
3. The Authority must be satisfied that:
   a. no reward has been or is to be given in contravention of section 32 of the Act (prohibition of commercial dealings in human material for transplantation), and
   b. when the transplantable material is removed –
      i. consent for its removal for the purpose of transplantation has been given, or
      ii. its removal for that purpose is otherwise lawful.
4. The Authority must take the report referred to in paragraph 6 into account in making its decision under paragraph 3.

---

5.   The authority shall give notice of its decision under paragraph 3 to:
   a.   the donor of the transplantable material or any person acting on his behalf
   b.   the person to whom it is proposed to transplant the transplantable material ('the recipient'), or any person acting on his behalf, and
   c.   the registered medical practitioner who caused the matter to be referred to the Authority under paragraph 2.
6.   Subject to paragraph 7 one or more qualified persons must have conducted separate interviews with each of the following:
   a.   the donor
   b.   if different from the donor, the person giving consent, and
   c.   the recipient,
   and reported to the Authority on the matters specified in paragraphs (8) and (9).
      Paragraph 6 does not apply in any case where the removal of the transplantable material for the purpose of transplantation is authorised by an order made in any legal proceedings before a court.
      The matters that must be covered in the report of each interview under paragraph (6) are:
   a.   any evidence of duress or coercion affecting the decision to give consent,
   b.   any evidence of an offer of a reward, and
   c.   any difficulties of communication with the person interviewed and an explanation of how those difficulties were overcome.
9.   The following matters must be covered in the report of the interview with the donor and, where relevant, the other person giving consent:
   a.   the information given to the person interviewed as to the nature of the medical procedure for, and the risk involved in, the removal of the transplantable material,
   b.   the full name of the person who gave that information and his qualification to give it, and
   c.   the capacity of the person interviewed to understand:
      i.   the nature of the medical procedure and the risk involved, and
      ii.   that the consent may be withdrawn at any time before the removal of the transplantable material.
10. A person shall be taken to be qualified to conduct an interview under paragraph 6 if –
   a.   he appears to the Authority to be suitably qualified to conduct the interview,
   b.   he does not have any connection with any of the persons to be interviewed, or with a person who stands in a qualifying relationship to any of those persons, which the Authority considers to be of a kind that might raise doubts about his ability to act impartially, and
   c.   in the case of an interview with the donor or other person giving consent, he is not the person who gave the information referred to in paragraph (9)(a).

The operation of Regulation 11 and the donation of a transplant by a person lacking mental capacity is shown in Scenario K5.

Under Regulation 12 the Authority's decision as to the matters specified in regulations 11(3) are to be made by a panel of no fewer than three members of the Authority, when the donor of the transplantable material is an adult who lacks capacity to consent to removal of the material, and the material is an organ or part of an organ if it is to be used for the same purpose as an entire organ in the human body.

The Authority has the right to reconsider its decision if it is satisfied that any information given for the purpose of the decision was in any material respect false or misleading, or there has been any material change of circumstances since the decision was made. The doctor who referred the case to the Human Tissue Authority and the donor or recipient also have the right to require the HTA to reconsider any decision it has made.

Information to be provided by a person who has removed transplantable material from a human body

Under regulations[5] which came into force in September 2006, a person who has removed transplantable material from a human body to be transplanted to another person must supply to NHS Blood and Transplant (a special health authority established by SI 2005 No 2529) the information set out in Schedule 1 to the Regulations (this includes information about the removal of the transplantable material and the donor). Under the same regulations a medical practitioner who receives transplantable material must supply to NHS Blood and Transplant the information set out in Schedule 2 to the regulations (this includes information about the receipt and the transplantable material).

Best interests and organ donation

Earl Howe in the House of Lords was anxious to prevent it being possible for the doctor of a client/patient to be allowed to agree to organ or tissue donation in his or her best interests.[6]

> Removing an organ, bone marrow or any other sort of tissue from a patient, whether mentally incapacitated or not, is an invasive process which is not without some risk. One cannot say that it will provide direct therapeutic benefit to the patient, although it is certainly possible to argue that looked at in a wider context it is in the person's best interests for the tissue to be removed. Indirectly, it may be of huge value to the person that a close relative, for example, will be given the chance of therapeutic treatment by virtue of such a transplant – a relative who may also be a carer, say.
>
> There are all kinds of scenarios that one can imagine in which the best interests of the person are best served by permitting the donation of tissue. But I am uncomfortable with the thought that a doctor, acting jointly with a relative or attorney, might take such a decision on his or her own.

Earl Howe's concerns should be answered by the provisions in the MCA and in the HTA and the regulations made under it, and the functions of the Human Tissue Authority. Clearly the principles of the MCA, the definitions of mental capacity and the criteria for determining best interests must all be applied in determining whether it is in the best interests of a person lacking the requisite capacity to become an organ or tissue donor. See Scenario K5 and Case Study K1.

Conclusions

It remains to be seen if the combined provisions of the Human Tissue Act 2004 and the Mental Capacity Act 2005 give effective protection to those lacking the requisite mental capacity where organs and tissue removal, storage and use are concerned. From 1 January 2007 the Human Tissue Authority and the Human Fertilisation and Embryology Authority were combined under the same Chair, and this may lead to further combined guidance covering this complex area.

References

1   Human Tissue Act 2004 (Persons who Lack Capacity to Consent and Transplants) Regulations 2006 (SI 2006/1659).
2   Ibid.
3   Human Tissue Authority (2006). Code of Practice on consent.
4   Human Tissue Act 2004 (Ethical Approval, Exceptions from Licensing and Supply of Information about Transplants) Regulations (SI 2006/1260).
5   Ibid.
6   House of Lords, 25 Jan 2005 Column 1239.

Scenarios K
Organ and Tissue Removal, Storage and Use

Introduction

These Scenarios should be read in conjunction with Chapter 14, which discusses the law relating to tissue and organ removal storage and use and transplants.

Removal of tissue for diagnostic purposes

Scenario K1: Removal of tissue for diagnostic purposes.

Rachel has severe learning disabilities and it is feared that she may be suffering from breast cancer. The doctor recommends that she should have a biopsy taken to determine whether it is malignant. Rachel is incapable of giving consent to the operation.

In Scenario K1 the Mental Capacity Act 2005 applies to the taking of the biopsy. It may come under the definition of serious medical treatment (see Chapter 5) and if there is no family member or friend who could be consulted over Rachel's best interests, an independent mental capacity advocate (IMCA) would be appointed to support Rachel and provide a report on what is in her best interests. Only if there were an appropriate person who could be consulted, or if it were an emergency situation and there was no time for the appointment of an IMCA, could the requirement to appoint an IMCA be dispensed with.

Storage and use of tissue or material taken from a living person

> **Scenario K2: Storage and use of tissue for a scheduled purpose.**
>
> On the facts of Scenario K1, medical staff asked if they could store the biopsy taken from Rachel and use it for clinical and research purposes. What are the legal requirements?

In Scenario K2, the storage and use of the tissue taken for the biopsy would come under the provisions of the Human Tissue Act 2004. This storage and use would come under the regulations for persons who lack capacity to give consent which came into force on 1 September 2006.[1] Regulation 3 provides for the storage and use of materials from adults who lack the capacity to give consent. The purposes for which it permits tissue to be stored and used without the consent of an adult lacking mental capacity include:

> Obtaining scientific or medical information about a living or deceased person which may be relevant to any other person (including a future person) if it is reasonably believed to be in P's best interests or its use for research purposes.

Further information would be required as to exactly what the doctors wish to do with the tissue. If the purpose is research which had begun before the research provisions of the Mental Capacity Act (MCA) came into force, and the research is ethically approved according to Regulation 8 (see Box 14.3 in Chapter 14, page 335), then its storage and use would appear to be legitimate and covered by the regulations. Scenario K3 provides an example of the workings of Regulation 8.

> **Scenario K3: An example of the workings of Regulation 8.**
>
> Ruth has had Alzheimer's for over fifteen years and is being cared for in a nursing home. Brian, a researcher into the chemistry of those suffering from Alzheimer's, is conducting research to ascertain if the disease can be accounted for by excess protein in the body. He therefore puts proposals before the research ethics committee to obtain approval for carrying out his research on those who suffer from Alzheimer's. He then approaches the manager of the nursing home to obtain consent for the taking of a blood sample from Ruth. What is the law?

Brian has to obtain the consent of the research ethics committee to undertaking the research in accordance with Regulation 8.[2] Box 14.3 in Chapter 14 sets out the wording of Regulation 8. The research ethics committee must have approved the research in the following circumstances:

- The research is in connection with disorders, or the functioning of the human body. This condition is satisfied since Alzheimer's disease is a disorder of the human body.
- There are reasonable grounds for believing that research of comparable effectiveness cannot be carried out if the research has to be confined to, or related only to, persons who have capacity to consent to taking part in it. This condition is also satisfied, since most people with Alzheimer's disease would not be able to consent.
- There are reasonable grounds for believing that research of comparable effectiveness cannot be carried out in circumstances such that the person carrying out the research is not in possession, and not likely to come into possession, of information from which the person whose body the defined material has come can be identified.

These conditions must apply to Ruth before the research can be deemed to come within the regulations and therefore be permissible.

Analysis of DNA

> **Scenario K4: An example of the analysis of deoxyribonucleic acid (DNA) and Regulation 5.**
>
> There is a dispute over the paternity of Elizabeth, who suffered severe brain damage at birth as a result of negligence by midwifery and obstetric staff. She was awarded compensation of £3 million. Her mother is in dispute with two men, both of whom claim to be the father of Elizabeth. The Social Services Department believe that there should be a DNA test to identify which of the two is the father of Elizabeth. Elizabeth is unable to consent to the DNA test. What is the law?

Scenario K4 comes under the Human Tissue Act 2004 and the regulations made under that Act.[3] Regulation 5 permits the DNA of a person incapable of giving consent to be analysed if one of the reasons is 'any purpose which the person carrying out the analysis reasonably believes to be in P's best interests'. If it is considered to be in Elizabeth's best interests for the DNA to be analysed, then permission can be given. This should clearly be documented. If there is a dispute as to whether it is in Elizabeth's best interests for the DNA to be analysed, then an order of the court could be sought, and if the court determined an analysis of DNA was in her best interests, consent would not be required, since a court order is an 'excepted' purpose.

Donation in the best interests

The difficulties of determining what is in the best interests of a person who has never had mental capacity are illustrated in the case shown in Case Study K1.

Case study K1: Best interests and bone marrow donation. Re Y [1997].[4]

The claimant, aged 36 years, sought a declaration from the court that two pre-liminary blood tests and a conventional bone marrow harvesting operation under general anaesthetic could be lawfully taken from and performed upon her sister Y. The facts were that the applicant was suffering from a pre-leukaemic bone marrow disorder. She had undergone extensive chemotherapy and a blood stem cell transplant. She had started to deteriorate and was likely to progress to acute myeloid leukaemia over the next three months. Her only realistic prospect of recovery was a bone marrow transplant operation from a healthy compatible donor. Preliminary investigations suggested that Y her sister would be a suitable donor. Y was 25 years and severely mentally and physically handicapped. She had lived in a community home for eight years. She was incapable of giving consent to the donation of bone marrow. The court had to decide whether it was in the best interests of Y for a declaration to be made for the blood tests and the bone marrow harvesting to take place.

The judge made it clear that it was the best interests of Y which were in dispute. The best interest of the sister were not relevant save in so far as they served the best interests of Y. The judge argued as follows: if the sister did not have the bone marrow transplant she would die. This would be a devastating blow to her mother, who suffered from ill health. They were a very close family. The mother would find it more difficult to visit Y in the community home, especially as after the death of Y's sister, the mother would then have to look after her only grand-child. Y would suffer as a result of the lack of contact with her mother. The risk of harm to Y from the blood tests was negligible. Although a general anaesthetic posed some risk, it was a low risk. She had already had a general anaesthetic for a hysterectomy without any apparent adverse ill effects. The bone marrow would regenerate. It was to Y's emotional, psychological and social benefit for her to be a donor.

It would, therefore, be in the best interests of Y for her to have the blood tests and be a donor for her sister. Clearly it was essential that in determining best interests there would have to be consultation with the carers and the wider family and her closeness to her sister would have to be determined. It would also have to be decided as to whether it was likely that she would wish to help her sister by the donation of tissue to her. The judge applied a best interests test to the decision making, taking into account what she would probably have wanted had she been able to make the decision.

There are dangers that a case such as that of *Re Y* could start a slippery slope. If bone marrow is justified, why not a kidney? It would be morally unacceptable for our community homes for those with learning disabilities to be seen as the source of spare parts and organ donations. Yet in an American case decided before *Re Y*, it was held that a mentally handicapped patient could be a live kidney donor for his brother.[5] It is to prevent any such slippery slope that there are now tighter pre-cautions to protect those who are incapable of giving consent to transplantation.

Present procedure

The case in Case Study K1 was decided before the Human Tissue Act 2004 and the Mental Capacity Act 2005 were enacted, and was decided upon principles of the common law. However if the same issue was to arise after the Human Tissue Act (HTA), whilst the actual proceedings would now be according to the new procedures, the actual decision would probably not be different. Scenario K5 looks at the situation under the Human Tissue Act 2004 and the regulations made under that Act.

Scenario K5: A request to use P as a transplant donor under Regulations 9–14 of the regulations.[6]

A request has been made to use the bone marrow of Julie, a person with severe learning and physical disabilities, for a transplant for her sister who has leukaemia. Julie is incapable of giving consent to the transplant.

Since Julie lacks the capacity to give consent then she is protected by the regulations issued under the Human Tissue Act (HTA). The Code of Practice on Transplants published by the HTA[7] notes that:

17. Where an adult lacks the capacity to consent and no decision was made while they were competent, then donation is lawful if it is:

- compliant with any regulations published by the Department of Health (DH) and
- approved by a panel of no fewer than three members of the HTA.

As a consequence of the regulations governing the use of tissue from persons who lack the capacity to give consent,[8] the procedure specified in Regulation 11 would have to be followed. Regulation 11 requires the Human Transplant Authority to ensure that:

- no reward has been or is to be given in contravention of Section 32 of the Human Tissue Act 2004
- either consent has been given or the removal is lawful
- a report has been provided by a qualified person who has conducted interviews with the donor, the person giving consent and the recipient, and the Authority takes this report into account. The report must cover any evidence of coercion or an offer of reward, any difficulties of communication and how these were overcome. In addition the report must also include details of the information given to the person who was interviewed on the risks involved, the full name of that person, and the capacity of that person to understand the nature of the medical procedure and the risk involved
- there must be at least three members of the Authority on a panel considering a case where the donor of the transplantable material lacks the capacity to give consent.

References

1   Human Tissue Act 2004 (Persons who Lack Capacity to Consent and Transplants) Regulations 2006 (SI 2006/1659).
2   *Ibid.*
3   *Ibid.*
4   *Re Y (adult patient) (transplant: bone marrow)* [1997] Fam 110; [1997] 2 WLR 556.
5   *Strunk* v. *Strunk* (1996) 445 SW 2d 145 (Ky CA).
6   SI 2006/1659 (see reference 1 above).
7   Code of Practice on donation of organs, tissue and cells for Transplantation (Code No 2, January 2006). HTA.
8   SI 2006/1659 (see reference 1 above).

15 The Informal Carer

Introduction

It is probable that the majority of adults who lack the mental capacity to make specific decisions are cared for by family and friends, rather than by paid care assistants or registered health and social services professionals. The question arises as to how much of the new legislation applies to the informal carer, and to what extent it affects their duties and responsibilities and their accountability for their actions or omissions. This chapter brings together a discussion on these various issues, and should be read in conjunction with Scenarios L.

Definition

The informal carer is the person close to the individual lacking mental capacity (P) who cares for, lives with or in some way takes responsibility for P. By definition this person is not paid, nor are they acting in a professional capacity towards P. Informal carers may include close friends, family members, neighbours or others who provide continuous or intermittent care for P. There is no statutory definition of an informal carer in the Mental Capacity Act 2005, so where this question arose reference would be made to earlier legislation such as the Carers (Recognition and Services) Act 1995 and the Carers and Disabled Children Act 2000. The Carers (Recognition and Services) Act 1995 defines a carer as 'an individual who provides or intends to provide a substantial amount of care on a regular basis for the relevant person' (S.1(1)(b)), and this same definition is used in the Carers and Disabled Children Act 2000 where the individual is over 16 years and provides a substantial amount of care on a regular basis for another individual aged 18 or over (S.1(1)(a)).

Duty of informal carer

Section 5 covering acts in connection with care and treatment brings the activities of the informal carer into the ambit of the Mental Capacity Act (MCA). Its provisions are discussed in Chapter 4, but effectively it means that any action taken by an informal carer in relation to a person who lacks mental capacity to make decisions must comply with the statutory provisions.

Section 5 states that:

If a person ('D') does an act in connection with the care or treatment of another person ('P'), the act is one to which this section applies if –

(a) before doing the act, D takes reasonable steps to establish whether P lacks capacity in relation to the matter in question, and

(b) when doing the act, D reasonably believes –

    (i) that P lacks capacity in relation to the matter, and

    (ii) that it will be in P's best interests for the act to be done.

(2) D does not incur any liability in relation to the act that he would not have incurred if P –

(a) had had capacity to consent in relation to the matter, and

(b) had consented to D's doing the act.

This section would appear to apply to all those making decisions on P's behalf including informal carers. It implies that the principles set out in Section 1 and discussed in Chapter 2 will apply to the role of the informal carer. In addition they should take into account all the considerations set out in Section 4 relating to best interests in deciding what should be done. Provided that they have complied with the statutory provisions, they will obtain the protection of the Act, just as if they had had the consent of a mentally capacitated adult when carrying out that activity or making that decision.

Scenario L1 illustrates the situation.

Standard of duty of care

Once a duty of care is assumed, even if it is on a voluntary basis, it must be carried out at a reasonable standard, and failure to comply with this duty could lead to an action for breach of the duty of care in the law of negligence. In addition, the informal carer may be liable to criminal proceedings as a result of Section 44. This section makes a person who has the care of P guilty of an offence if he ill-treats or wilfully neglects P (see Chapter 11). There is no definition of the words 'has the care of a person ('P')' in the MCA (but see the definitions above used in earlier legislation), and case law will develop following prosecutions of those who claim that they were not carers. It is probable that the words would not cover the neighbour who occasionally does some shopping for P, but would cover a person living with P or a person who is in regular contact with P and undertakes basic tasks of day-to-day living for P.

Informal carer as donee of a lasting power of attorney

P, before he or she lost mental capacity, may have appointed the informal carer as the donee of a lasting power of attorney. There must be clear evidence that the informal carer has explicitly accepted that appointment and that the provisions of the Act and the relevant Code of Practice have been followed (see Chapter 6). Failure by a donee of a lasting power of attorney to comply with the donor's instructions could lead to action being taken by the Office of the Public Guardian (OPG). See Scenario L2.

It is specifically stated in the MCA that the donee of a lasting power of attorney could be guilty of a criminal offence if he ill-treats or wilfully neglects P – S.44(1)(b) and (2). This would appear to apply whether the lasting power of attorney (LPA) is for personal welfare or for property and affairs.

Informal carer as a deputy appointed by the Court of Protection

Similarly the informal carer may be the person selected by the Court of Protection to be appointed as the deputy, in which case the carer would have to follow the statutory provisions and the relevant Code of Practice (see Chapter 7). See Scenario L3.

It is specifically stated in the MCA that a deputy appointed by the Court of Protection could be guilty of a criminal offence if he ill-treats or wilfully neglects P – S.44(1)(c) and (2).

Best interests

One of the basic principles of the Act is that an act done, or decision made under this Act for or on behalf of a person who lacks capacity must be done, or made, in his best interests (S.1(5)). (See Chapter 3.) When is an action or decision made under the Act as opposed to outside the Act? One view is that the Act applies whenever there is a decision that a person lacks mental capacity to make decisions and to all actions taken on his or her behalf. Another more restricted view is that the Act applies only to the more formal decision making by health or social service professionals, and those appointed in a formal capacity as donees of lasting powers of attorney, and deputies and officials of the Court of Protection.

The Code of Practice takes the interpretation of the wider remit of the impact of the Act in its first paragraph:[1]

> 1.1 The MCA 2005 (the Act) provides the legal framework for acting and making decisions on behalf of individuals who lack the mental capacity to make particular decisions for themselves. Everyone working with and/or caring for an adult who may lack capacity to make specific decisions must comply with this Act when making decisions or acting for that person, when the person lacks the capacity to make a particular decision for themselves. The same rules apply whether the decisions are life-changing events or everyday matters.

In paragraph 2.2 it states that:

> The statutory principles apply to any act done or decision made under the Act. When followed and applied to the Act's decision-making framework, they will help people take appropriate action in individual cases. They will also help people find solutions in difficult or uncertain situations.

It is therefore surprising that informal carers are not one of the categories of persons who are required to follow the Code of Practice.

It remains to be seen from the decisions of the Court of Protection and other civil or criminal proceedings the extent to which the courts hold that all carers, informal as well as professional, are bound by the Act and regulations made under it.

Decisions within their remit

Informal carers are only able to make decisions on behalf of a mentally incapacitated adult at a certain level. Serious decisions about health and accommodation would be made by others, probably registered health professionals, after, where appropriate, the instruction of an independent mental capacity advocate to advise the authority. For example, decisions relating to serious medical treatment and accommodation under Sections 37–39 would appear to have to be made by health or local social services authorities. Regulations define what is meant by serious medical treatment[2] and have extended the number of situations where an independent advocate must be appointed[3] (see Chapter 8).

Conflicts with statutory authorities and health and social services professionals

In the event of a dispute between an informal carer and a health or social services professional about either whether or not P lacks mental capacity or what is in P's best interests, every effort should be made to resolve the dispute through discussion or by more formal means of resolution, such as mediation or independent advocacy. If there is a dispute with the statutory services, it may be necessary to have recourse to the complaints procedure for the National Health Service or social services. (These procedures are different between England and Wales (see Chapter 16 on Wales).)

If all these methods of resolution fail, then eventually an application could be made to the Court of Protection to determine the issue. In such circumstances the Court of Protection could make a specific order, or appoint a deputy (see Chapter 7).

Code of Practice

The informal carer is not one of the persons who are required by the Act to follow the Code of Practice (see Section 42(4) and Chapter 17). This does not mean, however, that Codes of Practice are irrelevant to the informal carer. On the contrary the view was expressed by the Joint Committee that:

> We agree that only those acting in a professional capacity or for remuneration should be under a duty to abide by the Codes of Practice. However we believe that family members and carers should be strongly encouraged to follow the Codes of Practice.[4] [Authors note: originally it was envisaged that there would be several Codes of Practice].

The Joint Committee felt that it was inappropriate to impose upon informal carers a strict requirement to act in accordance with the Codes of Practice, but they did consider it essential that the informal carers have sufficient guidance and assistance, both to promote good practice and also to impress upon them the seriousness of their actions and the need to be accountable for them.[5]

Failure by informal carer to follow the Code of Practice

What would happen if the informal carer failed to follow the Code of Practice? What redress does P have?

The answer depends on the circumstances and the seriousness of the informal carer's conduct and failures in respect of P. For example a minor failure would probably have no consequences at all for P or for the carer, but a serious failure could lead to criminal or other proceedings (see Scenario L4).

Accountability

Informal carers may be held accountable for failures in fulfilling their duty of care to P. They could face civil and/or criminal proceedings.

Civil proceedings

In Chapter 11 on the protection of the vulnerable adult and accountability the law of negligence was discussed, and it was pointed out that health and social services professionals would be expected to provide the reasonable standard of care according to the Bolam Test.[6] The informal carer also owes a duty of care to P, who could be represented in a negligence action against the informal carer (see Chapter 11). The person alleged to be lacking the requisite mental capacity, represented by a litigation friend, would have to establish on a balance of probabilities that a duty of care was owed, that there had been a failure to follow a reasonable standard of care and therefore a breach of the duty of care, and that this breach had caused harm to the patient. How would the standard of care to be provided by an informal carer be measured?

In the past the courts have used the standard of the reasonable man on the Clapham omnibus. The question would be asked, what would a reasonable person, caring for the personal wellbeing and/or the property and finances of this person who lacked specific mental capacities, expect to undertake, and what risks would he or she be reasonably expected to anticipate and to take steps to guard against? See Scenario L5.

The harm could be personal injury or death or it could be loss or damage to property. Clearly there is little point in suing the informal carer, if the latter lacks the resources to pay any compensation awarded or is not insured for such compensation payment. However there may be advantages to P, if it were to be established that the informal carer was not acting in P's best interests so that others could be appointed to oversee his personal care and welfare and his property and finance.

Criminal proceedings

An informal carer could be guilty of a criminal offence in respect of his or her care and treatment of the patient. Obviously any theft of P's property could be followed by criminal prosecution. The new offence created by the MCA could also apply to the informal carer. Under Section 44(2), if a person D has the care of a person P who lacks, or whom D reasonably believes to lack, capacity, then it is an offence to ill-treat or wilfully neglect that person. The offence is considered in Chapter 11.

Scenario L6 provides an example.

Advance decisions

Where a person (P) has drawn up an advance decision, it is likely that he or she has told his or her closest relatives or friends of its existence. If P then loses his or her mental capacity to make treatment and care decisions, then the informal carer should ensure that the existence of this advance decision is drawn to the attention of the health and social services professionals. It may be that the advance decision nominates a specific person to act on behalf of P, should P lose the requisite mental capacity. It is important that the informal carer appreciates that he or she has no power to overrule the contents of the advance decision. In addition unless P specified that the advance decision was to apply to life-sustaining treatments, then life-sustaining treatment should be given. For P's prohibition on life-sustaining treatment to be valid, P must have specified this in writing and signed it (or another person has signed it in P's presence and by P's direction, and this signature must have been made or acknowledged by P in the presence of a witness who signs it or acknowledges his or her signature in P's presence – see Chapter 9).

See Scenario L7.

Research

Where a person lacks the requisite mental capacity to give consent to research, there is a statutory duty upon the researcher to consult the informal carer about

P's participation in the research. The informal carer should ensure that he or she is given all the relevant information about the research and any likely risks or discomfort to P in taking part. The informal carer will be the person most concerned at protecting P's interests, and should check against any advance decision or advance statement drawn up by P as to whether he has recorded a refusal to participate.

The informal carer would also need to be vigilant throughout the research process and ensure that, at any time when it would appear that P is showing signs of resistance and objection to the research, P's involvement ceases, unless it can be justified because it is intended to protect him or her from harm or to reduce or prevent pain or discomfort. Considerable responsibility would appear to rest on the informal carer where P is taking part in the research, to ensure P's rights are safeguarded (see Chapter 10 and Scenario L8).

Independent mental capacity advocate

There is a statutory duty upon NHS organisations and local authorities to ensure that P is receiving the support of an independent mental capacity advocate when decisions over serious medical treatment, accommodation and action are being taken to protect a vulnerable adult. However this is subject to the organisation concerned being

> satisfied that there is no person, other than one engaged in providing care or treatment for P in a professional capacity or for remuneration, whom it would be appropriate for them to consult in determining what would be in P's best interests (Ss.37(1)(b), 38(1)(b) and 39(1)(b)).

This means that where there is an informal carer, then that person would be expected to represent and support P.

What if there is a dispute between the informal carer and those employed by the statutory authority over what would be in P's best interests? Possibly in such circumstances it could be argued that it would not be appropriate for that person to be consulted over what was in P's best interests. This would enable the authorities to arrange for the appointment of the independent mental capacity advocate (IMCA), even though an informal carer existed. This is further discussed in Chapter 8 on the IMCA and Scenarios E.

In addition if for any reason the informal carer or other family member or friend refused to act as the representative of P, or was too ill or there were some other reason why it was not appropriate to rely upon them (for example they might live too far away), then in such circumstances it would be necessary for an IMCA to be appointed in the situations set out in the statute and the regulations (i.e. serious medical treatment, accommodation by NHS or LHA and care reviews). (Where an IMCA is required for protection purposes there is no requirement that there should be reliance upon a family member or friend or informal carer to act as an advocate, but an IMCA may be appointed.)

See Scenario L9.

Access to personal information

Frequently when an informal carer is the main person responsible for the personal welfare of a person lacking mental capacity, the informal carer will be the person from whom professionals seek information as to the personal history, health and financial situation. The informal carer would probably pass any necessary information on, if he or she is satisfied that that would be in the best interests of P. However there may be situations where the informal carer is seeking information from paid carers. What rules then apply? Scenario L10 explores a possible situation.

The basic principle is that health and social services professionals can disclose confidential information to informal carers if it is in the best interests of the person who lacks the requisite capacity to give consent. The disclosure would not include information which P has specifically asked not to be disclosed, and must be confined to what is relevant for the informal carer to have in P's best interests. There would be a duty on the informal carer to respect the duty of confidentiality so that this information was not passed on to anyone who did not need to have it in P's best interests (see **Principles of confidentiality and exceptions to that duty**).

The informal carer as donee of an LPA or deputy

Where the informal carer has been appointed as the donee of a lasting power of attorney or a deputy by the Court of Protection, and can therefore be viewed as the agent of P for specific purposes, then there are statutory provisions about the right of access to P's personal information under the Data Protection Act 1998. The deputy or a donee acting under a lasting power of attorney is able to obtain information as agent of P, which is relevant to the functions which he is undertaking and which is within the scope of his authority. The Information Commissioner has advised in the Legal Guidance which he has issued on the Data Protection Act 1998,[7] that an attorney acting under an enduring power of attorney or a receiver 'who has general authority to manage property and affairs' may make a subject access request. Therefore a deputy who has been granted authority to act only in relation to specific matters (rather than a general power) may make a subject access request on behalf of the person who lacks capacity, for such information as relates to the matter within his/her limited authority, without applying to the court.

The right of access would also be subject to those exceptions to subject access under the Data Protection regulations, i.e. access will be refused to information which could cause serious harm to the mental or physical health or condition of the applicant or another person, or which would disclose information about the identity of a third person, not being a health professional involved in the care of P, where the third person has not agreed to that identification.

Principles of confidentiality and exceptions to that duty

Any informal carer must ensure that P's right to a private life under Article 8 of the European Convention on Human Rights is respected, and also recognise the duty to respect the confidentiality of information which he or she obtains about the personal health and welfare or property and financial matters of P. This duty of confidentiality is subject to specified exceptions:

- disclosure with the consent of P (but this implies that P has the mental capacity to give consent)
- disclosure in the best interests of P
- disclosure required by court
- disclosure required by Act of Parliament (e.g. notification of infectious diseases, Prevention of Terrorism Acts, road traffic legislation)
- disclosure required in the public interest (e.g. if serious harm is feared to P or another person).

Any informal carer disclosing information confidential to the patient would be advised to keep details of what has been disclosed and the justification for the disclosure.

Documentation and the informal carer

It would be unfortunate if the effect of the MCA were to lead to a heavy burden of paperwork on the informal carer. However it is clear that in cases of potential dispute, an informal carer would need to keep some documents or records relating to the actions he or she had taken and discussions with others about whether or not P lacked the requisite mental capacity, and the factors which were taken into account in determining P's best interests. For example when determining what are in the best interests of P, the MCA requires the decision maker to take into account all the relevant circumstances as well as the list of criteria specified in Section 4. It would be of value if the informal carer made a note of the circumstances which had been taken into account in making any specified decision.

It is possible that some of the charities representing specific conditions and illnesses which could lead to impairment of mental capacity would design simple forms which an informal carer could keep (see list of websites setting out some of these organisations). Any informal carer who takes on a formal role such as the donee of a lasting power of attorney, or is appointed as a deputy by the Court of Protection, would be required to keep records of his or her actions. The deputy in particular may be required to provide the OPG with a report of the actions which have been taken.

The court may require a deputy to give to the Public Guardian such security as the court thinks fit for the due discharge of his functions and to submit to the Public Guardian such reports at such times or at such intervals as the court may direct (S.19(9)).

In addition since the deputy is entitled to be reimbursed out of P's property for his reasonable expenses in discharging his functions and can, if the court so directs, obtain remuneration out of P's property for discharging his functions, it is vital that the deputy keeps records of both expenses and remuneration, since these will be subject to scrutiny by the OPG.

See Scenario L11.

Record keeping guidance

In the absence of any advice from the Department of Health or organisations concerned with specific conditions where mental incapacity can arise, the following brief guidelines for records to be kept by an informal carer may prove useful.
Records should:

- identify problems that have arisen, the decisions made and the action taken
- be factual, consistent and accurate
- be written as soon as possible after an event has occurred
- be accurately dated, timed and signed
- not include meaningless phrases, irrelevant speculation and offensive subjective statements
- be readable on any photocopies
- be written, wherever possible, with the involvement of P.

where records include financial information about expenses of the carer or purchases made on behalf of P, a simple cash book should suffice with details and dates of entries.

How long should any such documentation be kept?

Where the carer is looking after P, a person who lacks mental capacity, then the time limits for court action on behalf of P do not start until P's death. The advice is therefore that any records should be kept for three years after P's death. This is specially so where he or she has suffered an injury for which compensation may be payable. Scenario L12 illustrates the effect of the time limits. Scenario L13 illustrates many of the issues faced by the informal carer.

Conclusions

Informal carers should be comforted by the fact that although the MCA would at first sight appear to be an overwhelming change in the lives of those who lack the requisite mental capacity, and therefore a huge burden on the informal carer, in practice many of the principles set down in the Act reflect the position which already existed at common law (i.e. judge made or case law). In addition many of the new tools such as the lasting power of attorney (LPA), the new Court of Protection with its jurisdiction to cover matters of personal welfare in addition to property and financial affairs and the power to appoint deputies, should make it easier for decisions to be made and disputes to be resolved. Most informal carers already act in the best interests of those they care for and who lack mental capacity. It is hoped that there will be monitoring of the Act following its implementation, to assess the extent to which the hopes of its supporters have been fulfilled and to identify any further measures which may be required.

References

1   Code of Practice for the Mental Capacity Act 2005. Department of Constitutional Affairs February 2007 para 1.1. TSO, London.
2   The MCA 2005 (Independent Mental Capacity Advocates)(General) Regulations 2006 (SI 2006/1832).
3   The MCA 2005 (Independent Mental Capacity Advocates)(Expansion of Role) Regulations 2006 (SI 2006/2883).
4   Joint Cttee Chapter 12 para 232.
5   *Ibid.* para 232.
6   *Bolam* v. *Friern Hospital Management Committee* [1957] 1 WLR 582.
7   See the Information Commissioner's website at www.informationcommissioner.gov.uk; and see para 4.1.7 of the Legal Guidance.

Scenarios L
The Informal Carer

Introduction

These Scenarios are designed to provide discussion of some of the areas of the Mental Capacity Act 2005 which may have an impact on the role of the informal carer. They should be read in conjunction with Chapter 15 and with the other specialist chapters.

Duty of care

> ### Scenario L1: Informal caring.
>
> Mavis is caring for her son, David, who has Down's syndrome. He hates having a bath or shower, but she insists that he has a bath or shower at least once a week. He complains to a young care assistant at the day centre, who says that he has rights under the Mental Capacity Act (MCA) and should seek legal advice.

It is unfortunate that the advice given to David is more likely to lead to dispute and disruption to the relationship of David and his mother, Mavis than to a resolution. The starting point of the problem must be the issue of competence. Does David have the mental capacity to make decisions about bathing and personal hygiene?

If the answer to that question is 'yes', then he should be left with that power, albeit his carers may impress upon him the benefits to himself and to others of his being clean and sweet smelling. Maybe something as simple as a choice of soap and other items may influence David's decision.

If the answer to the question is that David lacks the mental capacity to decide whether or not he should have a bath, then his mother has to act in his best interests, following the principles set out in Section 1 of the MCA (see Chapter 3) and applying the criteria for the best interests as set out in Section 4 (see Chapter 5). It is hopefully not an issue with which lawyers should be concerned. However if he resists bathing or showering, what action can his mother take? She may be able to obtain advice from the day centre on how to overcome David's reluctance to be washed. It may be that there is some specific fear which he has which can be assuaged. It may be that the day centre would be prepared to arrange for him to be bathed or showered at the day centre.

Could restraint be used?

Mavis may feel that she needs to use some form of restraint on David to encourage him to be bathed.

She would be bound by Section 6 of the MCA, which is considered in Chapter 5 on best interests.

If Mavis does an act that is intended to restrain David, as well as following the basic principles of the MCA and using the criteria of best interests as set out in Section 4 (see Chapter 5), she must satisfy two conditions:

1. she must reasonably believe that the restraint is necessary to do the act in order to prevent harm to David, and
2. the restraint which she uses must be a proportionate response to the likelihood of David's suffering harm, and the seriousness of that harm.

Mavis uses restraint on David if she either uses, or threatens to use, force to secure the doing of an act which David resists, or she restricts David's liberty of movement, whether or not David resists.

It may be that Mavis will need the assistance of another carer to ensure that David is bathed. If so they must ensure that only reasonable restraint is used and it is in proportion to David's suffering if he should be unwashed.

Informal carer as donee of a lasting power of attorney

Scenario L2: Informal carer as a donee of a lasting power of attorney.

Victoria appoints her son, John as the donee of a lasting power of attorney. He accepts the appointment for attorney of both personal welfare and finance and property. The respective forms are completed and executed by Victoria and John. Both powers of attorney give general powers to act in the best interests of Victoria. Subsequently Victoria suffers brain damage during a surgical operation and is transferred to a care home. John disputes with the care home manager as to whether his mother should be given antibiotics for a chest infection. He considers that she is unlikely to be discharged from the care home and return home, so he arranges for her house to be put up for sale. His sister, June, who disagreed that John should have had the power of attorney, believes that he is not acting in the best interests of their mother. She considers that the mother should receive active treatment and that the house should remain unsold, until such time as there was a clear prognosis of her mother.

Initially every effort should be made to resolve this dispute between brother and sister by discussion and counselling. The Code of Practice describes a similar disagreement where:

> Mrs Roberts has dementia and lacks capacity to decide where she should live. She currently lives with her son. But her daughter has found a care home where she thinks her mother will get better care. Her brother disagrees. Mrs Roberts is upset by this family dispute, and so her son and daughter decide to try mediation. The mediator believes that Mrs Roberts is able to communicate her feelings and agrees to take on the case. During the sessions, the mediator helps them to focus on their mother's best interests rather than imposing their own views. In the end, everybody agrees that Mrs Roberts should continue to live with her son. But they agree to review the situation again in six months to see if the care home might then be better for her.[1]

Another example of the use of informal methods of dispute resolution could be where parents of a person lacking the requisite mental capacity were divorced and were in disagreement over where their son should live. It may be possible for the social worker to resolve the dispute by arranging counselling, advice and mediation in order to reach a consensus decision. In this way the need to involve the Court of Protection or the appointment of a deputy could be avoided.

In contrast to these two situations, in the Scenario L2 John has a lasting power of attorney, with powers to make decisions on Victoria's personal welfare. He would have a duty to act according to the instructions in the LPA, and if these were only general then he would have to use the criteria of best interests as set down in Section 4 of the MCA (see Chapter 5). John cannot assume that it is in Victoria's best interests for her not to have life-sustaining treatment. If the dispute cannot be resolved, then the most appropriate action would be to contact the Office of the Public Guardian (OPG) for guidance and advice. Staff at the OPG should be able to provide advice and guidance on the appropriate steps to take. If the guidance fails to resolve the issue then an application could be made to the Court of Protection for a declaration as to what was in Victoria's best interests.

Informal carer as a deputy appointed by the Court of Protection

Scenario L3: Informal carer as a deputy appointed by the Court of Protection.

Stuart received compensation following a serious road traffic accident which left him with severe brain damage. He is living at home, supported by his parents and paid carers who provide 24-hour coverage. His father, Ralph, has been appointed as deputy by the Court of Protection to supervise payments from Stuart's trust fund and pay for his day-to-day care. Stuart's sister, Enid, believes that the father is not spending the money appropriately. Ralph has a gambling addiction and she considers that more could be done to improve Stuart's quality of life.

In the first instance Enid should check with her father on what is being spent on Stuart's behalf, and if she continues to be dissatisfied, then she could contact the Office of the Public Guardian for guidance. She could ask the OPG to investigate the role of the father as deputy. He would probably be asked to report on how Stuart's moneys were being spent and to produce an account. If Enid remained dissatisfied with the father's actions as deputy, the OPG might decide to appoint a visitor. Eventually it may be necessary for an application to go to the Court of Protection for an order replacing Ralph as deputy and making orders as to the future care of Stuart's finances.

Misappropriation of funds by a deputy could lead to criminal prosecution.

Informal carer and the Code of Practice

As discussed in Chapter 15, the informal carer is not one of the specified persons who is bound to follow the guidance in the Code of Practice under Section 42(4). However the general philosophy of those debating the Bill was that the informal carer would find the Code of Practice useful guidance, and therefore be inclined to follow it. What are the sanctions if they do not? Scenario L4 looks at a possible situation.

Scenario L4: Informal carer and the Code of Practice.

Brenda lived with her mother, Hilda, who had had multiple sclerosis for twenty years. Hilda was confined to a wheel chair and had had a lift installed in the house. Recently Hilda's condition had deteriorated, and there were times when she was unable to speak and make her views known. Prior to this she had been discussing with Brenda the possibility of her moving into a care home. Brenda was opposed to this, since the house was in her mother's name and she was concerned that if her mother moved to residential accommodation the house would have to be sold to pay the fees and she might be evicted. She considered therefore that it was better if Hilda was not encouraged to communicate and that the status quo was maintained for as long as possible. The district nurse who visited Hilda was concerned that a speech therapist had not been brought in to assist Hilda's communication. When she suggested this to Brenda, Brenda said that there was no need as she could understand Hilda and was meeting all her requirements.

In Scenario L4 it is clear that in failing to assist Hilda in making her own decisions and communicating, Brenda is failing to follow the basic principles of the MCA as set out in Section 1 (see Chapter 3):

A person is not to be treated as unable to make a decision unless all practicable steps to help him to do so have been taken without success. (S.1(3))

Brenda is also not facilitating Hilda's capacity to communicate and is therefore in breach of Section 3(2) of the MCA:

A person is not to be regarded as unable to understand the information relevant to a decision if he is able to understand an explanation of it given to him in a way that is appropriate to his circumstances (using simple language, visual aids or any other means).

In addition Brenda has failed to follow the guidance in the discussion of principle 2 (Paragraphs 2.6–2.9) and chapter 3 of the Code of Practice on the steps which can be taken in assisting Hilda to communicate and make her own decisions.

In particular Brenda has not done the following:

- Use any aids which might be helpful, such as pictures, photographs, pointing boards or other signalling tools, symbols and objects, videos or tapes.
- Find out what the person is used to – for example Makaton or some way of communicating that is only known to those who are close to them.
- If the person has hearing difficulties, consider using appropriate visual aids or sign language.
- Consider using any appropriate mechanical devices such as voice synthesisers or other computer equipment.
- In extreme cases of communication difficulties, consider other forms of professional help, such as an expert in clinical neuropsychology.[2]

What sanctions are available against Brenda?

Since Brenda appears to be the main carer, it would be difficult for health or social services to take action to protect Hilda's interests unless there was clear evidence that Brenda was acting contrary to Hilda's best interests. Unfortunately it may be easier to prove financial improprieties by an informal carer, than produce evidence of a failure to comply with the MCA statutory requirements. Her failure to follow the Code of Practice is unlikely to result in action being taken. Only if there were evidence of abuse or a breach of Section 44 of the MCA (ill-treatment or wilful neglect), is there likely to be intervention by the statutory authorities. If Hilda had other children or friends who were concerned about the fact that her communication skills were deteriorating and she was not therefore making her own decisions, then there is more likely to be intervention on behalf of Hilda. However the social services have a statutory duty to ensure that actions are taken in the best interests of Hilda and they will be required to monitor the situation, provide appropriate advice to Brenda and take action if necessary to secure the protection of Hilda.

Informal carer and civil proceedings

Scenario L5: Informal carer and civil proceedings.

On the facts of Scenario L4, Brenda left her mother locked in the living room when she went shopping. She argued that it was to protect the mother who might go into the kitchen and harm herself. The district nurse was concerned when visiting one day that she could not get into the house, but tried to talk to Hilda through the living room window. The district nurse considered that Brenda was acting illegally and if Hilda could not be safely left on her own then Brenda should arrange for carers to be present when she left the house. She felt that it was a breach of Hilda's human rights and also a breach of the duty of care which Brenda owed to Hilda.

In Scenarios L4 and L5 Brenda is in breach of the duty of care which she owes to her mother. She would also appear to be in breach of some Articles of the European Convention on Human Rights:

- Article 3   No one shall be subjected to torture or to inhuman or degrading treatment or punishment.
- Article 5   Everyone has the right to liberty and security of person. No one shall be deprived of his liberty save in the following cases and in accordance with a procedure prescribed by law.

However a civil action brought against Brenda is probably unlikely to be an effective remedy for Hilda. A basic principle of legal action is that there is little point in suing a person who would be unable to pay compensation, and it is not compensation which Hilda requires but a regime where her human rights are protected and her quality of life enhanced. Clearly a judgment has to be made on the balance of benefits and risks to Hilda in determining what action to take in relation to Brenda.

It may be that with help, support and advice, an agreement could be reached with Brenda to ensure that Hilda's quality of life was protected. For example it may be possible to point out that since Brenda lives in the house with Hilda, social services could not evict Brenda in order to fund the means tested benefits were Hilda to move to a care home. It may be a situation where social services might consider the benefits of the appointment of a deputy by the Court of Protection and make the appropriate application. If there were evidence of ill-treatment and wilful neglect by Brenda, then different considerations would apply (see Scenario L6).

Informal carer and criminal proceedings

Scenario L6: Informal carer and criminal proceedings.

Rachel lived with her sister, Mary, who had severe learning disabilities, with a mental age of 5 years. Mary attended a day centre on weekdays whilst Rachel was working. At weekends, other relatives would occasionally take Mary on outings, but usually Mary stayed at home. One morning when Rachel was out shopping, Mary used some matches and set fire to the living room sofa. Firemen were called, but Mary suffered burns and damage from smoke inhalation. Police are investigating the possibility of a criminal prosecution being brought against Rachel.

Section 44 creates a new criminal offence of ill-treatment and wilful neglect (see Chapter 11). Is Rachel guilty of a criminal offence under this section? Has she wilfully neglected Mary? Much of course would depend upon the details of Mary's condition which are not given in this Scenario. Should Mary have had a carer with her at all times? Was the failure to ensure that the matches were locked away from Mary's use evidence of wilful neglect? Was it reasonably foreseeable to Rachel that if Mary were left alone, harm could befall her? Wilful implies an intentional disregard for the possible consequences of Mary's being left on her own.

Informal carers and advance decisions

Scenario L7: Informal carer and an advance decision.

Harold drew up an advance decision following a diagnosis of multiple sclerosis. In this he said that were he to require ventilation, artificial nutrition or hydration, he would not wish to be given that and would prefer to be allowed to die. He told his wife, Angela, what he had done and asked her to witness the document. He carried a copy at all times in his wallet. He was injured in a shopping arcade when a ladder used by painters fell onto him. He was taken unconscious to hospital, accompanied by Angela. The nurses found the advance decision in his wallet. Angela said that it did not apply to this situation, since he was thinking of an intolerable state during the later stages of multiple sclerosis. The consultant said that he needed to be ventilated and said that he would have made preparations for him to be taken to intensive care, but in the light of the advance decision, he decided that he should be allowed to die. What is the legal situation?

Where there is a doubt as to whether an advance decision is applicable to a given situation, then there would have to be a referral to the Court of Protection for a declaration as to its applicability (see Chapter 9). Section 25(4)(c) states that an advance decision is not applicable to the treatment in question if there are reasonable grounds for believing that circumstances exist which P did not anticipate at the time of the advance decision, and which would have affected his decision had he anticipated them (see also Scenario F3). When Harold drew up the advance decision he was contemplating the final stages of multiple sclerosis, he was not contemplating being injured by a falling ladder. It is therefore likely that the Court of Protection would hold that the advance decision did not apply to his being ventilated at that time. Since the decision of the Court of Protection may take some time, the provisions of S.26(5) are extremely important, since this subsection states that:

Nothing in an apparent advance decision stops a person:

a. providing life-sustaining treatment, or
b. doing any act he reasonably believes to be necessary to prevent a serious deterioration in P's condition,

while a decision as respects any relevant issue is sought from the court.

Harold can receive all necessary life saving treatment whilst the validity is determined.

Informal carer and research

> **Scenario L8: Informal carer and research.**
>
> Margaret's son, Henry, has cerebral palsy. His speech therapist, Jenny, asks him if he would take part in a research project to test out new equipment for communicating. Margaret is unhappy at Henry's involvement and does not consider that he has the mental capacity to agree to participation in the research. What action can she take?

Margaret would first of all take her concerns to the researcher, Jenny. She would want to receive the details of the research project and details of its approval by the research ethics committee (REC). She would also want to know how, if at all, Jenny assessed Henry's ability to give consent to participation. If she were not satisfied with the answers she could endeavour to raise the issues with those responsible for the research project (if that were someone different from Jenny). Ultimately she could apply to the Court of Protection for a declaration on the capacity of Henry to give consent to research participation. Clearly it is open to Henry at any time to withdraw from the research project.

Informal carer and the independent mental capacity advocate

> **Scenario L9: Informal carer and independent mental capacity advocate.**
>
> Cathy and Mark care for their son, Andrew who has learning disabilities. Andrew attends a day centre and works on a project packaging screws, for which he is paid pocket money. Working with him is Sandra, who also has severe learning disabilities and lives at home with her parents. He and Sandra decide that they would like to live together and move out of their respective family homes. They are encouraged by the day centre manager to plan for this outcome and discussions commence with social services to find appropriate accommodation. When Cathy and Mark hear of the plan they are opposed to it. They consider that they are giving Andrew a good quality of life and that it would not be in his best interests to move out. The local authority knows that under Section 39 of the MCA (see Chapter 8) it has a responsibility to seek advice from an independent mental capacity advocate (IMCA), when it is considering the provision of residential accommodation for a person P who lacks capacity to agree to the arrangements. Cathy and Mark however claim that they are able to be consulted on the question of Andrew's accommodation and therefore an IMCA is not required.

In Scenario L9, the first question to be asked is: Does Andrew have the necessary mental capacity to decide if he wishes to move out of his parents' home and into alternative accommodation? If the answer to that question is 'yes', then there is no question of an IMCA being appointed and being consulted, though he may need the services of a solicitor to assist him in furthering his ambitions.

If however Andrew is assessed as lacking the requisite capacity, then the possibility of the appointment of an IMCA must be considered. The duty to seek the advice of an IMCA arises 'if the local authority is satisfied that there is no person, other than one engaged in providing care or treatment for P in a professional capacity or for remuneration, whom it would be appropriate for them to consult about P's best interests'. Would Cathy and Mark be seen as persons whom it would be appropriate to consult about Andrew's best interests? Even though they disagree with Andrew's wishes, they would still be able to provide the local authority with information about Andrew. They would probably not, however, be best placed to provide an independent view as to what would be in Andrew's best interests. However 'independence' from those consulted is not a requirement of the MCA. Case law will eventually determine whether people in Cathy's and Mark's situation come within the definition of 'appropriate for them to consult about P's best interests'.

Access to personal information and the duty of confidentiality

Scenario L10: Informal carer and confidentiality.

Tom was admitted to a care home with incipient Alzheimer's disease. He was visited regularly by his daughter, Janice who was concerned that he seemed to be getting very weak and lethargic. She made inquiries from the home manager and discovered that blood tests had been taken three months before and he had been found to be anaemic. He was given iron supplements and extra vitamins. She was concerned that she had not been told about this change in his condition and was anxious that further tests should be carried out to discover if there was any underlying cause of the anaemia. The home manager stated that since Tom was 92 years, it was not thought that any further tests were in his best interests, since it could reveal a chronic condition for which blood transfusions may be required and hospitalisation. Such further interventions would only cause him unnecessary discomfort and therefore were not felt to be in his best interests. Janice disagreed and considered that she should have been kept fully informed of his condition. In addition she believed that any underlying condition should be treated even if he had to be admitted to hospital. What is the law?

Two separate issues are raised by Scenario L10. The first is, what rights does Janice have as the daughter and possibly next of kin of Tom to be told confidential information about his condition? The second issue is that of the determination of Tom's 'best interests'.

a. Should Janice have been told about Tom's condition?

The care home staff have a duty of confidentiality towards Tom. If Tom had the capacity to give consent, then he could agree that personal information about his condition could be passed to his daughter, Janice. However he appears to lack the capacity to give consent to this (though this would have to be checked). The care home staff would be entitled to pass on to Janice any personal information about Tom if he lacked this requisite capacity, provided that it could be shown that it is in the best interests of Tom for Janice to be told.

The Code of Practice chapter 16[3] gives advice on confidentiality, and the National Health Service Code of Confidentiality[4] provides further guidance.

It is no easy task for the care home staff to determine what information should be given to Janice and what should be withheld, but they need to make this judgment and also document what information has been released and why. Clearly if Janice considers that Tom is not receiving the appropriate investigations into his condition, she would need to be given sufficient information to satisfy herself that the GP and the care home were acting in Tom's best interests.

b. What are Tom's best interests?

The definition of best interests is considered in Chapter 5, and the same criteria (set down in Section 4) would apply to decision making, whether by a professional or by an informal carer.

In answering the question 'What is in Tom's best interests?', account would have to be taken of his general health and well-being, overall prognosis and any beliefs and views he had expressed when he had the requisite mental capacity. Section 4(5) states that:

> Where the determination relates to life-sustaining treatment he (i.e. the decision maker) must not, in considering whether the treatment is in the best interests of the person concerned, be motivated by a desire to bring about his death.

In other words carers, whether professional or informal, cannot say to themselves that Tom would be better off dead and so it is not worth carrying out tests on him.

Documentation and the informal carer

Scenario L11: The informal carer and documentation.

Joan cares for her mother, Sarah, who lives alone. Joan regularly shops for her and collects her pension. Joan's brother, Malcolm is convinced that Joan is using Sarah's money for herself and not spending it on Sarah. Joan denies that.

If Joan were able to produce for Malcolm a cash book relating to the receipts and payments on Sarah's behalf, this might help convince him that Joan was not defrauding their mother. It may be that Joan has been appointed as an appointee by the Department for Work and Pensions (DWP) to claim, receive benefits and spend money on Sarah's behalf. If Malcolm is not satisfied by Joan's evidence he could apply to the DWP, stating that Joan is not acting in Sarah's best interests. If his allegations prove correct, then Joan could be removed as appointee.[5] Regulation 33 of the Social Security (Claims and Payments) Regulations 1987[6] enables the statutory appointment of an appropriate person to receive and deal with the pension.

Informal carer and time limits

> ### Scenario L12: Informal carer and limitation of time for bringing action.
>
> James, who is now 35, has Down's syndrome and has always lived in the family home with his widowed mother, Janice. When he was 22 he was accidentally scalded when Janice put him in a bath without checking the water first. She dressed the wounds herself and she did not think that he needed hospitalisation. Some years later a paid carer enquired about the scars on James' legs and Janice explained how it had happened. The care assistant felt that James should obtain some compensation from the insurance policy which covered the house. Janice felt that it was too long ago to bother about it.

The usual time limit for bringing a court action in respect of personal injury is three years from the injury occurring or three years from the knowledge that this has occurred. However there is an exception to this time limit in respect of children and those who are under a mental disability. The time limit within which children have to bring a legal action does not start to run until the child becomes an adult at 18 years. For those under a mental disability, the time limit within which the court action must be commenced does not start to run until the disability ends. Because James in Scenario L12 lacks the requisite mental capacity to bring a court action, there is no time limit on suing for compensation as long as he is alive. If Janice's insurance cover provides for accident insurance, then James could bring a claim on the basis of his mother's negligence in causing him to be scalded. The fact that the accident occurred over 13 years ago would not be a defence. Clearly any record made by Janice at the time would be essential evidence.

Multiple issues

Scenario L13 illustrates the multiple issues which an informal carer may face.

Scenario L13: Multiple issues.

Stan, aged 35 years, has Prader-Willi syndrome and is looked after by his elderly parents. He has the ability to make decisions about his clothes and activities, but his parents lock the fridge and the pantry and he has no choice over the food which he is given. They find him eating from a box containing a gross of chocolate bars and realise that he has stolen it from a nearby shop. They go to the shop to return the half eaten box and pay for the bars which Stan has eaten. They ask the shopkeepers not to report him to the police because he has stolen before and they are afraid of his being sent to prison.

The first question to be asked in Scenario L13 is the level of mental capacity of Stan. Does he have the capacity to make his own decisions? Whilst he was under a compulsion to eat, did he realise that stealing from the shop was a crime? It must also be established if it is in his best interests to face the consequences of his crime or to be protected as his parents wish. It may be for example that it would be in Stan's best interests to be cared for in a community home, where he was taught to control his eating, where he learnt to accept the consequences of his wrong doing and where he could become more independent. The key principles of *Valuing People*[7] (Rights, Independence, Choice and Inclusion; see Chapter 11) should be observed in developing a care plan for Stan. Whilst it is not impossible for these principles to be followed by informal carers, there may come a time where it is in the best interests of the person to move to a care home. If his parents opposed such a move then it may be appropriate for an independent mental capacity advocate to be appointed (see Chapter 8).

Check list for informal carer

- Is there a decision to be made?
- Can the assumption that P has the requisite mental capacity be followed?
- If not, how is P's capacity to make that specific decision assessed?
- Can the Code of Practice over what has to be taken into account in determining capacity be followed?
- If capacity to make that specific decision is lacking, how are P's best interests decided upon?
- Can the criteria set out in Section 4 (Chapter 5) be applied?
- Should others be involved in the decision making, such as NHS or local authority staff?
- What documentation for the basis for the decision making and the actions which have taken should be kept?

References

1 Code of Practice for the Mental Capacity Act 2005. Department of Constitutional Affairs February 2007 para 15.09. TSO, London.

2   Draft Code of Practice for the Mental Capacity Act 2005. Department of Constitutional Affairs 2006 para 3.35. TSO, London and see para 3.11 of finalised Code of Practice.
3   Code of Practice for the Mental Capacity Act 2005. Department of Constitutional Affairs February 2007 para 16.24. TSO, London.
4   Confidentiality: NHS Code of Practice, 7 November 2003. Available on the Department of Health website. Gateway reference 2003; product 33837.
5   www.dwp.gov.uk/publications/dwp/2005/gl21_apr.pdf
6   Social Security (Claims and Payments) Regulations 1987 (SI 1987/1968).
7   Department of Health (2001) *Valuing People: A New Strategy for Learning Disability for the 21st Century*. White Paper CM 5086.

16 Wales

Introduction

A referendum was held on 18 September 1997 which supported the devolution of specific powers to a Welsh Assembly. Subsequently the Government of Wales Act 1998 established the National Assembly for Wales (NAW). This is the representative body with legislative powers. It has 60 elected members and meets in the Senedd in Cardiff. Specific powers to make subordinate legislation, i.e. statutory instruments, were devolved to the NAW.[1] This meant that whilst the main legislative function still remained with the United Kingdom Parliament in Westminster, the NAW had the power to vary the details as to how that legislation will be implemented. For example the NAW set different rates for prescription charges from those which applied in England and from 2 April 2007 abolished them completely.

As a consequence of the Government of Wales Act 2006, from May 2007 the Welsh Assembly Government was established as an entity separate from but accountable to the National Assembly of Wales. This meant that all executive and regulatory functions transferred to the Welsh Assembly Government and are legally expressed as exercisable by the 'Welsh Ministers' and not by the NAW. The First Minister appointed by the Queen on the nomination of the Assembly appoints other Ministers and Deputy Ministers with her approval. These Ministers act on behalf of the Crown, but would have to resign if they lost the confidence of the Assembly. The Government of Wales Act creates a new executive structure for the Assembly, enhances the Assembly's law making powers and reforms the electoral system. The Welsh Assembly Government (WAG) is the devolved government for Wales. It is led by the First Minister and is responsible for health, education, economic development, culture, the environment and transport. The National Health Service (Wales) Act 2006 places the statutory responsibility for promoting and providing the health service in Wales on the Welsh Ministers.

Wales and the Mental Capacity Act 2005

It follows from the above that the Mental Capacity Act 2005 applies to Wales, but the Act recognises that there can be separate provisions in certain matters for Wales. These are collated briefly below. In particular the Mental Capacity Act 2005 enables certain regulations to be drawn up by the Welsh Assembly Government. These have therefore been subject to separate consultation in Wales. Wales uses the same Code of Practice for the Mental Capacity Act (MCA) as England. However the Lord Chancellor is statutorily bound to consult the NAW before preparing or revising a code.

The areas where Wales has its own Statutory Instruments are:

- definition of the Appropriate Body in research
- loss of capacity during research regulations
- Independent Mental Capacity Advocacy Service regulations

Research

Section 30(1) gives the 'appropriate authority' power to draw up regulations specifying who can give approval to a research project (other than a clinical trial research project). Appropriate authority includes the NAW. Consultation on the regulations to define the appropriate body which could give approval to research projects and on the regulations for arrangements where a person had given consent to a study but had lost capacity before the end of the project, commenced in August 2006.

The appropriate body in relation to a research project in the Welsh Regulations is:

A committee (or other body)

a. established to advise on, or on matters which include, the ethics of intrusive research in relation to people who lack capacity to consent to it; and
b. recognised for those purposes by the National Assembly for Wales.[2]

The appropriate body regulations came into force for the purpose of enabling applications for approval in relation to research to be made on 1 July 2007 and for all other purposes on 1 October 2007.

Loss of capacity during a research project

Section 34 of the MCA enabled regulations to be drawn up to cover the situation where P had consented to take part in a research project begun before the commencement of Section 30 (31 March 2008), but before the conclusion of the project lost capacity to consent to continue to take part in it, and research for the purpose of the project would be unlawful by virtue of Section 30 of the Act. The Welsh regulations[3] are almost identical to those applying to England but for convenience are given below.

The regulations provide that in such circumstances, despite P's loss of capacity, research for the purposes of the project may be carried out using information or material relating to him if:

(a) the project satisfies the requirements set out in Schedule 1,

(b) all the information or material relating to P which is used in the research was obtained before P's loss of capacity,

(c) information or material is either

i data within the meaning of Section 1 of the Data Protection Act 1998 or

ii material which consists of and/or includes human cells or human deoxyribonucleic acid (DNA); and

(d) the person conducting the project ('R') takes in relation to P such steps as are set out in Schedule 2.

Schedule 1 is shown in Box 16.1.

Box 16.1: Schedule 1 to the Regulations on loss of capacity during the research project.

Requirements which the project must satisfy:

1. A protocol approved by an appropriate body and having effect in relation to the project makes provision for research to be carried out in relation to a person who has consented to take part in the project but loses capacity to consent to continue to take part in it.

2. The appropriate body must be satisfied that there are reasonable arrangements in place for ensuring that the requirements of Schedule 2 will be met. [See Box 16.2 for Schedule 2.]

Box 16.2: Schedule 2 to the Regulations on loss of capacity during the research project.

Steps which the person conducting the project must take:

1. R must take reasonable steps to identify a person who – (a) otherwise than in a professional capacity or for remuneration, is engaged in caring for P or is interested in P's welfare, and (b) is prepared to be consulted by R under this Schedule.

2. If R is unable to identify such a person he must, in accordance with guidance issued by the appropriate authority, nominate a person who – (a) is prepared to be consulted by R under this Schedule, but (b) has no connection with the project.

3. R must provide the person identified under paragraph 1, or nominated under paragraph 2, with information about the project and ask him – (a) for advice as to whether research of the kind proposed should be carried out in relation to P, and (b) what, in that person's opinion, P's wishes and feelings about such research being carried out would be likely to be if P had capacity in relation to the matter.

4. If, any time, the person consulted advises R that in his or her opinion P's wishes and feelings would be likely to lead him to wish to withdraw from the project if he had capacity in relation to the matter, R must ensure that P is withdrawn from it.

5. The fact that a person is the donee of a lasting power of attorney given by P, or is P's deputy, does not prevent him from being the person consulted under paragraphs 1 to 4.

6. R must ensure that nothing is done in relation to P in the course of the research which would be contrary to – (a) an advance decision of his which has effect, or (b) any other form of statement made by him and not subsequently withdrawn, of which R is aware.

7. The interests of P must be assumed to outweigh those of science and society.

8. If P indicates (in any way) that he wishes the research in relation to him to be discontinued, it must be discontinued without delay.

9. The research must be discontinued without delay if at any time R has reasonable grounds for believing that one or more of the requirements set out in Schedule 1 is no longer met or that there are no longer reasonable arrangements in place for ensuring that the requirements of this Schedule are being met in relation to P.

10. R must conduct the research in accordance with the provision made in the protocol referred to in paragraph 1 of Schedule 1 for research to be carried out in relation to a person who has consented to take part in the project but loses capacity to consent to take part in it.

Independent mental capacity advocate (IMCA)

Section 35(1) requires the 'appropriate authority' to make arrangements for IMCAs to be available to represent and support persons who lack the capacity to make decisions relating to serious medical treatment, accommodation arrangements by the National Health Service and accommodation arrangements by the local authority. Section 30(7) defines 'the appropriate authority' in relation to the provision of the services of independent mental capacity advocates in Wales, as the National Assembly for Wales.

Under Sections 37 and 38, the NAW has the power to prescribe by regulations the definition of 'NHS body' in relation to bodies in Wales for the purposes of Section 37.

Consultation commenced in August 2005 on the Independent Mental Capacity Advocacy Service in Wales[4] and closed on 31 October 2005. It covered the following topics:

- operation of the IMCA service
- functions of the IMCA
- serious medical treatments – definition
- extending the IMCA service.

Different options were put forward for each topic.

The consultation paper stressed that the WAG did not regard the new IMCA service as a replacement or substitute for independent advocacy as it is commonly understood and practised in the social care sector. The aims of the WAG were to ensure that the IMCA:

- provides a seamless service
- does not overlap with other statutory services
- does not result in a client having to change advocates simply because they now qualify for 'statutory' advocacy.

The cost as calculated by the Regulatory Impact Assessment was an estimate of £390K for the running of the IMCA scheme in Wales. It was emphasised that this was a tentative figure based on several planning assumptions on the cost and frequency of cases and there were many uncertainties.

Operation of the IMCA service

The three options for commissioning the IMCA service were:

- WAG could directly commission a small number of organisations to provide the service.
- LAs or Local Health Boards (LHBs) could commission individual advocates.
- LAs or LHBs could commission independent organisations.

WAG also questioned whether there should be national standards and if so, whether they should apply to individual advocates, to organisations or to both.

WAG questioned what current training was considered to be most appropriate for the IMCA service, what learning should be covered, who should develop, deliver and accredit the training and to what extent should the IMCA training link with other programmes.

On the issue of independence WAG questioned how the independence of IMCAs could be built into the service and how should independence be built into any regulations and/or commissioning guidance or contracts.

On the topic of monitoring and accountability, WAG questioned whether the guidance should specify key objectives for monitoring the IMCA service or should this be left to the commissioning organisations, who should monitor compliance with the standards, what role, if any, should the Assembly Inspectorates play in monitoring the IMCA services, and how should complaints made against an IMCA service be investigated and by whom.

Functions of the IMCA

The key functions of the IMCA are set out in Section 36(2) of the MCA as follows:

- representing and supporting the person who lacks capacity
- obtaining and evaluating information
- ascertaining the person's wishes and feelings, as far as possible

- ascertaining alternative courses of action – for example looking at different care arrangements or residential homes
- obtaining a further medical opinion, if necessary.

The NAW is empowered under Section 36(1) and 36(2) to make regulations concerning the steps that the IMCA should take in undertaking these functions. WAG consulted on whether there were any steps which should be outlined and whether these steps should be in the regulations or in the Code of Practice. It also consulted on Section 36(3) (which enabled regulations to be drawn up to cover the IMCA challenging the decision maker) should be implemented and whether the IMCA should be able to bring simple cases before the Court of Protection without legal representation and be able to challenge the decision that P lacked the requisite mental capacity. WAG also consulted on what possible additional functions for the IMCAs could be included in the regulations, and whether local organisations should have discretion on how they use additional functions. The involvement of IMCAs in care reviews was also the subject of consultation.

Extending the IMCA service

Section 41(1)(a) gives power to the appropriate authorities to prescribe additional circumstances in which the IMCA's advice must or may be sought. WAG therefore consulted on six options:

- doing nothing
- revising the assumptions regarding the IMCA
- providing an IMCA in cases of dispute
- providing an IMCA where requested by one of the parties
- providing an IMCA for extra care housing
- allowing the commissioner of the service to determine priorities.

It also raised more general questions over:

- whether the groups who qualify for an IMCA should be broadened
- should additional situations and circumstances be covered
- how should they prioritise to meet those most in need, and
- what makes someone who lacks capacity but has family and friends particularly vulnerable.

The IMCA Regulations for Wales

The Mental Capacity Act 2005 (Independent Mental Capacity Advocate) Regulations for Wales[5] were approved by the National Assembly for Wales on 13 March 2007 and came into force on 1 October 2007. Unlike the two sets of English regulations there is one set only for Wales.

The regulations define an NHS body as a LHB (see **Local health boards** on page 380), an NHS trust (where all or most of its hospitals, establishments and facilities are situated in Wales), or a Special Hospital Authority performing functions only or mainly in respect of Wales.

Serious medical treatment

The NAW has the power under Section 37(6) and (7) to set the definition of serious medical treatments in its regulations. It consulted on three options: listing specific treatments; focusing on the characteristics of the decision to be taken, and a combination of those two. Eventually it defined serious medical treatment in the same way as the English regulations, i.e.:

Treatment which involves providing, withdrawing or withholding treatment in circumstances where:

a. in a case where single treatment is being proposed, there is a fine balance between its benefits to a person (P) and the burdens and risks it is likely to entail for P,
b. in a case where there is a choice of treatments, a decision as to which one to use is finely balanced, or
c. what is proposed would be likely to involve serious consequences for P.

The appointment of independent mental capacity advocates

Subject to any directions which it receives from the WAG, a LHB must make such arrangements as it considers reasonable to enable IMCAs to be available to act in respect of persons usually resident in the area for which the LHB is established and to whom acts or decisions proposed under Section 37 (serious medical treatment), Section 38 (accommodation by NHS) and Section 39 (accommodation by LA), or under the regulations, relate.

These arrangements can be made with a provider of advocacy services.

No person may be instructed to act as an IMCA unless that person is approved by the LHB or is employed by a provider of advocacy services to act as an IMCA.

The LHB must be satisfied that the person satisfies the appointment requirements before that person can be approved as an IMCA.

The LHB must ensure that any provider of advocacy services with whom it makes arrangements is required to ensure that any person employed by that provider of advocacy services and who is made available to be instructed as an IMCA satisfies the appointment requirements.

The appointment requirements are that a person:

a. has appropriate experience or training or an appropriate combination of experience and training;
b. is of integrity and good character; and
c. will act independently of any person who instructs him or her to act as an IMCA and of any person who is responsible for an act or decision proposed under sections 37, 38 and 39 of the Act or under these Regulations.[6]

In determining whether a person meets the appointment requirement of having the appropriate experience or training, regard will be had to standards in guidance that may be issued by the Assembly.

Before deciding if a person is of integrity and good character, an enhanced criminal record certificate issued under S. 113A or S. 113B of the Police Act 1997 (as amended by Section 163 of the Serious Organised Crime and Police Act 2005) is required. If the purpose for which the certificate is required is not one prescribed under Section 163(2), a criminal record certificate issued under Section 113B of the Police Act 1997 is required.

Functions of an independent mental capacity advocate

The IMCA must determine in all the circumstances how best to represent and support P and must act in accordance with the following requirements. The IMCA must:

a. verify that the instructions have been issued by an NHS body or local authority;
b. to the extent that it is practicable and appropriate to do so

    i. interview P in private, and
    ii. examine the records relevant to P to which the IMCA has access under Section 35(6) of the Act;

c. to the extent that it is practicable and appropriate to do so, consult

    i. persons engaged in providing care or treatment for P in a professional capacity or for remuneration, and
    ii. other persons who may be in a position to comment on P's wishes, feelings, beliefs or values; and

d. take all practicable steps to obtain such other information about P, or the act or decision that is proposed in relation to P, as the IMCA considers necessary.[7]

The IMCA must evaluate all the information he has obtained for the purpose of:

a. ascertaining the extent of the support provided to P to enable him to participate in making any decision about the matter in relation to which the IMCA has been instructed;
b. ascertaining how P would feel, what P would wish and the beliefs and values that would be likely to influence P, if he had capacity in relation to the proposed act or decision;
c. ascertaining what alternative courses of action are available in relation to P;
d. where medical treatment is proposed for P, ascertaining whether he would be likely to benefit from a further medical opinion.[8]

The IMCA is required to prepare a report for the NHS body or the local authority who instructed him or her (reg 6(5)) and may include in the report such submissions as he considers appropriate in relation to P and the act or decision which is proposed in relation to P (reg 6(6)).

Challenges to decisions affecting persons who lack capacity

Where an IMCA has been instructed to act and a decision (including a decision as to P's capacity) is made in relation to P, then the IMCA has the same rights to challenge the decision as if he or she were a person (other than an IMCA) who:

a. was entitled, in accordance with Section 4(7)(b) of the Act, to be consulted in relation to a matter about which the IMCA is now instructed; or
b. it would otherwise be appropriate for an NHS body or a local authority to consult.

Extension of remit of the IMCA

Like the English regulations the Welsh IMCA regulations extend the remit of the IMCA to include the review of arrangements as to accommodation and adult protection cases.

Review of accommodation arrangements by NHS body or LA ('care reviews')

The NHS body or LA **may** instruct a person to act as an IMCA in relation to P in the following circumstances where:

a. an NHS body or LA has made arrangements for the provision of accommodation in a hospital or care home for a person who lacks capacity
b. an IMCA has been instructed in relation to those arrangements in accordance with Sections 38 or 39 and
c. that accommodation has been provided for P for a continuous period of 12 weeks or more
d. the NHS body or LA propose to review P's accommodation arrangements (whether under a care plan or otherwise) and
e. they are satisfied that there is no person, other than a person engaged in providing care or treatment for P in a professional capacity or for remuneration, whom it would be appropriate to consult in determining what would be in P's best interests; and
f. they are satisfied that it would be of benefit to P to be so represented and supported.[9]

Like the English regulations this, unlike the duties under Sections 37, 38 and 39, is a discretionary duty, and the Code of Practice has given guidance on when the power to appoint an IMCA should be used in care reviews.[10] The power only applies where the person lacks the requisite mental capacity. The power does not apply where accommodation is provided under an obligation imposed by the Mental Health Act 1983 (see Chapter 13 and Scenario E6).

Adult protection cases

Where an NHS body or LA proposes to take or proposes to arrange to be taken, protection measures in relation to a person P who lacks capacity to agree to one or more of the measures, then the NHS or LA **may** instruct an IMCA to represent P if it is satisfied that it would benefit P to be so represented and supported. The Code of Practice gives guidance on when this discretionary power may be used.[11] The regulations do not require the person in an adult protection situation to have no friends or family to consult. The protective measures must be proposed or taken as a result of an allegation that P is being abused or neglected or is abusing or has abused another person. Protective measures includes measures to minimise the risk that any abuse or neglect of P, or abuse by P, will continue, and measures taken in pursuance of guidance issued under Section 7 of the LA Social Services Act 1970.[12]

This regulation does not apply where an IMCA has been instructed in accordance with Section 37 (serious medical treatment), and Sections 38 and 39 (accommodation provided by NHS or LA) or Regulation 8 (review of accommodation).

Lasting powers of attorney

The regulations drawn up in relation to LPAs, enduring powers of attorney and the Public Guardian apply to both England and Wales.[13] However provision is made for any of the forms set out in Schedules 1–7 to include a Welsh version of the form.[14]

Commencement of the MCA in Wales

For the most part Wales shares the same commencement dates for the provisions of the MCA (see Chapter 17) with a few differences. In Wales the IMCA service commenced on 1 October 2007. (In England it began on 1 April 2007.)

Local health boards

In Wales LHBs are the equivalent of the Primary Care Trusts in England. The NAW delivers the IMCA service through local health boards, who have financial responsibility for the service and work in partnership with local authority social services departments and other NHS organisations. The LHBs commission the IMCA service from independent organisations, usually advocacy organisations.

In England, a person can only be an IMCA if the local authority approves their appointment. In Wales, the LHB will provide approval.

The Commissioner for Older People in Wales

The Commissioner for Older People in Wales is established by an Act[15] of the same name and came into force on 16 February 2007.[16] An older person is a person over 60 years. The general functions are set out in Section 2 and include:

- promoting awareness of the interests of older people in Wales and of the need to safeguard those interests
- promoting the provision of opportunities for, and the elimination of discrimination against, older people in Wales
- encouraging best practice in the treatment of older people in Wales

- keeping under review the adequacy and effectiveness of law affecting the interests of older people in Wales.

The Commissioner also has the power to review the effect on older people of the discharge or failure to discharge of the functions of the Assembly. The Commissioner may review the arrangements for, and the operation of, advocacy, complaints and whistle-blowing arrangements, and can give assistance to older people in making a complaint. Assistance includes financial help as well as representation. The Commissioner may undertake or commission research. Powers of entry and of interviewing are given to the Commissioner or a person authorised by him. The Commissioner is required to work jointly with the Public Services Ombudsman for Wales where a case comes under both their jurisdictions. He is also required to establish a complaints procedure in relation to the discharge of his functions.

   Those organisations and persons whose functions are subject to review by the Commissioner are listed in Schedule 3 and include local authorities, health and social care bodes such as the Care Council for Wales, a LHB, NHS trust, the Wales Centre for Health, a family health service provider in Wales, an independent provider and the National Leadership and Innovations Agency for Healthcare. Education and training, arts and leisure, and environment organisations are also listed.

   Advice and support can be given for relevant older people in Wales which is intended to enable and assist them to express their views and wishes orally or using any other means of communication and the provision of advice (including information) about their rights and welfare.[17]

The Court of Protection

Section 45 states that there is to be a superior court of record known as the Court of Protection, which is to have an official seal and may sit at any place in England and Wales, on any day and at any time. The court is to have a central office and registry at a place appointed by the Lord Chancellor. The Lord Chancellor may designate as additional registries of the court any district registry of the High Court and any county court office. There will be a court of the Court of Protection in Cardiff but the administrative offices will be in England.

Section 63: international protection of adults

Schedule 3 –

(a) gives effect in England and Wales to the Convention on the International Protection of Adults signed at the Hague on 13th January 2000 (Cm. 5881) (in so far as this Act does not otherwise do so), and

(b) makes related provision as to the private international law of England and Wales.

Definitions of local authority

Section 64(1):
   'local authority' means –

(a)   the council of a county in England in which there are no district councils,
(b)   the council of a district in England,
(c)   the council of a county or county borough in Wales,

Complaints mechanisms

Wales also has different complaints and inspection mechanisms from those which exist in England. Further information on the NHS in Wales is available on its website.[18]

Community health councils (CHC)

Whilst CHCs were abolished in England in 2003 in favour of the establishment of the Patient Advocacy and Liaison Services (PALS), the National Assembly for Wales opted to retain them. The 20 CHCs in Wales are the only statutory lay organisations with rights to information about, access to and consultation with all NHS organisations. The Board of CHCs in Wales collates all the information about patients' concerns across Wales and ensures that it reaches the Health and Social Services Committee in the National Assembly. It also has links to the Department of Health if the issue is a joint concern with England, or it is a matter of funding beyond the scope of the Assembly.[19] In 2004 the powers and responsibilities of the CHCs in Wales were strengthened to give patients and families a stronger voice and better advice on NHS issues. The changes included:

- an independent complaints advocacy service across Wales
- the right to visit GPs, dental surgeries, opticians and pharmacies
- the right to visit private nursing homes where NHS patients are being treated
- setting up of a statutory all-Wales body to support and advise CHCs in their roles.

Healthcare Commission and Wales

The Healthcare Commission (the Commission for Health Audit and Inspection) was established under the Health and Social Care (Community Health and Standards) Act 2003, replacing the Commission for Health Improvement. It publishes an annual report on the state of healthcare in England and Wales, but the inspectorate role it has in England is carried out in Wales by Healthcare Inspectorate Wales. A concordat has been signed between bodies inspecting, regulating and auditing health and social care in Wales. This contains sets of principles and practices to support the improvement of services for patients, service users and carers and to eliminate any unnecessary burdens of external review. The concordat was published in May 2005 and is available from the Healthcare Commission website.[20]

Healthcare Inspectorate Wales (HIW)

Healthcare Inspectorate Wales is a department of the National Assembly for Wales, and is responsible for inspecting and investigating the provision of health care by and for Welsh NHS bodies. Since 1 April 2005 it has been responsible also for the regulation of the private and voluntary health care sector in Wales, having taken over this role from the Care Standards Inspectorate for Wales (see **Care Standards Inspectorate for Wales**). HIW's purpose is to promote continuous improvement in the quality and safety of patient care within NHS Wales. It undertakes reviews and investigations into the provision of NHS-funded care, either by or for Welsh NHS organisations.

Care Standards Inspectorate for Wales (CSIW)

The CSIW, set up in 2002 under the Care Standards Act 2000, regulates social care, early years and private and voluntary health care services in Wales, to ensure standards are enforced and vulnerable people are safeguarded. It is operationally independent of the National Assembly for Wales and it regulates the sector through a national office, eight regional and three local offices across Wales. It regulates approximately 7000 settings against the regulations and national minimum standards set by the NAW and the WAG. There are four specific aspects to its work:

- registration
- inspection
- complaints
- enforcement.

Its first priority is to provide protection for service users. It makes every effort to assist providers to meet their legal obligations and to maintain required standards, but will take firm enforcement action through criminal or civil proceedings against those providers who fail to comply with the requirements and law.[21]

It has published a booklet on the complaint procedure and guidance for handling complaints in regulated services, which is available on its website.[22] It was updated in 2007 to take account of any changes to the regulations.

The complaint process envisages the following stages: a local resolution procedure followed by a formal investigation procedure if the local resolution proves unsuccessful. However where there is a complaint about the registered person or manager, responsible individual or the person in charge, then the complaint will go straight to the formal investigation. This would be carried out by the CSIW. Where the complaint also involves the local authority or the NHS, then the local authority complaints procedure and/or the NHS complaints procedure will apply, and a joint investigation may be the outcome.

Regulations made under the Care Standards Act 2000 require that the complaints procedures operated by regulated services should consider complaints from any service user or any person – including relative or representative – who acts on their behalf.

Public Services Ombudsman for Wales

This office came into force in April 2006. It is a new office which replaces the previous offices of the Local Government Ombudsman for Wales, the Health Service Ombudsman for Wales, the Welsh Administration Ombudsman and Social Housing Ombudsman for Wales. Its role is to investigate complaints made by members of the public. The complaints are investigated independently and impartially, and when upheld, the Ombudsman states what the public body must do to make amends to the complainant and how the standard of service could be improved. The Ombudsman has issued as statutory guidance under Section 31 of the Public Services Ombudsman (Wales) Act 2005, *Guidance to Local Authorities on Complaints Handling.*

Conclusion

Divergences between Wales and England are likely to increase as the WAG progresses and the NHS (Wales) Act 2006 enables Wales to develop its own policies and practice in relation to healthcare.

References

1 www.walesoffice.gov.uk
2 The Mental Capacity Act 2005 (Appropriate Body)(Wales) Regulations 2007 (SI 2007/833).
3 The Mental Capacity Act 2005 (Loss of Capacity during Research Project) (Wales) Regulations 2007 (SI 2007/837).
4 Welsh Assembly Government (2005) *Mental Health Policy in Wales: Consultation on the Mental Capacity Advocacy Service in Wales.*
5 The Mental Capacity Act 2005 (Independent Mental Capacity Advocate) (Wales) Regulations 2007 (SI 2007/852 (W.77)).
6 *Ibid.* Reg 5(6).
7 *Ibid.* Reg 6(3).
8 *Ibid.* Reg 6(4).
9 *Ibid.* Reg 8.
10 Code of Practice for the Mental Capacity Act 2005. Department of Constitutional Affairs February 2007 para 10.62–65. TSO, London.
11 *Ibid.* para 10.66–68.
12 SI 2007/852 (see reference 5 above) reg 9.
13 The Lasting Powers of Attorney, Enduring Powers of Attorney and Public Guardian Regulations 2007 (SI 2007/1253).
14 *Ibid.* Reg 3(1)(a).

15   The Commissioner for Older People (Wales) Act 2006.
16   The Commissioner for Older People in Wales (Appointment) Regulations 2007 (SI 2007/396).
17   *Ibid.*
18   www.wales.nhs.uk/directory.cfm
19   www.wales.nhs.uk/chc/home.cfm@OrglD=236
20   www.chai.org.uk/aboutus.cfm
21   www.csiw.wales.gov.uk
22   Care Standards Inspectorate for Wales (2006) *Complaint Procedure and Guidance for Handling Complaints in Regulated Services*. WAG, Cardiff.

17

Implementation, Resources and Code of Practice

Introduction

Even before the passing by Parliament of the Mental Capacity Bill, steps were being taken in preparation for its implementation. The draft Code of Practice was prepared to assist Parliament in determining what was appropriately left for inclusion in a code and what should be part of the statutory provisions. In fact the Joint Houses of Parliament criticised the fact that it had not been prepared at an earlier time. The Department of Health was also asked for figures on the likely consequential costs of the new provisions, and in particular the provision of an Independent Mental Capacity Advocacy (IMCA) service. After the passing of the Act implementation teams were set up, a Best Practice tool for organisations likely to be involved developed, and the mental capacity implementation programme was established within the Department for Constitutional Affairs (DCA).[1] This chapter considers the legal significance of the Code of Practice and looks at some of the initiatives used in implementation. The chapter should be read in conjunction with Scenarios M1, M2 and M3, which consider implementation in a hospital context, a care home and by an informal carer.

Dates of bringing into sections into force

Certain sections of the Act dealing with the establishment of IMCA services were brought into force on 1 November 2006. Other sections dealing with research were brought into force on 1 February 2007, and it was proposed that the rest of the Act would be brought into force on 1 April 2007. However delays in establishing the new Court of Protection and the Office of the Public Guardian (OPG) led to a revised timetable (and an amending SI[2]) as follows:

1 November 2006   Sections 35–41 for the purposes of enabling the Secretary of State to make arrangements for independent mental capacity advocates and for local authorities to approve IMCAs.

1 July 2007   Sections 30–34 for the purpose of enabling applications for approval in relation to research to be made to and determined by an appropriate body.

1 October 2007   the other provisions of Sections 30–34 (research).

1 November 2006   Independent Mental Capacity Advocacy Service for purposes of enabling the Secretary of State to make arrangements.

1 April 2007   IMCA service in England for all other purposes apart from the making of arrangements (in Wales the IMCA service commenced on 1 October 2007 – see Chapter 16).

1 April 2007   Code of Practice.

1 April 2007   new criminal offence of ill treatment and wilful neglect (S.44).

1 April 2007   principles, assessing capacity, and determining best interests.

1 October 2007   Court of Protection, Public Guardian and Office of the Public Guardian and all other sections, except those below.

1 April 2008   Sections 30–34 in respect of any research which is carried out as part of a research project which began before 1 April 2007 and was approved before 1 April 2007 by a committee established to advise on, or on matters which include, the ethics of research in relation to people who lack capacity to consent to it.

Code of Practice

Introduction

For the early discussions of the Bill and the Joint Committee consideration, the DH had not at that time prepared a draft Bill, and this was criticised by the Joint Committee:[3]

> Although we re-iterate our anxiety to keep up the momentum and ensure that introduction of the Bill is not unduly delayed, we recommend that the Bill should not be introduced to Parliament until it can be considered alongside comprehensive draft Codes of Practice.[4]

As a consequence of these criticisms a draft code was prepared and made available for the later Parliamentary debates.

General principles are set out in the first section of the Mental Capacity Act which must be followed in the determination of mental incapacity and in making decisions on behalf of a person lacking the requisite capacity. In addition guidance is to be provided by the Secretary of State on a wide range of topics in one or more codes. A code is defined as a code prepared or revised under Section 42 (S.42(7)).

Subjects covered by codes

The Lord Chancellor has a statutory duty under Section 42 to prepare and issue one or more codes of practice on the following topics (S.42(1)):

a.   for the guidance of persons assessing whether a person has capacity in relation to any matter
b.   for the guidance of persons acting in connection with the care or treatment of
another person (see S.5)
c.   for the guidance of donees of lasting powers of attorney
d.   for the guidance of deputies appointed by the court
e.   for the guidance of persons carrying out research in reliance on any provision
made by or under the Act (and otherwise with respect to Ss. 30–34)
f.   for the guidance of independent mental capacity advocates
   fa.   for the guidance of persons exercising functions under Schedule A1
   fb.   for the guidance of representatives appointed under Part 10 of Schedule A1
   (added by the MHA 2007)
g.   with respect to the provisions of Ss. 24 to 26 (advance decisions and apparent
advance decisions), and
h.   with respect to such other matters concerned with the Act as he thinks fit.

The italicised subparagraphs fa and fb have been added by the Mental Health Act
paragraph 8(2) of Schedule 9.

The Lord Chancellor has the power to revise a code from time to time and may
delegate the preparation or revision of the whole or any part of a code so far as he
considers expedient (S.42(2) and (3)).

Legal force of codes

It is the duty of a person to have regard to any relevant code if he is acting in
relation to a person who lacks capacity and is doing so in one or more of the ways
set out in Box 17.1.

Box 17.1: Persons upon whom the Code of Practice is binding – S.42(4).

Those acting:
a.   as the donee of a lasting power of attorney
b.   as a deputy appointed by the court
c.   as a person carrying out research in reliance on any provision made by or
under the Act (see Sections 30–34)
d.   as an independent mental capacity advocate
   (da)   in the exercise of functions under Schedule A1
   (db)   as a representative appointed under Part 10 of Schedule A1 (added
   by the MHA 2007)
e.   in a professional capacity
f.   for remuneration (S.42(4)).

The italicised subsections (da) and (db) have been added by the Mental Health
Act 2007 paragraph 8(3) of Schedule 9.

It is interesting that the list set out in Box 17.1 omits the informal carer, i.e. the friend or relative who is caring for a person lacking mental capacity and is not paid. However it is hoped that in practice an informal carer will find codes of practice of considerable help to his or her decision making and activities on behalf of the mentally incapacitated person. Failure by an informal carer to follow code of practice guidelines would not have the implications that it does for those listed under Section 42(4) (see Chapter 15 and Scenarios L).

For those listed under Section 42(4) as shown in Box 17.1, the effect of failure to obey the code is that if it appears to a court or tribunal conducting any criminal or civil proceedings that a provision of a code or a failure to comply with a code is relevant to a question arising in the proceedings, the provision or failure must be taken into account in deciding the question (S.42(5)).

The explicit setting-out of the legal effect of the code was a recommendation of the Joint Committee. This stated that:

> The value of the Codes, [was] one essential means by which the State fulfils its obligations to ensure public authorities act in compliance with the Human Rights Act 1998. We seek reassurance that the wording used in the Bill will ensure that the Codes of Practice are afforded sufficient status to comply with human rights obligations.[5]

Guidance for deputies appointed by the court

A code provided for the guidance of deputies appointed by the court (S.42(1(d)) may contain separate guidance for deputies appointed by virtue of paragraph 1(2) of Schedule 5 (functions of deputy conferred on receiver appointed under the Mental Health Act) (S.42(6)).

Procedure to be followed in the preparation of codes

The Lord Chancellor has a statutory duty to consult the National Assembly of Wales (NAW) (see Chapter 16) and such other persons as he considers appropriate before preparing or revising a code (S.43(1)). In addition, the code cannot be issued unless a draft of the code has been laid by him before both Houses of Parliament and the 40-day period (further defined in Section 43(4) and (5)) has elapsed without either House resolving not to approve the draft (S.43(2)).

The Lord Chancellor must arrange for any code that he has issued to be published in such a way as he considers appropriate for bringing it to the attention of persons likely to be concerned with its provisions (S.43(3)).

Revision of codes

Under Section 42(2) the Lord Chancellor may from time to time revise a code of practice and must follow the same procedures set out under Section 43 for the preparation of the code. The Joint Committee expressed hopes that the DCA would make use of a wide range of expertise in the drafting etc., welcomed the consultation provisions and emphasised the use of the valuable experience from Scotland.

Assessment of capacity, supporting decision making and best interests

The Joint Committee was concerned that there needed to be more guidance on the assessment of capacity, and this was added to the subjects for which the Lord Chancellor should provide a code of practice – see Section 4(1)(a). (See Chapter 4.) Similar concerns were expressed about supported decision making[6] and determination of best interests,[7] and guidance was therefore included in the Code of Practice.

Decision makers acting under formal powers

In the Joint Committee discussions,[8] the Master of the Court of Protection suggested that there should be a number of obligations which should be imposed on decision makers, in addition to their specific duties, which might include obligations:

- to act reasonably
- to act diligently
- to act honestly and in good faith
- to act within the scope of his or her authority
- to limit interference in the life of the person without capacity to the greatest extent possible
- to protect him or her from abuse, neglect and exploitation
- to respect and advance his or her civil liberties and human rights
- to provide such assistance and support as is needed
- where appropriate, actively to help him or her resume or assume independent or interdependent living
- to involve him or her in all decision-making processes to the greatest possible extent
- to encourage such participation and to help him or her to act independently in the areas where he or she is able
- to encourage him or her to exercise whatever skills he or she has, and wherever possible to develop new skills
- to exercise substituted judgment by respecting and following his or her wishes, values and beliefs to the greatest possible extent, so far as these are known or can be ascertained, and will not result in harm or be contrary to his or her best interests.

The Joint Committee recommended that specific requirements of a standard of conduct be included in the codes of practice aimed at those exercising formal powers under the Act.[9]

Dilemma of inclusion in the Act or Code?

One of the significant dilemmas confronting the law makers and the Joint Committee was what provisions should be put into the Act (which would therefore have statutory force) and what provisions could be left to be included in the Code of Practice (which would have less weight). A similar discussion took place on the setting out of principles, and significant amendments were made to include the principles as Section 1 (like Scotland), rather than leave them to be incorporated in a Code of Practice.

Baroness Ashton of Upholland[10] stated that:

> One of the things that will happen when, as I trust, the Bill becomes law is that the code of practice, which I think I described earlier as the 'living document' upon which professional practice will be based within the framework of the Bill, will be out for consultation to enable us to engage with all those involved.

She also said:[11]

> For the decision-maker to gain the protection against liability offered by Clause 5, if it is an attorney, a deputy, or an independent consultee acting in a professional capacity or for remuneration, he must have regard to the code of practice, as Clause 40(4) [now section 42(4)] makes clear. It is important to be clear that any code of practice issue will be allowed to be used as evidence in court proceedings and could be taken into account by a court or a tribunal.

Similarly,[12] she said the Code of Practice could include what decisions doctors can make and what must be taken to court as being appropriate for the Code of Practice.

She also stated that: [13]

> Under the best interests criteria, professionals would be expected to consult fully about serious decisions, and it would be open to family or friends to ask for a second opinion, if that had not already happened. Any disputes that could not be resolved locally could ultimately be taken to the Court of Protection. We have also provided for an independent person to be consulted when serious medical decisions are taken for people who are 'unbefriended'. That independent person can ask for a second opinion if they have any concerns. I support the intention behind my noble friend's amendment – to make sure that right procedures are followed at all times, not left to individual good practice. I hope that Members of the Committee will recognise that, although we agree with the need to take certain cases to court and for a second opinion to be provided wherever it is asked for, it would be bureaucratic and inflexible to provide such safeguards in the Bill. It is the inflexibility about which I would be most concerned. We believe that **the best place is the code of practice**, which reflects existing best practice. On that basis, I hope that the noble Lord will feel able to withdraw his amendment.

The Joint Committee also voiced its concerns about getting the balance right between what was in the Act and what was left to the Code of Practice, and expressed concerns that too much was being put in the codes and insufficient in the legislation.[14]

Monitoring implementation of the Codes of Practice

The Joint Committee also recommended that the Codes of Practice should provide details of the OPG supervisory role and the sanctions which may apply in the event of non-compliance with the codes.[15]

> We recommend that the Court of Protection's powers should include the power to remove a donee or deputy who is acting incompetently or failing to comply with the guidance given in the Codes of Practice as to the expected standard of conduct. It should be made clear to decision-makers that if their behaviour falls below the standard of conduct set out in the Codes of Practice, the court has power to remove them as attorneys or deputies and if their conduct is criminal, they will face the prospect and consequences of prosecution.[16]

Best Practice Tool

This was published by the DH in August 2006 and provided guidance for local authorities, National Health Service trusts, foundation trusts and independent sector (private and voluntary) hospitals in England in preparation for the implementation of the Act in April 2007.[17] The Best Practice Tool sets down 37 statements for compliance, and suggests that the levels of compliance with these statements are coded red, amber or green according to the level of preparation. The required action on each statement should be recorded, and also the person to undertake the activity and the date by which it should have been completed.

The statements cover the following topics:

- meeting the five statutory principles
- availability of the Act, Explanatory Memorandum, regulations and Code of Practice for staff
- people who lack capacity
- information for service users who may lack capacity and their carers
- inability to make decisions
- best interests
- acts in connection with care and treatment – limitations on 'best interests' decision making
- paying for goods and services and handling money
- record keeping
- lasting powers of attorney
- resolving disputes
- declarations by the new Court of Protection
- deputies
- advance decisions
- excluded decisions
- interface with Mental Health Act 1983
- research
- Independent Mental Capacity Advocate (IMCA) Service
- criminal offences

- the new Court of Protection
- the Public Guardian
- enduring powers of attorney
- receivers
- Code of Practice
- implementation leads within organisations
- regional implementation leads
- awareness raising: brief summary of Act, easy read summary, regular newsletter, standard PowerPoint presentation
- education and training
- training materials
- commissioning IMCA services
- local implementation networks.

Implementation networks

The directors of adult social services were invited by the DH to nominate a contact person to liaise with the implementation programme via a Chief Executive Bulletin in March 2006. Care Services Improvement Partnerships (CSIP) nominated Regional Implementation Leads. These CSIP implementation leads will work with and support the work of the local implementation networks and agree regional plans that will provide a number of targeted regional awareness and education/ training events.

Local implementation networks

The suggested six tasks of the multi-disciplinary local implementation network put forward by the DH are:

- To ensure an independent mental capacity advocacy service is in place by April 2007.
- To disseminate information and publicity about the Act's implementation.
- To assist in awareness raising of health and social care staff, possibly via the dissemination and use of training materials, and by supporting a regional 'Training the Trainers' approach.
- To meet with an agreed frequency as a multi-agency local implementation with a Chair who attends a regional network meeting on its behalf.
- To sign off, along with directors of adult social services and social services' directors of finance, a local multi-agency agreed implementation plan that confirms how centrally provided training monies will be locally allocated.

Training materials and funds

The DH, in partnership with the Social Care Institute for Excellence, has commissioned the University of Central Lancashire to provide a range of training materials to support the Act's implementation. These will be provided in five modules to cover:

- generic, for all health and social care staff affected by the Act
- acute hospitals
- mental health services
- residential accommodation
- primary/community care.

Funds are available from the DH to support the implementation of the Act in 2006/7 and 2007/8.

Resources

The support and protection of mentally incapacitated adults is a resource-intensive service. The Joint Committee complained that no estimate of the cost of the full regulatory impact assessment of the Bill had been provided by the Department.[18]

Only late and highly provisional estimates were provided to the Joint Committee and the DH was criticised by the Joint Committee, especially in view of the fact that the Bill had been under consideration for so many years.[19] Possible costs were estimated at £171 million over ten years (but could possibly be lower if account were taken of the money already spent on mentally incapacitated decision making).[20]

Costs of training

The DH stated that these would be low cost, because the MCA simply builds on existing practice. However the Association of Directors of Social Services considered that the MCA had significant service delivery and implementation costs.

The Scottish experience suggested the need for a huge investment in training. There was a danger that, without that investment, a wide range of local interpretations would develop, inevitably leading to inequity.[21] The DH had estimated that about 100 000 professionals would need training under the MCA.[22]

Other costs included the support for the Court of Protection, the review of current assessment and care management practice, including risk assessment. The appointment of Directors of Social Services to make welfare decisions would result in additional demands on services which are already at capacity.

Legal aid

The cost implications of legal aid were disputed: on the one hand the DH considered them to be insignificant, because legal aid costs would be restricted to serious legal matters so should not increase costs significantly. On the other hand the Law Society said that the objectives of the MCA would be undermined by the lack of availability of public funding. The Scottish experience suggested that the legal aid costs were not too high.[23]

Savings

As far as savings were concerned the Joint Committee considered that local authorities may be able to levy charges on the property of mentally incapable people for whom they were acting as deputies. In addition if people made advance directions this might minimise the need for LA intervention.[24]

Cost of possible additions to the Bill

Advocacy

The DH was of the view that there was unlikely to be the necessary available resources to provide a facility for independent advocacy. The Joint Committee stated that although it supported some extra provision for advocacy, it thought that uncertainty about the extent of the DH's commitment to advocacy, and lack of any information about the possible costs entailed, further illustrated the problems of bringing the Bill forward before proper consultation on cost has been carried out.[25]

The uncertainties over whether there would be the resources to implement the Bill, and the fact that the DH had identified but not quantified the benefits, led the Joint Committee to vent its fury at being placed in the invidious position of having to carry out its duty of scrutiny without any detailed indications of what the Bill might cost or what the quantum of benefits might be.[26]

In the House of Lords Lord Carter sympathised with this dilemma over the resource implications of the Bill.[27] He warned against the dangers of double accounting and emphasised that marginal costs may only be involved in implementing the Bournewood safeguards:

> Many of the patients will already have costs attached to them, and it would be wrong to double-count the costs by including in the costs of Bournewood the costs which already apply.

Transitional arrangements

There are specific statutory provisions to allow for the transition between the situation before the Act came into force and the situation afterwards. Thus enduring powers of attorney executed before the Act came into force, will still be valid until such time as they are ended with the death of the donor or donee(s). Schedule 4 to the MCA covers the enduring powers of attorney. Research which has been undertaken prior to 1 April 2006 in which mentally incapacitated persons are participating can still be carried on, but only if the regulations are complied with.

Mental Health Act receivers

Schedule 5 of the MCA makes transitional provisions for those persons who have had a receiver appointed under Part 7 of the Mental Health Act 1983. From 1 October 2007 the Mental Capacity Act 2005 applies as if the receiver (R) were a deputy appointed for a person by the court, but with the functions that R had as receiver immediately before that day. The newly constituted Court of Protection will have powers over the deputies including the power to end the receiver's, (then known as the deputy's) appointment. If as a result of S.20(1) (necessity for the person to lack mental capacity) the receiver may not make a decision on behalf of P, R must apply to the court. If, on the application, the court is satisfied that P is capable of managing his property and affairs in relation to the relevant matter, then the court must make an order ending R's appointment as P's deputy in relation to that matter, but it may, in relation to any other matter, exercise in relation to P any of the powers which it has under Sections 15–19 (i.e. power to make declarations, decisions and appoint deputies, make decisions in relation to P's personal welfare, and in relation to property and affairs).

Interim procedural arrangements

A Practice Note was issued by the Official Solicitor[28] to cover the situation pending the coming into force of the Mental Capacity Act 2005. It set out the jurisdiction of the High Court in dealing with decisions and the lawfulness of proposed medical treatment or withdrawal of treatment, and decisions regarding welfare issues. It stated that court applications should be made:

1. where it was proposed to withdraw artificial nutrition and hydration from a patient in a permanent vegetative state;
2. in cases involving the sterilisation of a patient for contraceptive purposes where they could not consent;
3. in certain termination of pregnancy cases;
4. where there was any serious treatment decision and there was disagreement between those involved;
5. where the proposed treatment would involve the use of force or restraint, or where there were doubts or difficulties over assessment of either the patient's capacity or best interests.

In addition the Practice Note gave guidance on the test for capacity, the implications of advance directives and the relevance of a patient's best interests.

Proceedings would invariably be brought under the Civil Procedures Rules 1998 Part 8. The patient must always be a party. The claimant would usually be the NHS trust or local authority, but any properly interested person could bring proceedings. Incapacitated adults could be assisted by the appointment of the Official Solicitor.

Pilot IMCA schemes

Seven IMCA pilots were set up in January 2006, to help identify the practical issues involved in implementing the IMCA service. They are taking place in: Cambridgeshire; Cheshire & Merseyside; Croydon; Dorset; Hertfordshire; Newcastle; and Southwark.

The aim is to test the practicalities of providing advocacy services to particularly vulnerable people by helping them to make important decisions about medical treatment and changes of residence – for example moving to a hospital or care home. The results will be used when considering how to provide this service on a wider basis. Cambridge University will be evaluating the results of the pilots.

These pilot schemes were evaluated by the Learning Disabilities Research Group at the University of Cambridge, headed by Marcus Redley and its report is available on the DH website. It noted that decision makers were positive about their experience of working with the IMCA caseworkers and their involvement improved decision making by providing additional relevant information and kept the clients at the centre of the process. Many decision makers did not understand the purpose of the IMCA service and inappropriate referrals were made.

Recommendations included the need for adequate provision to be made for the supervision of caseworkers; IMCA caseworkers' skill and expertise should be recognised by the future national professional qualification, a national association and/or an appropriate salary. In addition to avoid an unnecessary strain on IMCA resources, good generic advocacy services may be a necessity.

Guidance from specific professional organisations and client-specific associations

The implications of the MCA are wide ranging, and many different organisations and associations have provided their members with specific guidance on the implications of the legislation for their specific needs. A direct web link between the DCA and many of these organisations is available,[29] including Age Concern, Alzheimer's Society, Care Services Improvement Partnership, Carers UK, Mencap, Mind and Scope. It also provides a direct link to the other relevant Government departments, including the IMCA service, the Office of the Official Solicitor and Public Trustee and the Public Guardianship Office. Health and social services professionals as well as carers and clients will find the various specialist sites of benefit in understanding the implications of the new legislation.

Disagreements and complaints

Many concerns on how the legislation is being implemented and how the vulnerable adults are being protected will initially be the subject of complaints and representations rather than legal action. The Code of Practice recommends that there should be attempts to resolve concerns initially through case conferences and discussions, mediation and the complaints procedures of the NHS, LA or independent sector. Chapter 15 of the Code of Practice considers the best ways to settle disagreements and disputes about issues covered in the Act.[30] In addition the pre-action protocol of the Court of Protection requires the parties concerned in a dispute to attempt to resolve the issues without an application to the court, where appropriate (some decisions have to go to the Court of Protection – see Chapter 7). Further guidance on how to deal with problems without going to court is provided in the Community Legal Services Information Leaflet, *Alternatives to Court*.[31] Information about mediation services can be obtained from the National Mediation Helpline[32] and the Family Mediation Helpline.[33]

In England new complaints regulations came into force on 30 July 2004.[34] These establish a statutory procedure for the handling of complaints about NHS services. Complainants could be assisted by representatives of the Patient Advice and Liaison Service, and if the complaint cannot be resolved speedily the Independent Complaints Advocacy Service could be a source of help and advice. If the complainant is dissatisfied by the attempt at local resolution, he or she can seek an independent review by the Healthcare Commission. Subsequently, if still dissatisfied, the complainant may be able to take the complaint to the Ombudsman or Health Service Commissioner. Patients detained under the Mental Heath Act can complain to the Mental Health Act Commission.

Complaints in Wales and the role of the Community Health Council are considered in Chapter 16.

Since 1 September 2006 social services departments must comply with the new procedures for the handling of complaints and ensure that the procedure covers the delivery of services, the types of services provided and failure to provide services.

Care homes in the independent sector registered with the Commission for Social Care Inspection are each required to have a complaints procedure.

Conclusions

Inevitably the full implementation will take several years and will be an ongoing process, as the Code of Practice is revised and as new guidance is published in the light of the feedback from the initial stages of implementation. Fundamental to the full implementation of the MCA are the resources which will be made available. It is possible that, like the London Olympics of 2012, the resource implications of the MCA are only the tip of the iceberg and some of the estimated savings have been greatly exaggerated. Much will depend upon the clarity of the legislation, the Code of Practice, the cost of the IMCA service and number of applications to the Court of Protection.

References

1   Mental Capacity Implementation Programme, Department for Constitutional Affairs, Steel House, Room 5.02, 11 Tothill Street, London SW1H 9LH. www.dca.gov.uk/legal-policy/mental-capacity/index.htm

2   Mental Capacity Act 2005 (Commencement Order No 1) 2006 (SI 2006/2814); Mental Capacity Act 2005 (Commencement No 1)(Amendment) Order 2006 (SI 2006/3473).

3   Joint Cttee Chapter 12 paras 228–254.

4   *Ibid.* para 229.

5   *Ibid.* para 231.

6   *Ibid.* para 241.

7   *Ibid.* para 247.

8   *Ibid.* paras 250–252.

9   *Ibid.* para 252.

10 House of Lords, 25 Jan 2005; Column 1230.

11 25 Jan 2005 House of Lords; Column 1241.

12 *Ibid.* p 4; Column 1243.

13 *Ibid.* p 6; Column 1244.

14 Joint Cttee paras 238–249.

15 *Ibid.* paras 253–254.

16 *Ibid.* para 252.

17 Department of Health (2006). Mental Capacity Act 2005: Best Practice Tool.

18 Joint Cttee Chapter 17 paras 309–341.

19 *Ibid.* para 315.

20 *Ibid.* para 317.

21 *Ibid.* para 320.

22 *Ibid.* para 321.

23 *Ibid.* paras 324–5.

24 *Ibid.* para 326.

25 *Ibid.* paras 328–9.

26 *Ibid.* paras 330–341.

27 House of Lords, 25 Jan 2005, doc 9 p 3.

28 Practice Note [2006] 2 FLR 373; Practice Note (Official Solicitor: Declaratory Proceedings: Medical and Welfare Decisions for Adults who Lack Capacity).

29 www.dca.gov.uk/legal-policy/mental-capacity/links.htm

30 Code of Practice for the Mental Capacity Act 2005. Department of Constitutional Affairs February 2007. TSO, London.

31 Community Legal Services Direct Information Leaflet Number 23, www.clsdirect.org.uk/legalhelp/leaflet23

32 National Mediation Helpline, Tel: 0845 60 30 809, www.nationalmediationhelpline.com

33 Family Mediation Helpline, Tel: 0845 60 26 627, www.familymediationhelpline.co.uk

34 The National Health Service (Complaints) Regulations 2004 (SI 2004/1768).

Scenarios M
Implementation, Resources
and Code of Practice

Implementation within a hospital context

> ### Scenario M1: Implementing the Act.
>
> Jake is chief executive of an National Health Service trust which includes two district general hospitals and a community unit. He asks Ken to take on the responsibility for ensuring the implementation of the Mental Capacity Act across the whole trust and allocates him a budget for the task. What are the significant changes which Ken will have to oversee and what aids are there for implementation?

It is probably true to say that every single section or specialty within a district general hospital and community will be affected by the changes brought about by the Mental Capacity Act 2005, though clearly some will be more influenced than others. Almost all hospital specialties will on occasions have patients who are incapable of making their own decisions. Although the Mental Capacity Act 2005 is concerned only with the person over 16 years, there are provisions which could apply to children younger than that, as Chapter 12 explains.

It is hoped that in scenario M1 the NHS trust is already part of the NHS implementation programme, which is explained on pages 292–4.

Key to Ken's work will be the following.

Training sessions and training materials on the impact of the legislation

A strategy to ensure that every employee has an understanding of the legislation and how it relates to their specific work must be drawn up, and Ken would be assisted by an implementation team covering all specialties and staff. Ken would need to access initial training sessions and ensure that those who receive the initial training are able to cascade the lessons to the rest of the staff, in the hope that eventually all staff will receive an initial training in the basic principles of the Act, definition of capacity and criteria for best interests and its relevance to their specific work.

Policies and procedures covering:

- consent procedures on behalf of a mentally incapacitated person who does not have the requisite capacity to give consent
- the use and legal significance of advance decisions
- research and the adult with specific mental incapacities
- applications to the Court of Protection
- property and finance of patients unable to take action on their own behalf
- Independent Mental Capacity Advocacy Service
- role and powers of donees of lasting powers of attorney
- role of deputies appointed by the Court of Protection.

The implementation team would be responsible under Ken for ensuring these policies were developed. However in preparing these policies for use across the NHS trust, the team would be wise to take advantage of policies and procedures produced nationally, by neighbouring trusts and other organisations, so that maximum use is made of all the available materials.

Implementation of the training and policies and procedures

Ken and his implementation team would probably also have the role of overseeing the implementation of the policies across the trust. This will be a slow process as new problems arise on the impact of the legislation, and a task force to advise on the questions and issues raised by individuals and specialties could be established. Lessons from these discussions could be spread across the trust. Perhaps a mental capacity newsletter may be of value for dissemination of the information.

Implementation in a care home

> ### Scenario M2: Implementation of the MCA in a care home.
>
> Justin, a Registered Nurse for Learning Disabilities, has been the manager of a care home for 30 elderly persons for over ten years. The home is owned by a private company. Justin had heard from a colleague working in the NHS that his NHS trust was setting up training sessions on the MCA. He asked his regional manager if the care home company was planning similar events to those in the NHS. The regional manager said he did not know anything about it and thought that the Act was only for the NHS.

The regional manager in Scenario M2 is of course completely wrong. As has been seen from this book, the MCA applies to every situation where decisions have to be made on behalf of an adult who lacks the requisite mental capacity. The decisions relate to care and treatment, property and affairs; in fact every possible decision that might have to be made.

Justin has a professional responsibility to keep up to date. He must therefore check the regional manager's statement and find out if the MCA does apply to his work in the care home. He could do this by looking at the many online information services about the MCA, including the Department of Health and Department of Constitutional Affairs websites. Once he has confirmed that the MCA is relevant to his work, he may be able to find a workshop or training session that he could apply to join. Since he would probably require the approval of the regional manager to attend such a seminar, he would need to give him evidence of the significance of such a session for the care home.

After attending a training session, Justin would have a responsibility to ensure that his staff understood the implications of the MCA for their work. Internal training, policies and procedures and monitoring of the implementation of the MCA would be required within his home. Justin should also attempt to persuade senior management within the company of the importance of the MCA, so that eventually all home managers and staff are trained in its implementation and significance.

Implementation for carers

Scenario M3: Carers and the MCA.

Jane was a social worker with responsibilities for the elderly. One of her clients was Olga, aged 85 years, with early stage Alzheimer's who lived with her daughter Avril and her son-in-law. Jane was concerned that Olga appeared to be having no say in some of the decisions which were being made. It seemed to Jane that Olga would have benefited from attending a day centre but Avril opposed this. Jane tried to explain to Avril the implications of the MCA but Avril did not consider that this was relevant to her or to Olga.

The task of ensuring that the family and friends and informal carers of those with limitations in mental capacity have instruction in the significance of the new legislation is huge. The DCA has published leaflets both for the informal carer and also for those with limited mental capacity. Inevitably the task of ensuring that this information is disseminated will fall upon the health and social services professionals and the voluntary and charitable organisations concerned. Whilst informal carers are not identified in the statute as being bound by the Code of Practice, there are many practical reasons why the Act and the Code of Practice should be brought to their attention, so that they can benefit from its guidance. Inevitably it will probably take a considerable time for the millions of people involved in making decisions on behalf of mentally incapacitated adults to be familiar with the new provisions, and in the meantime the professionals will have a duty to point out the implications.

In Scenario M3 Jane should obtain some of the leaflets produced by the DCA and the Alzheimer's Society and explain their significance to Avril, discussing with her what decisions Olga could make for herself and how other decisions which are outside her capacity could be made.

Conclusions

Alongside the Human Rights Act 1998, the Mental Capacity Act 2005 is one of the most important pieces of legislation to affect health and social care over the last half century. Inevitably there will be a period of uncertainty, since the MCA has such vast implications across every aspect of health and social care. There will also be resource pressures, since the assessment of capacity and the determination of what is in a person's 'best interests' will take longer than it has in the past. It is essential that those charged with the implementation of the MCA follow the philosophy which underpins the legislation, in ensuring respect and support for personal autonomy and a willingness to act in the best interests of those unable to make their own decisions. There is a danger that if the spirit of the MCA is not upheld, its implementation will descend to a bureaucratic nightmare of ticking boxes and paperwork.

18 Postscript

After the Human Rights Act 1998, the Mental Capacity Act 2005 can be seen as one of the most important pieces of legislation for the last two centuries. It is understandable that the implementation was delayed for over two years, since the training, organisational and management repercussions are immense. So too are the resource implications.

There are no clear figures on the numbers of those lacking the specific mental capacity who may therefore come within the provisions of the Act. *Valuing People*[1] calculated that there are about 210 000 people with severe learning disabilities in England and about 1.2 million with a mild or moderate disability. Numbers of those suffering from dementia are also uncertain. A study conducted by the London School of Economics and the Institute of Psychiatry Kings College London[2] suggested that at least 700 000 people suffered from dementia in Great Britain, and this figure is likely to increase to more than 1 million by 2025. The current costs of dementia were estimated at £17bn a year. Then there are the many other conditions which can lead to a lack of capacity: acquired brain injury, chronic psychiatric conditions, as well as motor neurone disease and other debilitating conditions. Nor is there any reliable estimate of the carers, both informal and paid, who are involved in their support and treatment.

It is obvious that there are many millions who directly or indirectly will be affected by the MCA, and the rules and regulations drawn up under it. For all of these the next few years are likely to present a steep learning curve as, inch by inch, they learn the basic principles and minutiae of the Act. The Government has promised ongoing monitoring of many of its provisions and the new institutions – the Court of Protection and the Office of the Public Guardian, together with Independent Mental Capacity Advocacy services – will be expected to make known their views on the effective implementation of the Act and any perceived weaknesses in its basic provisions, its Code of Practice and its implementation.

Inevitably there will be revisions, cases, and new Statutory Instruments to fine-tune and interpret some of the provisions. It is hoped that the Mental Capacity Act presents a stable and firm foundation on which the protection of the rights of those who lack the capacity to make their own specific decisions can be built.

References

1   Department of Health (2001) *Valuing People: A New Strategy for Learning Disability for the 21st Century*. White Paper CM 5086.
2   Bennett, R. Dementia care costs £17bn and will at least treble. *The Times*, 27 February 2007.

Websites

Action for Advocacy	www.actionforadvocacy.org
Action on Elder Abuse	www.elderabuse.org.uk
Age Concern	www.ageconcern.org.uk
Alert	www.donoharm.org.uk
Alzheimer's Research	www. Alzheimers-research.org.uk
Alzheimer's Society	www.alzheimers.org.uk
ASA Advice	www.advice.org.uk
Association of Contentious Trust and Probate Solicitors	www.actaps.com
Audit Commission	www.audit-commission.gov.uk
CARERS UK	www.carersonline.org.uk
	www.carersuk.org
Care Services Improvement Partnership	www.csip.org.uk
Citizens Advice Bureaux	www.citizensadvice.org.uk
Citizen Advocacy Information and Training	www.citizenadvocacy.org.uk
Civil Procedure Rules	www.open.gov.uk/lcd/civil/ procrules_fin/crules.htm
Commission for Equality and Human Rights	www.cehr.org.uk
Commission for Racial Equality	www.cre.gov.uk/
Community Legal Service Direct	www.clsdirect.org.uk
Contact the Elderly	www.contact-the-elderly.org
Convention on the International Protection of Adults	www.hcch.net/index_en.php?
Counsel and Care	www.counselandcare.org.uk
Court Funds Office	www.hmcourts-service.gov.uk/ infoabout/cfo/index.htm

Court of Protection	via the Office of Public Guardian or HM Courts Service (see below)
Dementia Care Trust	www.dct.org.uk
Department for Constitutional Affairs	www.dca.gov.uk
Department for Work and Pensions	www.dwp.gov.uk/
Department of Health	www.dh.gov.uk
Department of Trade and Industry	www.dti.gov.uk/
Disability Law Service	www.dls.org.uk/
Domestic Violence	www.domesticviolence.gov.uk
Down's Syndrome Association	ww.downs-syndrome.org.uk www.dsa-uk.com
Family Carer Support Service	www.familycarers.org.uk
Family Mediation Helpline	www.familymediationhelpline.co.uk
Foundation for People with Learning Disabilities	www.learningdisabilities.org.uk
General Medical Council	www.gmc-uk.org
Headway – brain injury association	www.headway.org.uk
Health and Safety Commission	www.hsc.gov.uk
Health and Safety Executive	www.hse.gov.uk
Help the Aged	www.helptheagedorg.uk
Help the Hospices	www.hospiceinformation.info
Health Professions Council	www.hc-uk.org
HM Courts Service	www.hmcourts-service.gov.uk
Home Farm Trust	www.hft.org.uk
Human Fertilisation and Embryology Authority	www.hfea.gov.uk/
Human Rights	www.humanrights.gov.uk
Independent Mental Capacity Advocacy	www.dh.gov.uk.imca
Law Centres Federation	www.lawcentres.org.uk
Law Society	www.lawsociety.org.uk/ choosingandusing/ findingasolicitor.law
Legislation	www.opsi.gov.uk/legislation or www.legislation.hmso.gov.uk
Linacre Centre for Healthcare Ethics	www.linacre.org
Making Decisions Alliance	www.makingdecisions.org.uk
Manic Depression Fellowship	www.mdf.org.uk
MedicAlert Foundation	www.medicalert.org.uk
Medicines and Healthcare Products Regulatory Agency	www.mhra.gov.uk
MENCAP	www.mencap.org.uk
Mental Capacity Implementation Programme	www.dca.go.uk/legal-policy/ mental-capacity/index.htm
Mental Health Foundation	www.mentalhealth.org.uk
Mental Health Lawyers Assoc	www.mhla.co.uk
Mental Health Matters	www.mentalhealthmatters.com/
Mind	www.mind.org.uk

Motor Neurone Disease Association	www.mndassociation.org.uk
National Audit Office	www.nao.gov.uk
National Autistic Society	www.nas.org.uk
	www.autism.org.uk
National Care Association	www.nca.gb.com
National Family Carer Network	www.familycarers.org.uk
National Mediation Helpline,	www.nationalmediationhelpline.com
National Patient Safety Agency	www.npsa.gov.uk
National Treatment Agency	www.nta.nhs.uk/
NHS	www.nhs.uk
NHS Direct	www.nhsdirect.nhs.uk
NHS Professionals	www.nhsprofessionals.nhs.uk
NICE	www.nice.org.uk
Nursing and Midwifery Council	www.nmc-uk.org/
Office of the Public Guardian	www.guardianship.gov.uk
Office of Public Sector Information	www.opsi.gov.uk
Official Solicitor	www.officialsolicitor.gov.uk
Open Government	www.open.gov.uk
Pain website	www.pain-talk.co.uk
Patient's Association	www.patients-association.org.uk
Patient Concern	www.patientconcern.org.uk
People First	www.peoplefirst.org.uk
Prevention of Professional	www.popan.org.uk
Abuse Network	
Princess Royal Trust for Carers	www.carers.org/
Relatives and Residents Association	www.releres.org/
RESCARE (the national society for	www.rescare.org.uk
mentally disabled people in	
residential care)	
Respond	www.respond.org.uk
Rethink (formerly the National	www.rethink.org
Schizophrenia Fellowship)	
Royal College of Nursing	www.rcn.org.uk
Royal College of Psychiatrists	www.rcpsych.ac.uk
SANE	www.sane.org.uk
Scope	www.scope.org.uk
Sense	www.sense.org.uk
Shipman Inquiry	www.the-shipman-inquiry.org.uk/ reports.asp
Solicitors for the Elderly	www.solicitorsfortheelderly.com
Speaking Up	www.speakingup.org/
Speakability	www.speakability.org.uk
Stroke Association	www.stroke.org.uk
Together: Working for Wellbeing	www.together-uk.org
Turning Point	www.turning-point.co.uk
UK Homecare Association	www.ukhca.co.uk
UK Parliament	www.parliament.uk

United Response	www.unitedresponse.org.uk
Values into Action	www.viauk.org
Veterans Agency	www.veteransagency.org.uk
VOICE UK	www.voiceuk.clara.net
Voluntary Euthanasia Society	www.ves.org.uk
Welsh Assembly Government	www.wales.gov.uk
World Medical Association	www.wma.net/e/policy/b3.htm

Recommended Further Reading

Richardson, J. (ed) (2007) *Archbold Criminal Pleadings, Evidence and Practice* 55th rev edn. Sweet and Maxwell, London.

Plant, C., Rose, W., Sime, S. and French, D. (2004) *Blackstone's Civil Practice*. Blackstone.

Brazier, M. (2007) *Medicine, Patients and the Law* 4th edn. Penguin, Harmondsworth.

British Medical Association. (2001) *Consent, Rights and Choices in Health Care for Children and Young People*. BMJ Books, London.

Dugdale, A.M. and Jones, M. (2006) *Clerk and Lindsell on Torts* 19th edn. Sweet and Maxwell, London.

Deakin, S., Johnston, A. and Markensinis, B. (2003) *Markensinis and Deakin's Tort Law* 5th edn. Clarendon Press, Oxford.

Dimond, B. (1997) *Legal Aspects of Care in the Community*. Macmillan Press, London.

Dimond, B. (2003) *Legal Aspects of Consent*. Quay Publications, Mark Allen Press, Salisbury.

Dimond, B. (2005) *Legal Aspects of Health and Safety*. Quay Publications, Mark Allen Press, Salisbury.

Dimond, B. (2005) *Legal Aspects of Medicines*. Quay Publications, Mark Allen Press, Salisbury.

Dimond, B. *Legal Aspects of Nursing* 5th edn. Pearson Education, Hemel Hempstead (in press).

Dimond, B. (2004) *Legal Aspects of Occupational Therapy* 2nd edn. Blackwell Scientific Publications, Oxford.

Dimond, B. (2002) *Legal Aspects of Pain Management*. Quay Publications, Mark Allen Press, Salisbury.

Dimond, B. (2002) *Legal Aspects of Patient Confidentiality*. Quay Publications, Mark Allen Press, Salisbury.

Dimond, B. (1999) *Legal Aspects of Physiotherapy*. Blackwell Scientific Publications, Oxford.

Dimond, B. (1999) *Patients Rights, Responsibilities and the Nurse: Central Health Studies* 2nd edn. Quay Publishing, Lancaster.

Eliot, C. (2007) *The English Legal System* 8th edn. Pearson Education, Harlow.

Glynn, J. and Gomez, D. (2005) *Fitness to Practise: Healthcare Regulatory Law, Principles and Process*. Sweet and Maxwell, London.

Hendrick, J. (2006) *Law and Ethics in Nursing and Healthcare* 2nd edn. Nelson Thornes Publishers.

Heywood Jones, I. (ed) (1999) *The UKCC Code of Conduct: a critical guide.* Nursing Times Books, London.

Holland, J. and Burnett, S. (2006) *Employment Law.* Oxford University Press, Oxford.

Howarth, D. and O'Sullivan, J. (2000) *Hepple, Howarth and Matthews Tort: Cases and Materials* 5th edn. Butterworths, London.

Jay, R. (2007) *Data Protection Law and Practice* 3rd edn. Sweet and Maxwell, London.

Jones, M. (2004) *Medical Negligence* 3rd edn. Sweet and Maxwell, London.

Jones, M. (2007) *Textbook on Torts* 9th edn. Oxford University Press, Oxford.

Jones, M. and Morris, A. (2005) *Blackstone's Statutes on Medical Law.* 4th edn. Oxford University Press, Oxford.

Jones, R. (2006) *Mental Health Act Manual* 10th edn. Sweet and Maxwell, London.

Keenan, D. (2007) *Smith and Keenan's English Law* 15th edn. Pearson Longman, London.

Kennedy, I. and Grubb, A. (2000) *Medical Law and Ethics* 3rd edn. Butterworths, London.

Leach, P. (2005) *Taking a Case to the European Court of Human Rights* 2nd edn. Blackstone Press Ltd, London.

Maclean, A. (2001) *Briefcase of Medical Law.* Cavendish Publishing Ltd, London.

Mandelstam, M. (1998). *An A-Z of Community Care Law.* Jessica Kingsley Publishers, London.

Mandelstam, M. (2005) *Community Care Practice and the Law* 3rd edn. Jessica Kingsley Publishers, London.

Mason, J. and McCall-Smith, A. (2005). *Law and Medical Ethics* 7th edn. Butterworths, London.

McHale, J. and Fox, M. (2006) *Health Care Law: Texts and Materials.* Sweet and Maxwell, London.

McHale, J. and Tingle, J. (2001) *Law and Nursing* 2nd edn. Butterworth-Heinemann, Oxford.

Montgomery, J. (2003) *Health Care Law* 2nd edn. Oxford University Press, Oxford.

Mowbray, A. (2007) *Cases and Materials on the European Convention on Human Rights* 2nd edn. Butterworths, London.

Murphy, J. (2006) *Street on Torts* 12th edn. Butterworths, London.

Rogers, W. (2006) *Winfield and Jolowicz on Tort* 17th edn. Sweet and Maxwell, London.

Selwyn, N. (2004) *Selwyn's Law of Employment* 3th edn. Butterworths, London.

Sime, S. (2006) *Practical Approach to Civil Procedure* 5th edn. Blackstone Press Ltd, London.

Slapper, G. and Kelly, D. (2006) *The English Legal System* 7th edn. Routledge-Cavendish, London.

Stauch, M., Wheat, K. and Tingle, J. (2006) *Text, Cases and Materials on Medical Law.* 3rd edn. Routledge-Cavendish, London

Storch, J. (2004) *Towards a moral horizon, Nursing ethics for leadership and practice.* Pearson Education, Toronto.

Taylor, S. and Emir, A. (2006) *Employment Law: An introduction.* Oxford University Press, Oxford.

Tingle, J. and Foster, C. (2002) *Clinical Guidelines: law, policy and practice.* Cavendish Publishing, London.

Tschudin, V. (2003) *Ethics in Nursing: The Caring Relationship* 3rd edn. Butterworth-Heinemann, Oxford.

Wilkinson, R. and Caulfield, H. (2000) *The Human Rights Act: a Practical Guide for Nurses.* Whurr Publishers, London.

Index